Smart Healthcare for Sustainable Urban Development

Rosy Madaan
Manav Rachna International Institute of Research and Studies, India

Komal Kumar Bhatia
J.C. Bose University of Science and Technology, YMCA, India

Supriya P. Panda
Manav Rachna International Institute of Research and Studies, Faridabad, India

Vishal Jain
Sharda University, India

Payal Gulati
J.C. Bose University of Science and Technology, YMCA, India

A volume in the Advances in Medical Technologies and Clinical Practice (AMTCP) Book Series

IGI Global
PUBLISHER of TIMELY KNOWLEDGE

Published in the United States of America by
IGI Global
Medical Information Science Reference (an imprint of IGI Global)
701 E. Chocolate Avenue
Hershey PA, USA 17033
Tel: 717-533-8845
Fax: 717-533-8661
E-mail: cust@igi-global.com
Web site: http://www.igi-global.com

Library of Congress Cataloging-in-Publication Data

Names: Madaan, Rosy, 1983- editor. | Bhatia, Komal, 1979- editor. | Panda, Supriya, 1963- editor. | Jain, Vishal, 1983- editor. | Gulati, Payal, 1984- editor.
Title: Smart healthcare for sustainable urban development / Rosy Madaan, Komal Bhatia, Supriya Panda, Vishal Jain, Payal Gulati, editors.
Description: Hershey, PA : Medical Information Science Reference, [2022] | Includes bibliographical references and index. | Summary: "The book outlines many current challenges to digital health-care adoption and how IoT and big data technologies can help promote digital health-care adoption and improve health-care efficiency, discussing how IoT, Big data, and Deep learning techniques can together help improve the adoption of smart health which will result in improved health-care delivery and access"-- Provided by publisher.
Identifiers: LCCN 2021044614 (print) | LCCN 2021044615 (ebook) | ISBN 9781668425084 (hardcover) | ISBN 9781668425091 (ebook)
Subjects: MESH: Medical Informatics | Artificial Intelligence | Internet of Things | Big Data | Urban Renewal | Sustainable Development
Classification: LCC R859.7.A78 (print) | LCC R859.7.A78 (ebook) | NLM W 26.55.A7 | DDC 610.285/63--dc23
LC record available at https://lccn.loc.gov/2021044614
LC ebook record available at https://lccn.loc.gov/2021044615

This book is published in the IGI Global book series Advances in Medical Technologies and Clinical Practice (AMTCP) (ISSN: 2327-9354; eISSN: 2327-9370)

British Cataloguing in Publication Data
A Cataloguing in Publication record for this book is available from the British Library.

For electronic access to this publication, please contact: eresources@igi-global.com.

Advances in Medical Technologies and Clinical Practice (AMTCP) Book Series

Srikanta Patnaik
SOA University, India
Priti Das
S.C.B. Medical College, India

ISSN:2327-9354
EISSN:2327-9370

Mission

Medical technological innovation continues to provide avenues of research for faster and safer diagnosis and treatments for patients. Practitioners must stay up to date with these latest advancements to provide the best care for nursing and clinical practices.

The **Advances in Medical Technologies and Clinical Practice (AMTCP) Book Series** brings together the most recent research on the latest technology used in areas of nursing informatics, clinical technology, biomedicine, diagnostic technologies, and more. Researchers, students, and practitioners in this field will benefit from this fundamental coverage on the use of technology in clinical practices.

Coverage

- Clinical High-Performance Computing
- Clinical Studies
- Diagnostic Technologies
- Medical Imaging
- Neural Engineering
- Clinical Nutrition
- Patient-Centered Care
- Biomedical Applications
- Biomechanics
- Telemedicine

IGI Global is currently accepting manuscripts for publication within this series. To submit a proposal for a volume in this series, please contact our Acquisition Editors at Acquisitions@igi-global.com or visit: http://www.igi-global.com/publish/.

The Advances in Medical Technologies and Clinical Practice (AMTCP) Book Series (ISSN 2327-9354) is published by IGI Global, 701 E. Chocolate Avenue, Hershey, PA 17033-1240, USA, www.igi-global.com. This series is composed of titles available for purchase individually; each title is edited to be contextually exclusive from any other title within the series. For pricing and ordering information please visit http://www.igi-global.com/book-series/advances-medical-technologies-clinical-practice/73682. Postmaster: Send all address changes to above address.

Titles in this Series

For a list of additional titles in this series, please visit: www.igi-global.com/book-series

The Internet of Medical Things (IoMT) and Telemedicine Frameworks and Applications
Rajiv Pandey (Amity University, India) Amrit Gupta (MRH, SGPGI, Lucknow, India) and Agnivesh Pandey (C.S.J.M. University, India)
Medical Information Science Reference • © 2022 • 325pp • H/C (ISBN: 9781668435335) • US $380.00

Leveraging AI Technologies for Preventing and Detecting Sudden Cardiac Arrest and Death
Pradeep Nijalingappa (Bapuji Institute of Engineering and Technology, Davangere, India) Sandeep Kautish (Lord Buddha Education Foundation, Nepal) Mangesh M. Ghonge (Sandip Institute of Technology and Research Centre, India) and Renjith V. Ravi (MEA Engineering College, India)
Medical Information Science Reference • © 2022 • 263pp • H/C (ISBN: 9781799884439) • US $435.00

Advancement, Opportunities, and Practices in Telehealth Technology
S.N. Kumar (Amal Jyothi College of Engineering, India) Sundaravaradhan Suresh (KPR Institute of Engineering and Technology, India) Padmanabhan Vivekananth (ISBAT University, Uganda) and Sherin Zafar (Jamia Hamdard University, India)
Medical Information Science Reference • © 2022 • 335pp • H/C (ISBN: 9781668452318) • US $380.00

Principles and Methods of Explainable Artificial Intelligence in Healthcare
Victor Hugo C. de Albuquerque (Federal University of Ceará, Brazil) P. Naga Srinivasu (VNR Vignana Jyothi Institute of Engineering and Technology, India) Akash Kumar Bhoi (KIET Group of Institutions, India & Sikkim Manipal University, India) and Alfonso González Briones (University of Salamanca, Spain)
Medical Information Science Reference • © 2022 • 347pp • H/C (ISBN: 9781668437919) • US $435.00

Big Data Analytics and Artificial Intelligence in the Healthcare Industry
José Machado (Centro ALGORITMI, Universidade do Minho, Portugal) Hugo Peixoto (Centro ALGORITMI, Universidade do Minho, Portugal) and Regina Sousa (Centro ALGORITMI, Universidade do Minho, Portugal)
Medical Information Science Reference • © 2022 • 360pp • H/C (ISBN: 9781799891727) • US $435.00

Computational Intelligence and Applications for Pandemics and Healthcare
Sapna Singh Kshatri (Bharti Vishwavidyalaya, India) Kavita Thakur (Pt. Ravishankar Shukla University, India) Maleika Heenaye Mamode Khan (University of Mauritius, Mauritius) Deepak Singh (NIT, Raipur, India) and G. R. Sinha (Myanmar Institute of Information Technology, Mandalay, Myanmar)
Medical Information Science Reference • © 2022 • 357pp • H/C (ISBN: 9781799898313) • US $380.00

IGI Global
PUBLISHER of TIMELY KNOWLEDGE

701 East Chocolate Avenue, Hershey, PA 17033, USA
Tel: 717-533-8845 x100 • Fax: 717-533-8661
E-Mail: cust@igi-global.com • www.igi-global.com

Table of Contents

Detailed Table of Contents

The growing development of deep learning and its increasingly widespread use signals a trend to convert to a new standard in each application area, consolidating itself as a general purpose technology. In the general analysis of innovations based on the use of deep learning on different applications of medical images, it can be inferred that its use is increasingly widespread and that it is driving greater innovations and transformations at an increasingly greater speed. Additionally, it is evident that the use of deep learning in medical imaging for the diagnosis of various anomalies incorporates a significant number of the elements and methodological and organizational aspects identified under this study (e.g., invention methods from the perspective of application of deep learning). Therefore, this study emphasizes various aspects of deep learning models to have opted as a ready reference while examining the medical images as a de-facto standard.

Hepatitis is inflammation of the liver most often caused by a viral infection. The supervised data mining technique diagnosed hepatitis using a dataset. Data mining methods have been widely used to analyze biomedical information. This chapter sheds light on the severe viral hepatitis which is spreading around the world at an alarming rate. It is necessary to diagnose such a disease at an early stage to reduce suffering. Early diagnosis of hepatitis is difficult because of the different characteristics associated with it. Artificial intelligence has gained an extensive recognition in medical applications with its growing contribution in interpretation of medical images, diagnosis, design, and development of expert frameworks to assist the practitioners, design of prosthetics, and design of drugs for diverse phases of medicine. A model needs to be created that can be used to visualize life in hepatitis. This chapter uses the Naïve Bayes classifier and provides an improved Naïve Bayes classifier to provide more precision.

millions of people globally, and the number is growing every day. COPD, for example, afflicted roughly 251 million individuals worldwide in 2016, and claimed the lives of 3.17 million people (i.e., 5% of the population). There are many distinct sorts of the pulmonary diseases: COPD, pulmonary fibrosis, asthma, and lung cancer, to name a few. This chapter explains the three machine learning algorithms that helped to diagnose pulmonary diseases based on the dataset.

Hypertension is known to be one of the most common medical and lifestyle disorders, signalized by the elevated levels of blood pressure, that is systolic and diastolic blood pressures more than 140 mm/Hg and 90 mm/Hg, respectively, associated with the various risk factors for cardiovascular diseases, chronic kidney disease, and some of the neurodegenerative diseases. Major lifestyle parameters such as lack of physical activity, high concentration of salt in diet, alcohol consumption, smoking, stress, and high weight are significantly related to this disease. Computational models of physiological frameworks can significantly help with our comprehension of the frameworks under study and can likewise be utilized in educating and examination apparatuses. Computational models can supplement exploratory and clinical investigations, yet additionally challenge flow standards, reclassify our comprehension of systems driving lifestyle, and shape future research.

Remote monitoring is a healthcare tool that enables physicians to stay connected to their patients from afar and offer treatment anytime it is needed. The sensing devices may be worn, implanted, or sensors in the surrounding environment can be linked to the internet, allowing physicians and caregivers to deliver patients with effective and timely medicine. This application is used to remotely monitor the patient's vital parameters using sensors, gadgets, and items in their environment. The patient's essential data is transferred and exchanged in real time between the patient and the caretakers. Its primary use is in the treatment of chronic diseases such as diabetes, heart disease monitoring, asthma, and so on. In many sectors, recent technological advancements and connectivity have resulted in the rise of internet of things (IoT) and artificial intelligence (AI) applications.

The healthcare system is transforming from traditional medication to smart healthcare. Smart healthcare plays a vital role in urban development. Medicines and injections are the key building blocks of the healthcare system. Environmental conditions like temperature, pressure, and humidity can adversely affect the quality of medicines and injections. So, maintaining proper temperature and humidity is a must to keep them safe. There is need of continuous monitoring of medicines and injections during their supply chain. The wireless sensor network (WSN) strives to detect surrounding parameters and relay sensed data to the base station without any human deployment. Supply chain management (SCM) in healthcare system is also one of the applications, which requires a different type of monitoring, supervision, and handling at different levels. WSN adds a contribution in the making of smart healthcare, as it uses the smart way (sensors) of monitoring the medicines and injections in the supply chain.

Vijayakumari B., Mepco Schlenk Engineering College, India
Benitha V. S., Mepco Schlenk Engineering College, India
Shabna R. M., Mepco Schlenk Engineering College, India
Siva Sundari T., Mepco Schlenk Engineering College, India
Manonmani T., Mepco Schlenk Engineering College, India

In modern India, with the government surveys, it is clearly agreed upon that still women are the major victims of violent crimes and harassment. Since most of the women employees are there in all the fields, women have to travel a long distance lonely and during late hours also. Thus, women's safety is a much desired need of this hour. This chapter focuses to provide safety for women and to reduce the number of crimes to some extent and provides security exclusively for women employees. The ultimate aim of the device is to transmit the emergency situation of the victim along with their current location to parents and the police for help. The location is traced using GPS and a message is sent via GSM to the predefined numbers. When women sense that they are in danger they can manually press the button so that their current location along with an alert message is sent to the predefined numbers. The device can involuntarily detect the emergency situation by fall detection sensor and heart rate sensor. This module can also send an alert using medical emergency.

Rohan Saini, J.C. Bose University of Science and Technology, YMCA, India
Sonali Gupta, J.C. Bose University of Science and Technology, YMCA, India

The deaf face far more difficulties than normal people in day-to-day life, and sign language acts as the most important communication tool for them. Though a lot of books are available as a learning resource for this language, it's not common amongst a major section of the Indian population. An important area of concern is when they need to seek healthcare facilities. The doctors and other hospital staff struggle to understand their issues, and they themselves also put in much effort and time to communicate it to the doctors. Irrespective of joint efforts put in by both the communities, they are unable to get proper health benefits and the services of world-class doctors. In order to solve this problem, SISD, which is a smart interactive system for differently abled persons, based on Indian Sign Language has been proposed. It works similarly to the interactive voice response (IVR) system. SISD provides the user with choices (animations/videos of signs) and recognizes the user's choice via a sign language recognition system.

The COVID-19 pandemic has been an eye-opener towards human lifestyle and the healthcare sector. During this phase, a new factor witnessed by humankind is the economic and social impact of the healthcare sector. Due to this rising concern in the healthcare sector, new market segments, niches, and micro-niches are created, which have given some abundant opportunities for entrepreneurs to execute new business models, ideas, and technological implementations. This definitely will add uniqueness and will revolutionize the healthcare sector. Adding up, the new normal at this moment is artificial intelligence, machine learning, and virtual reality, which together have changed the perspective of the healthcare sector. So, keeping all these factors in mind, this chapter focuses on transformations in the healthcare sector during the pandemic followed by discussing various innovations and entrepreneurial ideas in the same with all the overcoming challenges. Furthermore, the significant innovations which have improvised the understanding of novel biological threats will also be discussed.

In this chapter, electrical activity in the brain is measured with the help of brain sensors. Further, electrical activity is stored and analyzed for two different datasets: first, for the epileptic seizure, and second, for brain activity. Next, both epileptic seizure and brain activity datasets are used for deep learning models interfacing with Apache Spark. The deep learning model has a feed-forward neural network, which helps determine features from the epileptic seizure dataset that are important and fit in the hidden patterns among them. Further, FFNN is interfaced with Apache Spark to analyze how it can be beneficial with processing of the deep learning model. The results of the accuracy of deep learning model and processing time caused by Apache Spark help determine how effective the FFNN is for predicting the seizure activity in the brain and how Apache Spark can be applied with a deep learning model to increase its effectiveness for different types of datasets.

Human emotions like neutral, sad, happy, and others reveal the state of the mind of a person. This information is useful and thus finds its technical, interpersonal, and societal applications in various areas like surveillance, suicide prevention, marketing and strategy, entertainment, etc. The espousal of data science peaked the scientific interest in the detection of human emotions in the late 2000s and early

Preface

With the development of information technology, the concept of smart healthcare has been evolving gradually. New generation of information technologies have come into picture. Technologies, such as the internet of things (loT), cloud computing, big data, and artificial intelligence has come into picture for the transformation of the old medical system making healthcare better in terms of efficiency, convenience, and personalization. Such variations are required for coping up with the requirements of individual people along with improvement in the efficiency of medical care, which largely enhances the experience of medical and health services. This also stands in the direction of future development of modern medicine.

The book basically discusses about current challenges to digital health-care adoption and how IoT and big data technologies can help promote digital health-care adoption and improve health-care efficiency. It also discusses some of the ways in which IoT, Big data and Deep learning techniques can together help improve the adoption of smart health which will result in improved health-care delivery and access. It also presents the concept of "Smart hospitals are those that optimize, redesign or build new clinical processes, management systems and potentially even infrastructure, enabled by underlying digitized networking infrastructure of interconnected assets, to provide a valuable service or insight which was not possible or available earlier, to achieve better patient care, experience and operational efficiency."

This book is mainly targeted at researchers, undergraduate students, postgraduate students, academicians, and scholars working in the area of data science and its application in health sciences. Also, the book is beneficial for engineers who are engaged in developing actual healthcare solutions. Some unique features of the book are listed below:

- The book can help promote digital health-care adoption and improve health-care efficiency
- The book presents a discussion on Smart Healthcare based on the latest data-driven medical technologies. It includes a discussion on how Artificial Intelligence, Big Data Analytics, Machine Learning, and Precision Medicine can be used for healthcare solutions
- Some case studies have been discussed concerning real-world applications and systems so that the reader can have a clear understanding

One can gain a thorough understanding of new upcoming technologies and applying these technologies for smart healthcare like edge cognitive computing, big data management, and the cognitive Internet of Things for digital governance. M.Tech and Ph.D. scholars can work in the direction of providing healthcare solutions. They can learn the basics of the establishment of Smart hospitals for sustainable urban development. Interested researchers can gain an understanding of how the upcoming technologies can be used for dealing with diseases like Alzheimer's disease, cardiovascular diseases, diabetes mellitus, and tuberculosis.

Chapter 1

This chapter presents a study on medical image detection using Deep Learning. It emphasises on various aspects of Deep Learning models that can be adopted as a ready reference while examining the medical images as a de-facto standard.

Chapter 2

This chapter presents a novel hybrid method based for Hepatitis disease diagnosis using Naïve Bayes and Decision. This chapter uses the Naïve-Bayes as a classifier and provides an improved-Naïve-Bayes is developed to provide more precision.

Chapter 3

This chapter presents a Breast Cancer Detection system using Different Classification and Ensemble Methods and also emphasizes on how healthy life style can be maintained.

Chapter 4

This work presents nine machine learning techniques for identifying stress using the SWELL dataset. Automated classifiers have been used to predict working circumstances and stress-related mental states and their performance has been compared for three stress conditions (no stress, interruption and time pressure).

Chapter 5

This chapter focusses on Smart Prediction of Pulmonary Diseases using Artificial Intelligence and Deep Learning. Various technologies such as the Internet of Things (IoT), Artificial intelligence (AI), and Deep Learning (DL) that play an important role in improving disease detection without causing pain to patients are discussed.

Chapter 6

The objective of this chapter is to design a mathematical model that depicts the change in blood pressure levels in consideration to different controlled lifestyle factors like salt consumption, physical exercise, stress and to optimize the mathematical model using Genetic Algorithm, the approach that is highly effective in diagnosing medical conditions.

Chapter 7

This chapter presents some recent developments of Smart Hospitals and the associated challenges. It focusses on the recent technical improvements and connectivity that has led in the emergence of new businesses in a variety of industries.

Chapter 8

The proposed chapter will highlight the smart way of monitoring the SCM in healthcare with the incorporation of WSN. The initial part of work will be a survey of sensors' deployment in various levels of the supply chain in healthcare system. The next part will emphasis on enhancing the network lifetime through effective utilization of energy resources.

Chapter 9

This chapter focusses to provide safety for women and to reduce the number of crimes to some extend and provides security exclusively for women employees. The ultimate aim of the device is clannish the emergency situation of the victim along with their current location to parents and the police for help. The location is traced using GPS and a message is sent via GSM to the pre-defined numbers.

Chapter 10

In this chapter, an automatic sign language recognition system SISD that can help deaf patients to express their issues to the doctor has been designed. SISD is a machine consisting of a camera for capturing sign language data and a touch screen that can assist the user by showing sign videos and other information. It also generates the transcript at the end of the conversation. The main aim of SISD is to provide deaf and dumb patients with an automatic recognition system that can understand their problem and save their time and efforts in emergency situations. This is the first novel approach for creating a healthcare interaction system using a concept of IVR.

Chapter 11

Innovations are crucial key to providing the best to them while fighting the novel biological threats. Adding on with life sciences and health care is entrepreneurship that is accelerating the bedding ideas into notions. Even the government is financing and finding such projects to deliver products and services that could be a helping hand in a medical emergency. This chapter focusses on reformation of the healthcare sector with innovation and entrepreneurial approaches.

Chapter 12

Due to seizure activity, anxiety becomes part of a patient's life and affects them in their routine activities. Seizure activity is so harmful that it causes irreversible changes in the brain, which remains unprovoked after sometimes. Consequently, this had been a significant concern among clinical researchers and a substantial area of interest in epileptic disorder. This chapter focusses on Spark based deep learning for recognition of epileptic seizure with multimodal brain waves.

Chapter 13

The chapter lists methods for the Recognition of Human Emotions based on Physiological Response and(or) Facial Expressions. Detection of human emotions is a key area of research. The findings of the research are utilized by various industries for business purposes and by civic bodies for administration purposes.

Chapter 14

This chapter focusses on Transport Data Analytics with selection of tools and techniques for emergency medical services. Emergency Medical Services (EMS) is inevitable in urban transport. The objective of this chapter is to present the use of transport data analytics in sustainable mobility and transport.

Chapter 15

The chapter is dedicated to a different implementation of the method of collection of features. Creating a ML model is basically a technique for extracting all the elements applicable to a query. A function must be declared vital because it is useful for creating a ML model of the issue under investigation.

Rosy Madaan
Manav Rachna International Institute of Research and Studies, India

Komal Kumar Bhatia
J.C. Bose University of Science and Technology, YMCA, India

Supriya P. Panda
Manav Rachna International Institute of Research and Studies, India

Vishal Jain
Sharda University, India

Payal Gulati
J.C. Bose University of Science and Technology, YMCA, India

Acknowledgment

The editors would like to acknowledge all the people involved in this project and more specifically, to IGI Global team, the authors and reviewers that were involved in the process.

First, the editors would like to pay sincere gratitude to the authors of the chapters for contributing their time and expertise to this book.

Second, the editors wish to acknowledge the valuable contributions of the reviewers regarding the improvement of quality, coherence, and content presentation of the chapters.

Above all, to the Great Almighty, the author of knowledge and wisdom, for his countless love and blessings. We would like to thank our family and friends who have always been a support for us.

Chapter 1
Study on Medical Image Detection Using Deep Learning

Ruchi Garg
J.C. Bose University of Science and Technology, YMCA, India

Sushil Kumar
J.C. Bose University of Science and Technology, YMCA, India

Sonali Gupta
https://orcid.org/0000-0001-5885-0612
J.C. Bose University of Science and Technology, YMCA, India

ABSTRACT

The growing development of deep learning and its increasingly widespread use signals a trend to convert to a new standard in each application area, consolidating itself as a general purpose technology. In the general analysis of innovations based on the use of deep learning on different applications of medical images, it can be inferred that its use is increasingly widespread and that it is driving greater innovations and transformations at an increasingly greater speed. Additionally, it is evident that the use of deep learning in medical imaging for the diagnosis of various anomalies incorporates a significant number of the elements and methodological and organizational aspects identified under this study (e.g., invention methods from the perspective of application of deep learning). Therefore, this study emphasizes various aspects of deep learning models to have opted as a ready reference while examining the medical images as a de-facto standard.

1. INTRODUCTION

Advances in AI in recent years make it possible to create new technologies and have more and more applications in various fields. Its foundations, complex algorithms, are intended to solve all kinds of intuitive and subjective problems that until now, computers were not capable of solving, and were the domain only of human beings, capable of solving them automatically i.e. recognizing someone in a photo, or the medical field, detect the presence of an abnormality in an image or a signal (Galaz et al., 2021).

DOI: 10.4018/978-1-6684-2508-4.ch001

To achieve good performance by computers in these problems, it is sought to make them learn from experience, to learn reality in the form of simple concepts that are related to each other forming more complex ones, so that there is a hierarchy of concepts, with many layers. From this learning model, with multiple levels of representation and abstraction, what is known as Deep Learning arises (Athanasios et al., 2018). Computers that work with Deep Learning algorithms have to be able by themselves to acquire their knowledge, extract their deductions, their patterns from the data provided. This learning capacity is what is known as Machine Learning. (Machine Learning), and encompasses the aforementioned Deep Learning (Linardatos et al., 2020).

However new this field may seem, Deep Learning has been around for quite some time. The lack of fame for these techniques is mainly due to two reasons: 1) the unavailability of large amounts of data to train the models, and 2) not having enough hardware (HW) or software (SW) in the computers. powerful as for the execution of the models. In recent years, both problems have been solved, and their multiple applications have motivated growing interest in this field. From image classification and structure segmentation to speech recognition or object detection, the possibilities are many. For this reason, today it is being used by technology companies, SW infrastructure companies, and for scientific applications, among others (Ching et al., 2018).

The infinite scientific and medical applications of Deep Learning algorithms i.e. for computer-aided diagnosis, for making predictions from large amounts of data, for processing images in medicine, for designing drugs, or for constructing 3D maps of the brain are precisely the motivation for this work, as they can help improve patient health care, in terms of both precision and speed. A specific medical task where these algorithms are achieving very good results is the classification of lesions and tumors, that is, given a certain image, and based on its characteristics, assign the image one of the two possible output classes (i.e. malignant or benign tumor). In particular, helping the specialist to make better decisions or to look at certain parts of the image where the anomalies may be (Ker et al., 2017).

For this reason, because it is a very widespread application, and also because various tumors are spreading most frequently worldwide, in this study we want to pay special attention to Deep Learning techniques that can be used for diagnosis, monitoring, and evolution of tumors. Furthermore, after studying the state of the art in depth, a methodology based on a Deep Learning algorithm will be designed, the purpose of which is to classify these tumors.

Main Methods of Deep Learning

With the growing interest in this field, there are more and more types of Deep Learning algorithms, which are emerging as modifications of others for specific and concrete objectives. It is not possible to make a classification in a strict and closed way, because depending on the context of the problems and the various approaches to solving the problems, these classifications vary. For this reason, the classification that has been most suitable for this work has been chosen, following the one presented in (Guo et al., 2015). The revised algorithms are thus grouped into the following four categories: 1) Convolutional Neural Networks, 2) Restricted Bolztmann Machines, 3) Auto coders, and 4) Sparse Coding; which are reflected in a more clarifying way, together with their variants, in Figure 1 of these four categories, the main notions will be explained and both their contributions and their limitations will be analyzed.

On the other hand, special attention will be paid to explain the CNN (Guo et al., 2015), (https://cs231n.github.io/convolutional-networks/) as they are the ones that have the most applications in medical image analysis and in particular in mammography analysis as follows:-

Figure 1. Various models and specifications under deep learning methods

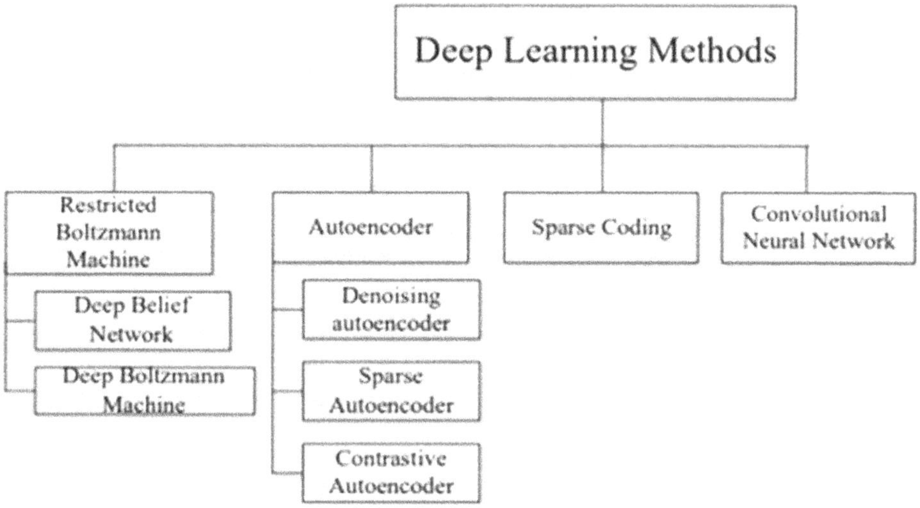

Convolutional Neural Networks (CNNs)

Convolutional neural networks or CNNs, from their English name, are perhaps the part of AI that has been most inspired by Biology, specifically by Neuroscience, since they work in an analogous way to how the cortex would Primary visual (i.e. In both cases the information stored in 2D feature maps is defined, and the CNNs are made up of individual basic units grouped in clustering layers, emulating the cells of the cortex that are grouped together in the form of complex cells).

CNNs represent a very successful deep model, and today they are used in a large number of applications, generally obtaining very good results. In particular, they are widely used in computer vision tasks, and therefore also in medical image analysis, which is why they are of great interest for this work. It is verified that for this type of images they are the most robust and successful networks that exist for now, as it was demonstrated in 2012, when a CNN won the challenge of recognition of objects of ImageNet (Krizhevsky et al., 2012) moment from which only improvements have been achieved (Guo et al., 2015).

When defining a CNN, it can be said that it is the type of neural network for data processing with a known and gridded topology, such as the data of an image that make up a 2D grid made up of pixels. In this definition a great advantage is intrinsic, the fact that the inputs can be of different sizes, something especially very useful when working with images.

Regarding its structure, CNNs are made up of three different types of layers; those of convolution (CONV), those of grouping and those totally connected (fully-connected layers, FC). A very typical scheme is the one that can be seen in Figure 2, where the network is made up of 5 CONV layers with several clustering layers followed by 3 FC layers, although these numbers may change (https://cs231n.github.io/convolutional-networks/) . Each of these layers is explained in detail below.

Figure 2. CNN network formed by 5 convolutional layers with max_pooling
Obtained from (Szegedy et al., 2015).

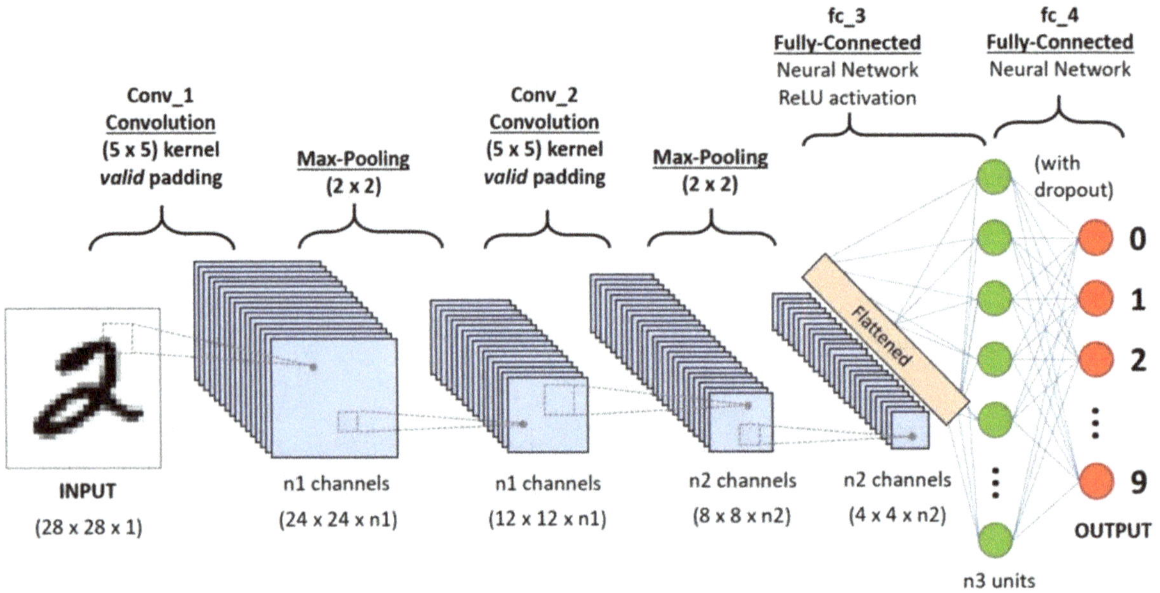

Convolutional Layers (CONV)

The convolution operation is what gives the architecture its name and is used in at least one of its layers, both the complete image and the intermediate feature maps, generating new feature maps. It has three main advantages that make the Deep Learning system more efficient:

a. The connectivity or dispersed interactions. Instead of having one parameter for each interaction between each input and each output, these parameters are shared, so there are fewer parameters than interactions. In this way the memory requirements are lower, in addition to learning correlations between neighboring pixels.
b. The sharing of parameters. It is linked to the previous concept; various functions of the model use the same parameters. Memory is saved.
c. The invariance to the location of the object. Derivative of equivariance, which refers to the fact that if the input changes, the output changes to the same extent.

Due to these advantages, the FC layers are sometimes replaced by CONV layers, to speed up the learning process. This happens for example in NIN techniques(Network to Network) (Hinton et al., 2012).

Layers of Grouping or Pooling

Clustering layers are very useful as they provide the location of features in images when it is not necessary to know the pixels corresponding to these features exactly.

They are generally placed after each CONV layer in order to reduce the dimensions of the feature maps. To do this, they apply a function to the outputs closest to the output of the network, modifying the latter. Different functions can be used (average_ pooling, norm_ pooling, etc.), but the most widely used by far is that of max_ pooling (Guo et al., 2015), which reduces the dimensionality of the input by taking for each rectangular set of fixed and chosen size, the maximum value of the pixels in that region, and making that value the new value of the output pixel. This can be done in 1D, as in the case of Figure 3 (a), where a 4x4 feature map is reduced to 2x2 by applying a max_pooling of 2x2; or in 2D, very useful for subsampling images and patches, represented in Figure 3 (b), and where it can be seen that the number of layers (64) remains intact.

Figure 3. Operation of the operator max-pooling on a 1D (a) and 2D (b) feature map

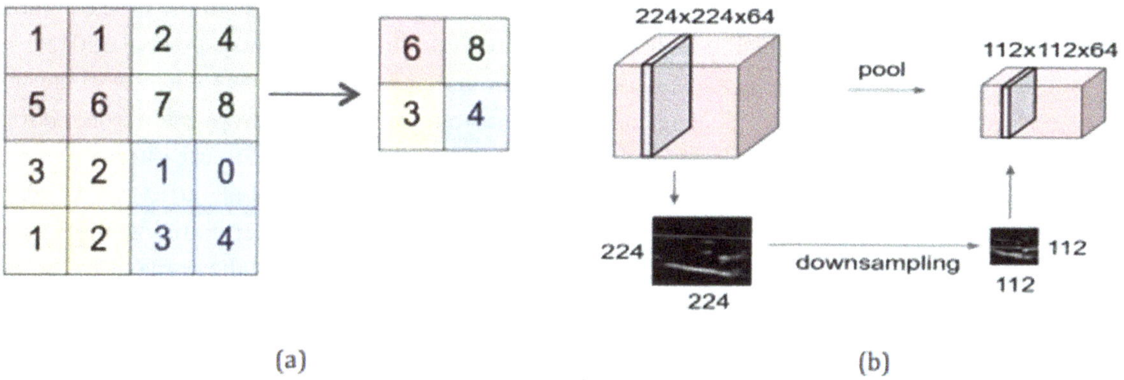

Due to their multiple uses in images and their advantages in reducing dimensions and invariance, grouping layers are the most studied of the three types of layers. From this intense study three different approaches are born, each one with different purposes and for different procedures, although it is argued that the best practice is to combine the three to achieve a good performance of CNN (Guo et al., 2015).

a. Pooling stochastic. Equivalent to max pooling, but many copies of the input image are generated, each with small local deformations. Its stochastic nature, randomly choosing the activation within each region of neurons, solves the problem of overfitting that many times causes the max_ pooling.
b. Spatial grouping of pyramids (Spatial Pyramid Pooling, SPP). In this case the last grouping layer is replaced by an SPP, capable of extracting fixed-length representations of images, so that the limitation of requiring a fixed-size input image is omitted. It is a strategy that is generally applied to CNNs to increase their performance.
c. Def-pooling. It is a type of layer that is introduced at some point in the network to be able to work with the deformations of the objects more efficiently, which is a challenge in the field of vision by computer, and particularly in the recognition of objects.

Fully Connected Layers (FC)

These types of layers are placed after the last of the grouping layers to convert 2D feature maps into a 1D vector, much more useful for representing these features later. The FC layers work like a traditional neural network and contain approximately 90% of the parameters of the network (https://cs231n.github.io/convolutional-networks/) .

The 1D vector of the output of the network is usually of predefined length, for example for an image classification task it will be of length equal to the number of categories that are had. Another common option in image analysis is to take it as a 1D feature vector for further processing (later called feature extraction).

The main disadvantage of these layers is the great computational load that they generate when training them, due to the amount of parameters they handle. For this reason, many authors defend reducing the connections between the neurons of these layers using some type of method, as in the case of Google LeNet (Szegedy et al., 2015), reducing them in number, or even eliminate them (Guo et al., 2015).

Finally, the training of CNNs is explained, as it is the most complicated part when working with this type of architecture. If you decide to use a supervised strategy, having to propagate throughout the network back and forth requires very powerful computers. Thus, it is suggested to use alternatives such as Dropout (Hinton et al., 2012; Srivastava et al., 2014) Drop Connect (Wan et al., 2013), in which the algorithm omits half of the feature detectors so that the model generalizes better, initialize the network with pre-trained parameters instead of random ones, adjust the parameters of the network to the task for which it is used, and finally apply data augmentation techniques, widely used when working with medical images as they alleviate the need to have large amounts of labeled data. Due to the multiple uses that CNNs are given in the domain of computer vision, there are different models of very popular CNNs, of which the following are highlighted:

AlexNet It is one of the best known CNN architectures, which follows the typical 5 CONV and 3 FC layer structure. This model was responsible for the rise of CNNs when they trained in ImageNet obtaining remarkable results (Krizhevsky et al., 2012) and today it is still used for the task of image classification. In it you can find different data augmentation techniques based on geometric transformations. Still, it does have the drawback that it requires a fixed input image resolution (224x224, specifically), plus there's still no clear understanding of why it works so well.

Clarifai is another model that emerged when trying to explain how the intermediate layers of CNN architectures functioned internally. Its structure is the conventional one and it also achieves very good results, better than the AlexNet in the classification of images, as for ImageNet.

SPP or Network with Spatial Clustering of Pyramids is another model whose motivation is to avoid the requirement of a fixed resolution of input images, for which it uses SPPs. By introducing the SPP layers in different models of CNNs (He et al., 2014). The precision of these has been increased, which is why this grouping strategy has achieved great popularity.

VGG It is a deep CNN used for image recognition, which instead of using 5 uses between 13 and 15 CONV layers, hence its depth. VGG obtains very good results when classifying images, thus demonstrating that increasing the depth of the network can go hand in hand with increasing its precision. In the case of VGG this is possible because it uses very small convolutional filters in all layers. Another advantage it brings is a greater generalizability to other data sets (Simonyan et al., 2014).

GoogLeNet it's another CNN even deeper than VGG. It is made up of 22 CONV layers, and a single FC layer. When using this network in image classification tasks, an increase in the precision of the results is also observed.

Although the results obtained by these CNNs in terms of image classification are very satisfactory, in the last two years other deep architectures have emerged that seek to improve them, such as Inception (Szegedy et al., 2015; Szegedy et al., 2016), Res Net (He et al., 2016), and Dense Net (Huang et al., 2017). These three models are particularly interesting for this work, since the architecture to be designed is based on them. Therefore, the structure of these networks will be detailed in Chapter 4.

Finally, comment on two other types of networks that derive from the previous ones, and that have other applications, specifically object detection and semantic segmentation. The RCNN (regions with CNN characteristics) are a combination of CNNs with a linear SVM (Support Vector Machine) used to detect objects. They start by generating multiple proposals for objects or candidates, from which they extract their characteristics using CNN, and finally they classify each candidate with the SVM into categories. This strategy of recognition by regions achieves very good results, and for this reason it is widely used in computer vision and also in medical imaging. However, its performance is limited both by the fact that the network needs the location of the object in the image and by the large number of candidates it generates. Unlike RCNNs, FCNs (fully convolutional network) are used primarily for semantic segmentation, and are useful for removing the restriction on image resolution.

Restricted Boltzmann Machines (RBMs)

RBMs are a type of generative stochastic neural networks. They are models based on "energy", models with an energy function composed of several terms, where each term corresponds to a factor in the probability distribution. Each of these terms can be understood as an "expert" who determines whether a specific restriction is satisfied. They are, therefore, probabilistic models in which the output is expressed as a function of probabilities, which is advantageous for human interpretation (Zhang et al., 2017).

Today the term RBM is used in a generalized way, to name any model with latent variables, which are grouped into a single layer and interact with the rest of the layers parameterized by matrices, thus learning the representation of the input. They can be understood more as graphical models used to compose and train other deep learning models, and not as such, although they share several characteristics with them (i.e. their units are organized in layers, the connectivity between layers is described by means of a matrix, connectivity is relatively dense, etc (Fischer et al., 2014).

Regarding the applications of RBMs, facial/image segmentation and recognition stand out, although their uses in medical imaging and in general in computer vision are much smaller than in the case of CNNs.

All RBMs belong to the set of Boltzmann Machines, with the main modification that they require that the visible units be in the same proportion as the hidden ones, thus forming a bipartite graph. This division is imposed to make the algorithms more efficient. The main variants of RBMs to consider, the ones most used in computer vision tasks, are the three that follow, the main difference being the type of connections between the units that make up the different layers.

Deep Belief Networks (Deep Belief Networks, DBNS)

DBNs were one of the first non-convolutional models that showed good performance when training deep architectures. Since then, it has been investigated how to work with them and improve their results, but the constant difficulties encountered in their training stage have caused their use to decline over the years (Webb et al., 2010; Lopes et al., 2015).

The architecture of DBMs is characterized by being made up of several layers with latent variables, which are the hidden layers, and typically binary, in addition to the input and output layers, which can be binary or real. These layers are connected only between neurons in neighboring layers, but never between units of the same layer, and are undirected between the first two layers and directed toward the layer closest to the data for all others. The output of these networks is always in the form of a joint probability distribution over observable data and labels.

To train them, you must first initialize the network layer by layer, and then adjust all the weights together with the desired outputs. This unsupervised procedure has two advantages; first that the network is always initialized in a proper way, and second, that no tagged data is required for training. On the contrary, it has the disadvantage of involving a high computational cost. In addition, if you think about the tasks related to computer vision, you also have to consider the problem that they do not take into account the 2D structure of the input image, and for these two reasons is why their use is minimal in the newer models (Webb et al., 2010; Lopes et al., 2015).

Deep Boltzmann Machines (DBMs)

DBMs, unlike DBNs, are totally undirected models and always with more than one hidden layer or latent variable, each one of them being mutually independent and conditioned by neighboring layers (even layers are conditionally independent of odd layers and vice versa). The units that make up these layers are usually binary but there is also the possibility that they are real. The training of these networks is analogous to that of the RBMs, by layers, although thanks to their structure improvements are achieved in the classification task, which can be even more increased if modifications are made at the time of pre-training and training. The disadvantage of this variant is its temporal complexity, something undesirable when working with large data sets (Salakhutdinov et al., 2009).

Deep Energy Models (DEMs)

The three variants of RBMs explained as under, DEMs are the most recent. Unlike the previous ones, it only presents a layer of latent hidden units, in order to achieve a faster and more efficient training, training all the layers at the same time and not layer by layer. This results in qualitative and quantitative ranking improvements (de Giorgio & Andrea, 2015).

Auto Encoders (AEs)

The easiest way to understand an autoencoder is to think of a very simple network. simple, made up of three layers, one input, one hidden, and one output, and trained to copy its inputs to its outputs. Logically, its design does not seek make an exact copy. On the contrary, the hidden layer imposes restrictions for that only relevant input information is copied, prioritizing some aspects of the data, those that are more useful, over others. Although at first glance the output looks identical to the input, it has been reduced, Features that were not relevant have been removed. More specifically, to produce this reconstruction, a two-stage process is followed, one encoder and another decoder, and as the process is executed it goes optimizing by minimizing the reconstruction error, to finally obtain the new function learned. It should be noted that due to the fact that the auto coder seeks to copy the input to the output, both have to be the same dimensions (de Giorgio & Andrea, 2015) (Almeida et al., 2020).

Sparse Coding

Sparse coding models seek, like autoencoders, to extract characteristics from input data to describe them completely. They are linear unsupervised learning models, which work by adding noise, usually Gaussian, to the input data, to obtain reconstructions of the same. The training that is usually applied is in phases, alternating those that encode the data with others for the reconstruction of the data given the encoding (Földiák et al., 2008; Rangamani et al., 2018).

The main advantage of these methods is that they do not cause generalization errors, and therefore they are better generalizers when used as feature extractors, including in cases where very little tagged data is available to train. This is very useful when working with medical images, since they are not always accompanied by labels. On the contrary, disadvantages are the large amount of time it takes to do the calculations and the difficulty of its training stage (Földiák et al., 2008; Rangamani et al., 2018).

Characteristics extraction is the main application of sparse coding models, since in addition to the advantage of not requiring only labeled data, it has many others, such as: it better reconstructs descriptors by capturing correlations between similar descriptors; effectively captures salient image properties; It works in the same way as the biological visual system; works very well with patches of images, a deep network training strategy to detect objects that will be discussed later, as these signals are scattered; and patterns with sparse features are more linearly separable (Földiák et al., 2008; Rangamani et al., 2018).

Finally, and without going into detail, some of the most representative algorithms of sparse coding are mentioned (Gao et al., 2012).

1. Sparse Coding SPM (Sc SPM): It is an extension of the already mentioned SPMs. With them it is achieved that the reconstruction error is much lower, but the mutual dependence between the local characteristics is also ignored, since it treats them separately, which is not advantageous.
2. Laplacian Sparse Coding (LSC): This variant improves the Sc SPM by selecting the centers of the clusters so that they are similar, achieving a more robust solution.
3. Hyper-graph Laplacian Sparse Coding (HLSC): The HLSC is an extension of the LSC where the similarity between the different instances is defined by a hyper graph, achieving greater robustness with this improvement.

2. LITERATURE REVIEW

In medical imaging, the segmentation of organs and other substructures is essential to be able to make a quantitative analysis of clinical parameters in relation to the shape and volume of the same structures i.e. for brain, breast, chest or cardiac analyzes. In addition, segmentation is a first step in computer detection systems, gaining even greater importance.

Due to this importance of correctly segmentation of the structures of interest, there are many models that propose different approaches to address the problem, from specific CNN architectures to RNNs of the specific CNNs it is worth mentioning U-Net, published in 2015 (Ronneberger et al., 2015). Its main novelties are the combination, in equal amounts, of layers of upsampling and layers of downsampling, and the presence of connections between opposite convolution and deconvolution layers, which allow characteristics of these layers to be concatenated. With these two improvements, and from a training perspective, this means that the medical images can be processed by the network in a single forward step, resulting in the segmentation map directly. Furthermore, thanks to this structure, the U-net takes into account the global context of the image, something that as has been discussed continuously is a great advantage compared to standard CNNs. From the model of U-Net other authors have implemented other architectures that provide certain improvements.

On the other hand, to avoid, or at least reduce, the redundant computation caused by the use of sliding windows to classify pixels, there are authors who propose using FCNNs. The performance of these networks is very satisfactory since they can be applied to multiple targets at the same time (i.e. with the same trained FCNN, both the brain in MRIs, the pectoral muscle in MRIs and the coronary arteries in CTAs are segmented from different images) (Moeskops et al., 2016).

For imaging, 2D or 3D CNNs are used to convert one input image to another. These architectures usually lack grouping layers and therefore require training with a set of data in which the desired input and output are included, and in which the differences between them are defined, as well as the loss function. An example of its use in medical imaging is shown in (li et al., 2014) where a series of images were generated and used in CAD for the diagnosis of Alzheimer's in cases where the original data were not available, because they had been acquired or because they were not available.

On the other hand, it should be mentioned that even though brain images are 3D volumes, most of the methods work in 2D, and consequently analyzing 3D volumes slice by slice. This is done so that the computational cost is lower, or because in many cases the volumes are too thick for analysis. Even so, the most recent publications have used networks that operate in 3D (Hosseini asl et al., 2016; Payan et al., 2015).

Mammography is undoubtedly the most widely used imaging modality for these tasks in breast cancer, because it is the most commonly performed study and therefore from which more data is available, not annotated, but above all annotated, which it is very useful for training deep learning models. Even though most of the articles reviewed use mammograms, they do find others that propose using other imaging modalities, such as US (Jamieson et al., 2012; Kisilev et al., 2016; Zhang et al., 2016), MRI (Dalmış et al., 2016), and TS volumes (Fotin et al., 2016; Samala et al., 2016; Samala, Ravi et al., 2016).

CAD computer-based decision support systems (to generalize and not just CADx or CADe) usually perform tasks in three steps. The most general scheme begins with a stage of obtaining, processing and adapting the data, which can be manual or automated. Next, there is a stage of detection and localization of lesions, which can be more or less automated as well, and finally there is the classification stage. Different types of models are required for the different tasks, and the works analyzed here focus either on some of them or on the overall process. For the second stage, which is where deep models have more weight, in recent years there is still a lot of work that proposes CNNs for the stages of extraction of characteristics, detection and localization of the lesions (Fonsecaetal., 2015; Arevalo et al., 2015).

Thus, returning to CNNs, the typical way of operating for the detection of abnormalities, either in a mammogram or in another type of medical image, is divided into a series of steps. To begin with, a series of candidates are generated that can be different types of abnormalities, generally masses or microcalcifications, defined by their coordinates, and then all of them are passed through an extractor of characteristics that have been defined and extracted manually in a previous phase (Dhungel et al., 2015), leaving the system only with some of them that will be the output of this network and the input of the next layer, the one in charge of the classification (if the purpose of the system is to classify and not just detect and locate).

Regarding the extraction of characteristics, when it is manual, it has to be carried out from a theoretical and verified knowledge, that is, an expert radiologist, or more than one, has to work in choosing these characteristics and in noting the images, to pixel or region level, so that it can be used as a basis for learning. Some examples of characteristics used are histograms of intensity values, morphology characteristics and texture descriptors: shape, border type or density (Kisilev et al., 2016), although it is often It is useful to add other characteristics such as location and context, and even not inherent to the injury itself, such as patient data (Kooi et al., 2016) But this extraction of characteristics is linked to the need to have a set of data annotated by a very large expert. Obviously, this is very complicated because to do it correctly, more than one radiologist would be needed to evaluate and label the images, in addition to having to reach a confidentiality agreement on the part of the doctors and patients, who they are usually opposed to data sharing (Akselrod-Ballin et al., 2016).

Once all these systems have been proposed and built, it is vital to analyze their performance in terms of effectiveness and precision, in addition to comparing their results with those of specialist radiologists and against older traditional CAD systems (less automated, with manual extraction of features for example). Typically, on the one hand, systems with automatic characteristics provide results similar to the old ones, but if they are combined with some characteristics extracted manually and always chosen with criteria, pointing to the weak points of the neural network, the results usually improve a lot (Arevalo et al., 2015; Kooi et al., 2016), and in fact in many situations it is a much more effective strategy to follow than looking for larger amounts of samples to add to the training set. On the other hand, the proposed systems improve precision with respect to that of individual specialists, but not with respect to that of media specialists (Kooi et al., 2016).

Although significantly better results than humans have not yet been achieved, work must continue to build and improve these networks. There are numerous factors that greatly influence the quality of the results, and these are usually pre-processing or post-processing methods of the images. The pre- processing includes different techniques for improving image quality and eliminating noise, and if they are not applied, they cause the precision of the network to drop significantly (Dhungel et al., 2015). Although they are usually steps that are applied separately, there is a system that already proposes integrating them as a first part of it, thus achieving an automatic pre-processing, as can be seen in (Akselrod-Ballin, et al.2016), where a series of regions are proposed having already segmented, removed the background of the image and cut the region automatically. The different forms of image pre-processing will be explained in detail later when the methodology designed in this work is explained. Another stage prior to feeding the network that can be considered pre-processing is the selection of the ROI, which has already been discussed previously.

Data augmentation strategies, widely used in medical imaging to achieve a larger data set, should also be taken into account within the pre-processing.

The data augmentation usually follows two lines; a more classical one based on geometric transformations, whether they are rotations, translations, inversions and changes of scale (Samala et al., 2016; Samala, Ravi et al., 2016; Dhungel et al., 2015) and another associated with the works already reviewed that use patches to train their networks, cutting sub- images that can be superimposed, from each one of the images, in such a way that a multitude of sub-images with different combinations of pixels are obtained. Together with the increase in data, the need arises to make the classes to which the data belong patches are balanced, to achieve a good training of the net. To achieve this, a quantity of patches of the class greater in number, equating the sets (Samala et al., 2016) or the inequality is maintained but in the training it is corrected by showing the patches in less quantity a greater number of times (Kooi et al., 2016). The patches also usually have subsampling techniques associated to reduce their size and make them all the same dimension or post-processing techniques to reconstruct the original image from them.

Consequently, summary of the various works that use Deep Learning models for the analysis of mammograms. For each of them, the most relevant system components are detailed, along with the image modality, the purpose of the system and the results obtained are depicted as under:-.

Table 1. Summary of the various works that uses deep learning models

Reference No.	Modality and [Database]	Pre-Processing	Obtaining Parameters	Method & Results
(Selvathi et al., 2017)	Classification by DM scores (dense tissue/woven fat/ bottom) MT [Mini-MIAS]	Noise removal by filtering Suppression of radio paque artifacts by thresholding Fund segmentation	Obtaining ROIs by growth of regions	Autoencoder + Softmax Classifier Accuracy=98.5%
(Wang et al., 2017)	Detection of BACs (Chest Arterial Calcifications) [840 FFDMs from 210 cases from different centers]	Segmentation and Scaling	Subimages of 95x95 pixels Data augmentation (Rotation of 90º, 180º and 270º and flippings)	DCNN Identification of BACs similar to that of human readers
(Kooi et al., 2016	Discrimination of isolated benign cysts and malignant masses [1000 images with malignant masses and 600 images with cysts]	Log-transformed, inverted, and segmented images Augmentation of tissue-level data	Manual extraction of 260x260 patches Extraction of 5 manual features. Rear combination with automatic features. Pre-trained network with normal mass patches	DCNN AUC=0.80 AUC=0.87 if only lesions larger than 20 mm are used
(Zhang et al., 2016)	Automatic selection of characteristics Classification of malignant / benign tumors [227 SWE images]	Sub-sampling of images to a fixed size and resolution	Automatic feature selection (no segmentation or annotated data) Manual extraction of 286 simple features for comparison	PGBM + RBM + SVM Precision=93.4% Sensitivity=88.6% Specificity=97.1% AUC=0.947
(Sun et al., 2016)	cancer diagnosis [1,874 pairs of mammograms (one CC slice and one MLO slice)]	Sub-region segmentation, bilateral feature extraction, feature selection, classification, etc. Augmentation of data by geometric transformations	Semi-supervised learning (Few labeled ROIs + many unlabeled ROIs) 21 features manually annotated and others obtained a posteriori	DCNN AUC=0.8818 Precision=0.8243
(Samala et al., 2016)	Microcalcification detection and true/false classification [64 DBT cases with microcalcifications (64 CC views +63 MLO views)]	Pre-processing of volumes to obtain the images Filtering of high-frequency noise Geometric transformations to increase the data set Data balancing	Manually annotated true microcalcifications and 16x16 ROI in the center of each FP removal by another CAD Detection by iterative thresholding and region growth, clustering, and reduction of FPs	DCNN AUC=0.93 (Compared to a CNN with AUC=0.89)
(Akselrod-Ballin et al., 2016)	Detection of abnormalities and classification into normal, benign, malignant [(BI-RADS score 1-5) 850 mammograms]	Automatic pre-processing for breast tissue segmentation	Automatic candidate region proposal and automatic selection Data augmentation	DBN + RCNN + Random Forests Accuracy of 0.775% AUC = 0.66

3. CONCLUSIONS AND FUTURE WORK

In the present work we have studied the bases of Deep Learning as well as the different models that are used, and the applications of these techniques. With this, it has been learned what this field consists of, which has recently gained so much attention, with the aim of awakening interest in these techniques. The work has been focused on the analysis of medical images, discovering the surprising number of applications in different organs and with different purposes that these deep models are covering.

Starting from the good results they achieve, the growing importance of aid systems for detection and decision in medical applications is highlighted once again which, without totally replacing the professional, can be of great help, facilitating their work as well as providing better diagnostics and other services to patients.

Specifically, the study of these algorithms on mammographic and tumor images, seeing that it was one of the lines with more research. For this, a thorough bibliographic review of the articles considered most relevant has been carried out, with which it has been possible to have a complete vision of what and how the detection of lesions and the classification of tumors in images of the various parts of human body. It has been learned how algorithms are implemented and that there is no rule for them to work, but that a heuristic study is necessary; the importance of studying the whole of images and of adapting them to the network to obtain good results; how to read the results, what to do to improve them, etc.

In addition, the articles related to the models of deep convolutional networks most used in computer vision have been reviewed. From the lack of application of this type of network to medical image analysis, and understanding the problems faced by more traditional neural networks, the motivation for this work has arisen: to design a deep convolutional network that can be used for analysis of lesions on mammography. This type of network would alleviate the problems of required extensive annotated databases, of physicians having to pinpoint lesions on images before or locating regions of interest as a pre-algorithm training phase, of high computational costs, or of imprecise locations of images with the lesions; all of them commented throughout this work.

The network that has been designed, although based on theoretical concepts and other works, is only a schematic, and therefore it would be a good future work and of great interest to be able to implement and test it. Given that the database and the necessary software are available, it is intended to leave it as an open line to be continued, so that from this work the implementation of this network and the interpretation of the results is feasible, seeking how improving them and comparing them with those of other works.

Thus, it can be concluded by saying that the results obtained in this study are very satisfactory, because even though the designed network has not been implemented, deep learning in medical imaging has been exhaustively studied, a field that is still very new and that arouses great interest, learning a multitude of concepts about it and currently having the necessary bases to develop more studies in relation to Artificial Intelligence, both theoretical and practical.

REFERENCES

Akselrod-Ballin, A., Karlinsky, L., Alpert, S., Hashoul, S., Ben-Ari, R., & Barkan, E. (2016). *A Region Based Convolutional Network for Tumor Detection and Classification in Breast Mammography.* . doi:10.1007/978-3-319-46976-8_21

Almeida, I., & Barros, P. (2020). *Denoising Autoencoder - Deep Learning*. Academic Press.

Arevalo, J., González, F., Ramos, R., Oliveira, J., Lopez, G., & Angel, M. (2015). Representation learning for mammography mass lesion classification with convolutional neural networks. *Computer Methods and Programs in Biomedicine*, *127*, 248–257. Advance online publication. doi:10.1016/j.cmpb.2015.12.014 PMID:26826901

Ching, T., Himmelstein, D. S., Beaulieu-Jones, B. K., Kalinin, A. A., Do, B. T., Way, G. P., Ferrero, E., Agapow, P. M., Zietz, M., Hoffman, M. M., Xie, W., Rosen, G. L., Lengerich, B. J., Israeli, J., Lanchantin, J., Woloszynek, S., Carpenter, A. E., Shrikumar, A., Xu, J., ... Greene, C. S. (2018). Opportunities and obstacles for deep learning in biology and medicine. *Journal of the Royal Society, Interface*, *15*(141), 20170387. doi:10.1098/rsif.2017.0387 PMID:29618526

Dalmış, M., Gubern-Mérida, A., Vreemann, S., Karssemeijer, N., Mann, R., & Platel, B. (2016). A computer-aided diagnosis system for breast DCE-MRI at high spatiotemporal resolution. *Medical Physics*, *43*(1), 84–94. doi:10.1118/1.4937787 PMID:26745902

de Giorgio, A. (2015). *A study on the similarities of Deep Belief Networks and Stacked Autoencoders*. . doi:10.13140/RG.2.1.3502.8883

Dhungel, N., Carneiro, G., & Bradley, A. (2015). Deep Learning and Structured Prediction for the Segmentation of Mass in Mammograms. *Deep Learning and Structured Prediction for the Segmentation of Mass in Mammograms.*, *9349*, 605–612. Advance online publication. doi:10.1007/978-3-319-24553-9_74

Fischer, A., & Igel, C. (2014). Training restricted Boltzmann machines: An introduction. *Pattern Recognition*, *47*(1), 25–39. doi:10.1016/j.patcog.2013.05.025

Földiák, P., & Endres, D. (2008). Sparse coding. *Scholarpedia.*, *3*(1), 2984. doi:10.4249cholarpedia.2984

Fonseca, P., Mendoza, J., Wainer, J., Ferrer, J., Pinto, J., Guerrero, J., & Castaneda, B. (2015). *Automatic breast density classification using a convolutional neural network architecture search procedure*. doi:10.1117/12.2081576

Fotin, S., Yin, Y., Haldankar, H., Hoffmeister, J., & Periaswamy, S. (2016). *Detection of soft tissue densities from digital breast tomosynthesis: comparison of conventional and deep learning approaches*. . doi:10.1117/12.2217045

Galaz, V., Centeno, M., Callahan, P., Causevic, A., Patterson, T., Brass, I., Baum, S., Farber, D., Fischer, J., Garcia, D., McPhearson, T., Jiménez, D., King, B., Larcey, P., & Levy, K. (2021). Artificial intelligence, systemic risks, and sustainability. *Technology in Society*, *67*, 101741. doi:10.1016/j.techsoc.2021.101741

Gao, S., Tsang, I., & Chia, L.-T. (2012). Laplacian Sparse Coding, Hypergraph Laplacian Sparse Coding, and Applications. *IEEE Transactions on Pattern Analysis and Machine Intelligence*, *35*(1), 92–104. Advance online publication. doi:10.1109/TPAMI.2012.63 PMID:22392702

Guo, Y., Liu, Y., Oerlemans, A., Lao, S.-Y., Wu, S., & Lew, M. (2015). Deep learning for visual understanding: A review. *Neurocomputing*, *187*, 27–48. Advance online publication. doi:10.1016/j.neucom.2015.09.116

He, K., Zhang, X., Ren, S., & Sun, J. (2014). Spatial Pyramid Pooling in Deep Convolutional Networks for Visual Recognition. *IEEE Transactions on Pattern Analysis and Machine Intelligence*, *37*(9), 1904–1916. Advance online publication. doi:10.1109/TPAMI.2015.2389824 PMID:26353135

He, K., Zhang, X., Ren, S., & Sun, J. (2016). Deep Residual Learning for Image Recognition. *2016 IEEE Conference on Computer Vision and Pattern Recognition (CVPR)*, 770-778. 10.1109/CVPR.2016.90

Hinton, G., Srivastava, N., Krizhevsky, A., Sutskever, I., & Salakhutdinov, R. (2012). *Improving neural networks by preventing co-adaptation of feature detectors*. arXiv preprint. arXiv.

Hosseini asl, E., Gimel'farb, G., & El-Baz, A. (2016). Alzheimer's Disease Diagnostics by a Deeply Supervised Adaptable 3D Convolutional Network. *Computational and Mathematical Methods in Medicine*.

Huang, G., Liu, Z., & Weinberger, K. Q. (2017). Densely Connected Convolutional Networks. *2017 IEEE Conference on Computer Vision and Pattern Recognition (CVPR)*, 2261-2269. 10.1109/CVPR.2017.243

Jamieson, A., Drukker, K., & Giger, M. (2012). Breast Image Feature Learning with Adaptive Deconvolutional Networks. *Proc SPIE, 8315*. . doi:10.1117/12.910710

Ker, J., Wang, L., Rao, J., & Lim, T. (2017). Deep Learning Applications in Medical Image Analysis. *IEEE Access*. . doi:10.1109/ACCESS.2017.2788044

Kisilev, P., Sason, E., Barkan, E., & Hashoul, S. (2016). *Medical Image Description Using Multi-task-loss CNN*. . doi:10.1007/978-3-319-46976-8_13

Kooi, T., Litjens, G., Ginneken, B., Gubern-Mérida, A., Sánchez, C., Mann, R., Heeten, G., & Karssemeijer, N. (2016). Large Scale Deep Learning for Computer Aided Detection of Mammographic Lesions. *Medical Image Analysis*, *35*, 303–312. Advance online publication. doi:10.1016/j.media.2016.07.007 PMID:27497072

Krizhevsky, A., Sutskever, I., & Hinton, G. (2012). ImageNet Classification with Deep Convolutional Neural Networks. *Neural Information Processing Systems.*, *25*. Advance online publication. doi:10.1145/3065386

Li, R., Zhang, W., Suk, H.-I., Wang, L., Li, J., Shen, D., & Ji, S. (2014). *Deep Learning Based Imaging Data Completion for Improved Brain Disease Diagnosis*. doi:10.1007/978-3-319-10443-0_39

Linardatos, P., Papastefanopoulos, V., & Kotsiantis, S. (2020). Explainable AI: A Review of Machine Learning Interpretability Methods. *Entropy (Basel, Switzerland)*, *23*, 18. doi:10.3390/e23010018

Lopes, N., & Ribeiro, B. (2015). *Deep Belief Networks (DBNs)*. doi:10.1007/978-3-319-06938-8_8

Moeskops, P., Wolterink, J., Van der Velden, B., Gilhuijs, K., Leiner, T., Viergever, M., & Išgum, I. (2016). Deep Learning for Multi-Task Medical Image Segmentation in Multiple Modalities. *LNCS*, *9901*, 478–486. doi:10.1007/978-3-319-46723-8_55

Payan, A., & Montana, G. (2015). Predicting Alzheimer's disease: a neuroimaging study with 3D convolutional neural networks. *ICPRAM 2015 - 4th International Conference on Pattern Recognition Applications and Methods, Proceedings, 2*.

Rangamani, A., Mukherjee, A., Basu, A., Arora, A., Ganapathi, T., Chin, S., & Tran, T. (2018). *Sparse Coding and Autoencoders*. Advance online publication. doi:10.1109/ISIT.2018.8437533

Ronneberger, O., Fischer, P., & Brox, T. (2015). U-Net: Convolutional Networks for Biomedical Image Segmentation. *LNCS, 9351*, 234–241. doi:10.1007/978-3-319-24574-4_28

Salakhutdinov, R., & Hinton, G. (2009). Deep Boltzmann Machines. *Proceedings of AISTATS 2009.*

Samala, R., Chan, H-P., Hadjiiski, L., Cha, K., & Helvie, M. (2016). *Deep-learning convolution neural network for computer-aided detection of microcalcifications in digital breast tomosynthesis.* doi:10.1117/12.2217092

Samala, R., Chan, H.-P., Hadjiiski, L., Helvie, M., Wei, J., & Cha, K. (2016). Mass detection in digital breast tomosynthesis: Deep convolutional neural network with transfer learning from mammography. *Medical Physics, 43*, 6654. doi:10.1118/1.4967345]

Selvathi, D., & AarthyPoornila, A. (2017). *Performance analysis of various classifiers on deep learning network for breast cancer detection.* doi:10.1109/CSPC.2017.8305869

Simonyan, K., & Zisserman, A. (2014). *Very Deep Convolutional Networks for Large-Scale Image Recognition.* arXiv 1409.1556.

Srivastava, N., Hinton, G., Krizhevsky, A., Sutskever, I., & Salakhutdinov, R. (2014). Dropout: A Simple Way to Prevent Neural Networks from Overfitting. *Journal of Machine Learning Research, 15*, 1929–1958.

Sun, W., Tseng, B., Zhang, J., & Qian, W. (2016). Enhancing deep convolutional neural network scheme for breast cancer diagnosis with unlabeled data. *Computerized Medical Imaging and Graphics, 57*. Advance online publication. doi:10.1016/j.compmedimag.2016.07.004

Szegedy, C., Liu, W., Jia, Y., Sermanet, P., Reed, S., Anguelov, D., Erhan, D., Vanhoucke, V., & Rabinovich, A. (2015). Going deeper with convolutions. *The IEEE Conference on Computer Vision and Pattern Recognition (CVPR)*, 1-9. 10.1109/CVPR.2015.7298594

Szegedy, C., Vanhoucke, V., Ioffe, S., Shlens, J., & Wojna, Z. (2016). Rethinking the Inception Architecture for Computer Vision. *2016 IEEE Conference on Computer Vision and Pattern Recognition (CVPR)*, 2818-2826. 10.1109/CVPR.2016.308

University of Stanford. (n.d.). *Convolutional Neural Networks for Visual Recognition.* https://cs231n.github.io/convolutional-networks/

Voulodimos, A., Doulamis, N., Doulamis, A., & Protopapadakis, E. (2018). Deep Learning for Computer Vision: A Brief Review. Computational Intelligence and Neuroscience. doi:10.1155/2018/7068349

Wan, L., Zeiler, M., Zhang, S., Lecun, Y., & Fergus, R. (2013). *Regularization of Neural Networks using DropConnect*. Academic Press.

Wang, J., Ding, H., Azamian, F., Zhou, B., Iribarren, C., Molloi, S., & Baldi, P. (2017). Detecting Cardiovascular Disease from Mammograms With Deep Learning. *IEEE Transactions on Medical Imaging*. doi:10.1109/TMI.2017.2655486

Webb, G., Fürnkranz, J., Hinton, G., Sammut, C., Sander, J., Vlachos, M., Teh, Y., Yang, Y., Mladenić, D., Brank, J., Grobelnik, M., Zhao, Y., Karypis, G., Craw, S., Puterman, M., & Patrick, J. (2010). *Deep Belief Networks*. doi:10.1007/978-0-387-30164-8_209

Zhang, N., Ding, S., Zhang, J., & Xue, Y. (2017). An overview on Restricted Boltzmann Machines. *Neurocomputing*, *275*. Advance online publication. doi:10.1016/j.neucom.2017.09.065

Zhang, Q., Xiao, Y., Dai, W., Suo, J., Wang, C., Shi, J., & Zheng, H. (2016). Deep learning based classification of breast tumors with shear-wave elastography. *Ultrasonics*, *72*. Advance online publication. doi:10.1016/j.ultras.2016.08.004

Chapter 2
Hepatitis Disease Diagnosis Using a Novel Hybrid Method Based on Naïve Bayes and Decision Table

Pooja
Sharda University, India

Kulwinder Kaur
Independent Researcher, Australia

ABSTRACT

Hepatitis is inflammation of the liver most often caused by a viral infection. The supervised data mining technique diagnosed hepatitis using a dataset. Data mining methods have been widely used to analyze biomedical information. This chapter sheds light on the severe viral hepatitis which is spreading around the world at an alarming rate. It is necessary to diagnose such a disease at an early stage to reduce suffering. Early diagnosis of hepatitis is difficult because of the different characteristics associated with it. Artificial intelligence has gained an extensive recognition in medical applications with its growing contribution in interpretation of medical images, diagnosis, design, and development of expert frameworks to assist the practitioners, design of prosthetics, and design of drugs for diverse phases of medicine. A model needs to be created that can be used to visualize life in hepatitis. This chapter uses the Naïve Bayes classifier and provides an improved Naïve Bayes classifier to provide more precision.

1. INTRODUCTION

Since the last few decades, Artificial Intelligence has gained an extensive recognition in medical applications with its growing contribution in interpretation of medical images, diagnosis, design and development of expert frameworks to assist the practitioners, developing prosthetics, and drugs designs during diverse phases in medical science. The accessibility of enormous medicinal information in hospitals

DOI: 10.4018/978-1-6684-2508-4.ch002

and other health organizations prompts the requirement for effective data analysis tools to extract useful knowledge. Several techniques and data mining tools have been developed till date for data classification. In the last few years, Data Mining and Knowledge Discovery have captivated quite a recognition in the information industry and medical industry due to the paramount requirement of converting huge data into knowledge and information(Mohammed Abdullah Al-Hagery et.al, 2015).

Liver is considered as the powerhouse of the body as it contributes highly to process nutrients and metabolize medication. It expels out all toxic waste products from the body. Hepatitis is a standout amongst the most essential reasons for chronic liver infection and a huge number of individuals are at risk for its complications (S Pushpalatha and Dr. Jagdesh Pandya, 2014).

The word hepatitis is a combination of two words with the Ancient-Greek word "hepar" which means 'liver', and the Latin "it" means inflammation/swelling. Numerous circumstances are responsible for this inflammation including a viral or bacterial contamination, liver damage due to any poisonous consumption, and attack by the immune system of the body. There exist several forms of hepatitis, and the malady is typically brought on by one of three viruses: hepatitis A, hepatitis B, or hepatitis C virus. The hepatitis infection is a transforming infection that adjusts with the progressions after some time and can be hard for the body to battle. The side effects incorporate the aggravation of the liver portrayed by disquietude, joint hurts, stomach torment, retching 2-3 times each day, crap, loss of craving, dull pee, fever, augmented liver and/or jaundice. Some persistent types of hepatitis give not many of these indications and are possibly present when the prolonged irritation has prompted the substitution of liver-cells through connected tissue; this infection cycle is mentioned as cirrhosis-of-liver. Since the symptoms do not usually appear earlier the delay in diagnosis leads to a very serious stage. Hence it is mandatory to have a system that is efficient enough to predict the earlier diagnosis of hepatitis accurately by detailing down the type of the virus found in the patient's body.

With the constantly increasing scientific knowledge, it will become very tough for physicians to stay abreast of drugs beyond their specialized field. In case the medical hassle lies past the physician`s competence, the answer is to seek advice from a specialist, that's generally both unavailable or now no longer to be had in that instant. The diagnosis done by a physician depends upon his experience, his training, and his observations. But the results cannot be considered reliable due to limitations of human memory, lack of adequate experience. Hence it becomes severely important for the patients to consult an expert system that deals with them like a human being but promises to produce most accurate results computationally and logically with minimum percentage of errors.

1.1 Background

(Mohammed Abdullah Al-Hagery et.al, 2015) explains the importance of statistical methods and Data Mining tools to enhance the data analysis in large historical data sets. Since hepatitis has been considered as the major cause of the most of the deaths per year and is accounting for liver cancer in majority, hence there is an immediate need of an effective data analysis tool for medical information analysis to perform a better diagnosis for better treatment purposes. In this paper, the authors have come up with three independent classification models, one for each hepatitis type able to cover all possible conditions that come under each virus type for efficient prediction of patient status. It contributes highly to help the physicians in earlier diagnosis by implementing data mining tools. The data analysis is achieved in two steps, initiating with the recognition of data contents to form the clusters and further applying the NN classifier to diagnose the type of virus in the patient.

(Huda Yasinet. et.al, 2011) have investigated the factors that highly increase the risk of hepatitis C virus.It is a massive issue and cannot be afforded to be tested only by physicians as it may involve some inaccuracy. As the symptoms remain unnoticed for years hence the damage caused by it is extremely serious. Hence understanding the need of an accurate expert diagnosis system, the authors have proposed to make the understanding of a regression base logistic model to check all those factors that marks the importance of HCV cases. Logistic Regression Modeling involves making the chances of an event as a couple of linear set of variables and is described as:

$$\mathrm{E}\left(\frac{Z}{X}\right)=\frac{S^{T}}{1+S^{T}}=\prod(X)=\frac{S^{T}}{1+S^{T}} \tag{1}$$

Where $\prod(X)$ represents the expected value of the response variable, natural logarithms base is e.

T can be further described as:

$$\mathrm{T}=p_0+p_1x_1+p_2x_2+\ldots\ldots p_nx_n \tag{2}$$

Where, p_i and x_i are coefficients and predictors respectively for n predictors.

To manage the missing values issue, data normalization techniques have been favored. Beginning with the trimming down of dimensions of the problem and further applying the binary logistic regression to categorize and manage all the cases by making the use of all conditional and countable measures for reducing the data.

(T.Karthikeyan and P.Thangaraju, 2013), analyzes the data of hepatitis patients with various classification algorithms with an aim to classify and scale the accuracy of the hepatitis database. The final effects for those classification tasks are being depicted on the basis of accuracy and time. The existence of various independent features makes the prognosis of hepatitis very challenging in an early stage which can be performed hence with the aid of a model. In this paper, the biomedical data has been analyzed with data mining used in bioinformatics as the data mining algorithms produce reliable outcomes in forecasting and differentiation of inter related data. The dataset considered in the work consists of 155 instances and 19 attributes, and the class shows the prognosis of life Yes (or) No while it consists of 14 nominal attributes and 6 multi-valued attributes. This analysis is very time consuming which is overcome by using WEKA data mining tool. The experimental result tells that algorithm Naïve Bayes takes a reduced amount of time in Weka .

(Ghumbre Shashikant Uttreshwar et.al, 2009), understands the necessity of an expert diagnosis system to avoid any kind of uncertainty. Comprehensibility is highly needed in any machine learning technique. Encouraged with this advancement, the authors have investigated the use of AI in depicting Hepatitis B prediction. For the use of it, a very smart model has been produced based upon the two important domains of AI. The logical inference depicts the type of hepatitis present in the patient along with a generalized regression neural network to make predictions about the severity level of the disease.

(Dakshata Panchal and Seema Shah, 2011) emphasizes on the need of an intelligent diagnosis system which is able to process huge medical data and is much more reliable than human experts' decision. In this paper an intelligent system is made to diagnose Hepatitis B virus at an earlier stage. Hepatitis B is a liver disease brought about by the hepatitis B infection (HBV). It can transmit to others by means of sexual contact, illegal usage of medicines and drugs, introduction to blood that is infectious and the result of effects of vaccination of newborn babies. The most preferable solution for diagnosis includes an expert system where the knowledge base includes implementation of human reasoning and use of a set of decision rules including physical symptoms and laboratory analysis that lead to suggestions.

(Dr. S. Vijayarani and Mr.S.Dhayanan, 2015), supported the involvement of the data mining techniques in the health care systems for efficient knowledge discovery. Classification is the widely used data mining technique, the authors have also used Naïve-bayes and Support Vector Machine (SVM) for liver-disease prediction. Naïve-bayes is a probability model where it expects that the presence of a specific element of a class is disconnected to the presence of some other element and that a limited quantity of preparing information is expected to appraise the methods and changes of the factors additionally taken for classification. SVM techniques can be used for characterization of direct and non-straight information and here the first preparing information is changed into higher measurement utilizing non-linear mapping. Both the algorithms have been simulated and their performance has been compared with respect to classification accuracy and execution time. SVM classifier proved to be best in terms of highest classification accuracy while the Naïve Bayes classifier resulted in minimum execution time.

(Nahid Khorashadizade and Hassan Rezaei, 2015), highlighted the immediate importance of rapid diagnosis of the hepatitis disease to curb the serious effects of this virus at the earlier stage. For a smart diagnosis, the authors have developed a new technique involving Principal Component Analysis (PCA) and Error Minimized Extreme Learning Machine (EMELM)PCA algorithm is the most common method of feature extraction where data is mapped from a complex and multi-dimensional space into a simple space keeping the same dimensions. It is an orthogonal linear conversion in vector space with ordered dimensions in such a way that the data components are placed according to the maximum possible variance. SLFNs are feed forward neural networks with only one hidden layer and Extreme Learning Machine (ELM) is an enhanced learning algorithm which selects the parameters of hidden layer at random and subsequently leading to cut the learning time. The proposed algorithm includes two phases: the feature reduction by PCA in phase 1and the classification by EMELM in phase 2 where records with missing values of data set hepatitis are removed and then the data set is normalized in [0,1] range.

2 PROPOSED METHODOLOGY

2.1 Naive Bayes Classification

The essential necessity of Artificial Intelligence oriented methodology is a dataset. The classifier is displayed with the named information. This paper includes the utilization of multinomial gullible Bayes as a gauge classifier because of its proficiency. The component words are thought to be free and further every event is utilized to plan down the features into its proper notion class. Innocent Bayes is utilized on the grounds that this is anything but difficult to assemble and execute and to appraise the boundaries it requires a limited quantity of preparing information.

The posterior decision rule is represented as follows for a classifier based on maximum:

$$c = \arg\max \ c \in C(P(\frac{c}{m})) \tag{3}$$

$$= \arg\max \ c \in C \ P(c) \prod_{1 \le k \le n_d} P(\frac{t_k}{c}) \tag{4}$$

Where t_k represents the words contained in each important and C embodies the usual of segments used in the cataloging, the previous likelihood of a class C text and the class C conditional probability is represented by P(c) and $P(\frac{c}{m})$ respectively, and $P(\frac{l_k}{c})$ denotes the conditional probability of word l_k in class c. The equation (1) can be reduced to

$$C = (\arg\max \ c \in C \log P(c) + \sum_{1 \le k \le n_d} \log\log P(\frac{l_k}{c})) \tag{5}$$

2.2 Proposed Algorithm

The information to be put away in decision table calculation is recovered from the chosen set of characteristics and that model is utilized as a query table while making the expectations for the information. Every entry in the table is related to a class likelihood. It is exceptionally testing to choose a part of a set with profoundly discriminative attributes in the decision table. Naive Bayes depends on Bayes' hypothesis with independence assumptions between indicators. The Naive Bayesian classifier has a number of advantages, one of which is its ease of use. This is due to the fact that it is the most basic categorization method. It can easily manage a data collection with multiple properties due to its simplicity. Furthermore, estimating the means and variances of the variables required for classification needs just a modest quantity of training data.

1) In our new discoveries, the decision table portrays the contingent likelihood table for naive bayes calculation i.e naive bayes likelihood is approved utilizing decision table standards.
2) The calculation assesses the qualities, at each point in the inquiry, by grouping the characteristics of traits into two disjoint subsets: one for each of naive Bayes and decision table.
3) At first all ascribes are shown by the choice table. At each movement, forward determination search is used, and the characteristics browsed this are shown by Naive Bayes and the rest by the choice table.

At every progression in this investigation, it appraises the legitimacy connected with classifying the attributes within two different sets. The estimation for class should be made to develop base class probability checks.

We can divide the features into two distinct areas which must be based upon finding at every point, then every feature which is ordered using NB and the leftover is controlled by DT. Then finally the conclusions for each work is calculated and estimations for probability are found.

Step 1. For each occasion in dataset,

In the event that (numeric) Throws special case

Else

Assess benefits of parting the trait into naive-bayes and choice table utilizing forward AS search.

Step 2. Discover the probabilities of each attribute utilizing NB as:

a. Let M be training-set containing tuples of data/features and their respective class labels as represented below:

$$Y= (y_1, y_2, y_3, \ldots, y_n) \tag{6}$$

b. If a tuple Y is given, the classifier will predict that Y belongs to the class having the highest posterior probability, conditioned on Y. That is, the naive Bayesian classifier predicts that tuple Y belongs to class Ci if and only if

$$P(Y) > P(C_j|Y) \text{ for } 1 \leq j \leq m, j \neq i \tag{7}$$

Thus, we maximize $P(Y)$. According to the Bayes- theorem

$$P(Y) = \frac{P(C_i)P(C_i)}{P(Y)} \tag{8}$$

The term P(Y) is constant for all classes, only $P(C_i)P(C_i)$ needs to be maximized. If the class prior probabilities are not known, then the classes are equally likely, that is,

$$P(C_1) = P(C_2) = = P(C_m) \tag{9}$$

c. Reducing computation in evaluating $P(C_i)$, the naive assumption of class-conditional independence is made. Thus,

$$P(C_i) = \prod_{k=1}^{n} P(y_k \mid C_j) \tag{10}$$

$$= P(y_1|C_i) \times (y_2|C_i) \times \ldots \times P(y_n|C_i) \tag{11}$$

d. Predicting the class label of Y, $P(C_i)P(C_i)$ is calculated for all class C_i.

$$P(C_i)P(C_i) > P(C_j)P(C_j) \; 1 \leq j \leq m, j \neq i \tag{12}$$

The predicted class label is the class C_i for which $P(C_i)P(C_i)$ is the maximum.

Step 3. Calculate the probabilities using decision-table as:

a. Decision table consists of:
   - Schema R ($B_1, B_2, \ldots, B_n$, Class, Sup, Con).
   - Rows $Ro_i = (b_{1i}, b_{2i}, \ldots, b_{ni}, cl_i, su_i, con_i)$ in table R represents a classification rule, whereas b_{ij} ($1 \leq k \leq p$) can be either from DOM(B_i) or a special value ANY,

$d_i \in \{d_1, d_2, ..., d_m\}$

msup $\leq supp_i, \leq 1$; mcon $\leq con_i \leq 1$, Where msup and mcon are predetermined threshold .for dataset Q with n attributes $B_1, B_2, ..., B_n$

The interpretation of the rule is if (E_1=e_1) and (E_2=e_2) and … and (E_n=e_n) then class = d_i with probability con_i and having support sup_i, where ak[1] ANY, 1≤ k≤ p.

Finding rows whose attribute values are either ANY or equal to the corresponding attribute values of u($b_{1u}, b_{2u}, ..., b_{nu}$), searching for the matches in a decision table could result in following:

1. Matched-row found:
2. More than one matched-row found:
    a. based on confidence and support:

$$kR_u j = 1 = \{Conf_i = k \max i\, j = 1 Conf_j\} \tag{13}$$

    b. based on weighted 'confidence' and 'support':

$$kR_u j = 1 = \{R_i | Conf_i * Sup_i = k \max i\, j = 1(Conf_j * Sup_j)\} \tag{14}$$

The class of the primary coordinating line can be essentially relegated to the example to be grouped.

3. No coordinating column is discovered: The strategy utilized for grouping such examples is to utilize the default class.

Step 4. The general class likelihood is figured as
P (Decision-Table) * (P (Naive-Bayes)/earlier likelihood of class)
Expecting X (Decision-Table) = set of qualities in the Decision-Table
X (Naive-Bayes) =set of properties in Naive-Bayes

The Bayes measure, which is used to build decision trees, can handle continuous attributes directly and automatically select the most appropriate discretization and interval numbering limits. The Naive Bayes node assists in the resolution of overgeneralization and overspecialization issues that are common in decision trees.

3 PERFORMANCE PARAMETERS

The assessment parameters considered for performance evaluation of the proposed system are: The evaluation parameters include various terms such as true-positive, true-negative, false-negative and false- positive. Confusion-Matrix contains these terms that are utilized for assessment.

1. **Precision and Recall:** It checks how many patients are correctly classified to have hepatitis disease among those all that are classified as having hepatitis.

$$\text{Precision} = \frac{n_{s\rightarrow s}}{n_{s\rightarrow s} + n_{h\rightarrow s}} \tag{15}$$

$$\text{Recall} = \frac{n_{s\rightarrow s}}{n_{s\rightarrow s} + n_{s\rightarrow h}} \tag{16}$$

$$\text{F-measure} = \frac{2 * recall * precision}{precision + recall} \tag{17}$$

3. **Accuracy:** Accuracy is the percentage of correctly identified patients to have hepatitis disease or not. It can be measured as the number of correctly classified hepatitis patients to the total number of patients.

$$\text{Accuracy} = \frac{n_{s\rightarrow s} + n_{h\rightarrow h}}{n_{s\rightarrow s} + n_{s\rightarrow h} + n_{h\rightarrow s} + n_{h\rightarrow h}} \tag{18}$$

Table 1. Contingency table

		Correct Labels	
		Positive	**Negative**
Classified Labels	**Positive**	True Positive ($n_{s\rightarrow s}$)	False Positive ($n_{h\rightarrow s}$)
	Negative	False Negative ($n_{s\rightarrow h}$)	True Negative ($n_{h\rightarrow h}$)

(S Pushpalatha and Dr. Jagdesh Pandya, 2014)2. **F-measure:** is the harmonic-mean of 'precision' and 'recall'.

Table 2. Naïve bayes

Training Set Evaluation Results			Testing Set Evaluation Results	
Correct-Classified Instances	150		Correct-Classified Instances	44
Incorrect-Classified Instances	5		Incorrect-Classified Instances	2
Accuracy	96.7742		Accuracy	95.6522

Table 3. Improved naïve bayes

Training Set Evaluation Results			Testing Set Evaluation Results	
Correct-Classified Instances	151		Correct-Classified Instances	45
Incorrect-Classified Instances	4		Incorrect-Classified Instances	1
Correct-Classified Instances	97.4194		Accuracy	97.8261

4. RESULTS AND DISCUSSIONS

This section presents the simulation results and the evaluation parameters. The data is divided into training split and testing split sets. The improved algorithm is providing more accuracy.

Figure 1. Accuracy comparison of proposed with the existing Naïve Bayes

Contingency Table		Correct Labels	
		Positive	Negative
Classified Labels	Positive	**True Positive** ($n_{i \to i}$)	**False Positive** ($n_{k \to i}$)
	Negative	**False Negative** ($n_{i \to k}$)	**True Negative** ($n_{k \to k}$)

5. CONCLUSION

Nowadays, hospitalized treatments have become highly attributed to the recent growth in technology in recent times. In addition, IT and communication tools have further improved the implementation of medical practice improving the performances for the diagnosis of hepatitis is the major onus which can be performed by the data mining. This paper reviews disparate relevant data mining tools which are very helpful for the hepatitis diagnosis.

In this work, we have proposed the research work by skillfully improving the existing naïve bayes algorithm just to achieve better performance. And the final overall results depict more accuracy rate.

REFERENCES

Afif, M. H., Hedar, A.-R., Abdel Hamid, T. H., & Mahdy, Y. B. (2013). SS-SVM (3SVM): A new classification method for hepatitis disease diagnosis. *International Journal of Advanced Computer Science and Applications*, *4*(2), 53–58.

Al-Hagery, Alfaiz, & Alorinim, & Althunayan. (2015). Knowledge discovery in the data sets of hepatitis disease for diagnosis and prediction to support and serve community. *International Journal of Computer and Electronics Research*, *4*(6), 118–125.

Ba-Alwi, F. M., & Hintaya, H. M. (2013). Comparative study for analysis the prognostic in hepatitis data: Data mining approach. *International Journal of Scientific and Engineering Research*, *4*(8), 680–685.

Ghumbre & Ghatol (2009). Hepatitis B Diagnosis Using Logical Inference AndGeneralized Regression Neural Networks. *Proceedings of IEEE International Advance Computing Conference (IACC 2009).*

Karthikeyan & Thangaraju. (2013). Analysis of classification algorithms applied to hepatitis patients. *International Journal of Computer Applications*, *62*(15), 25-30.

Khorashadizade, N., & Rezaei, H. (2015). New method for rapid diagnosis of hepatitis disease based on reduction feature and machine learning. *Journal of Advanced Computer Science & Technology*, *4*(1), 148–155. doi:10.14419/jacst.v4i1.4353

Panchal, D., & Shah, S. (2011). Artificial intelligence based expert system for Hepatitis B diagnosis. *International Journal of Modeling and Optimization*, *1*(4), 362–366. doi:10.7763/IJMO.2011.V1.61

Pushpalatha, S., & Pandya, J. (2014). Comparison of data models for hepatitis diagnosis - data mining technique. *International Journal of Advanced Research in Computer Science and Software Engineering*, *4*(1), 1092–1095.

Vijayarani & Dayananda. (2015). Liver disease prediction using SVM and Naïve Bayes algorithms. *International Journal of Science, Engineering and Technology Research, 4*(4), 816-820.

Yasin, Jilani, & Danish. (2011). Hepatitis-C classification using data mining techniques. *International Journal of Computer Applications*, *24*(3), 1-6.

Chapter 3
Breast Cancer Detection Using Different Classification and Ensemble Methods

Tanisha Gupta
J.C. Bose University of Science and Technology, YMCA, India

Piyush Gupta
J.C. Bose University of Science and Technology, YMCA, India

Ved Pal
J.C. Bose University of Science and Technology, YMCA, India

Komal Kumar Bhatia
J.C. Bose University of Science and Technology, YMCA, India

ABSTRACT

Breast cancer causes the cells in the breast to grow in an uncontrolled manner. Countless research has been conducted to enhance the timely diagnose of breast cancer, which expands the likelihood of survival and hence the survival rates. Mammography photographs were the focus of the majority of the investigation. Early detection of cancer is frequently delayed because symptoms are frequently not visible during the early stages of cancer. Mammography scans, on the other hand, can sometimes produce false positives, putting the patient health in danger. Different techniques, which are simpler to implement and perform better with different data sets, are needed to develop more reliable and safer forecasts. Healthcare data is huge and unstructured. Machine learning has long been the methodology of choice in breast cancer pattern classification and forecast modelling because of its distinct benefits based on feature identification from a comprehensive breast cancer dataset. The study evaluates and compares the results of seven different ML algorithms based on different performance metrics.

DOI: 10.4018/978-1-6684-2508-4.ch003

1 INTRODUCTION

The presence of new emerging technologies in the medical field and the massive amount of patient data have made way for new strategies to develop for cancer prevention and detection. Whenever the cells present in the breast develop a malignant tumor, this is referred to as breast cancer. The human body has an enormous cell count. Cells grow when they are needed by the human body and die once they're no longer needed. This is the natural process of cells. The cells that develop in cancer even though they aren't needed by the body. These aberrant cell growths generate a lump, which is commonly referred to as a tumor Partial or complete timely detection and diagnosis can benefit cancer patients. Most frequent cancer in females is Breast Cancer, which can be cured if found early and treated appropriately with conventional treatments, but there is no natural cure for cancer. One in every two Indian females diagnosed with breast cancer dies, resulting in a 50% probability of fatality in India (Erlay et al., 2012; Bray et al., 2013). Early or timely detection of breast cancer is impossible since no signs are visible during the early stages of the disease. A regular mammogram test is the first and best tool for doctors to find out about early symptoms. Breast cancer can be prevented if a healthy lifestyle is maintained from a young age, which includes being physically active, limiting the use of alcohol, and proper food intake.

Artificial intelligence includes machine learning (ML). Because of its specific benefits based on feature identification from a large breast cancer dataset, ML has been a popular choice among researchers for breast cancer prediction. A dataset is provided for the learning, as a contrast to the normal approach, where results for all the cases are provided beforehand. The major objective of machine learning is to enable computers to understand themselves. Various machine learning methods are utilized to develop tools that aid in the detection and, ultimately, the reduction of patient mortality rates. The primary goal of these tools is to provide faster analysis of large amounts of data while avoiding potential diagnostic and detection errors.ML algorithms are widely utilized in the creation of prediction models to enhance successful decision-making. Cancerous cells can form lumps of tissue, also referred to as tumors. Benign tumors are non-cancerous, which means they do not spread and grow at a slow pace, whereas malignant tumors are cancerous, which means they grow rapidly, destroying nearby tissues and spreading at a higher pace.

Tumors are classified as benign or malignant using the Wisconsin Diagnostic Breast Cancer (WDBC) dataset. The dataset comprise of a repository with 569 data points separated into 212 malignant (M) and 357 benign (B) categories. The classification is based on ten separate features. In real-world data, there are large groupings of missing and noisy data. To eliminate these errors and produce confident forecasts, the data is preprocessed. When cleaning acquired data, noise and missing values are prevalent. To generate an accurate and useful output, the noise in the data must be removed, and missing values must be filled in. The method includes smoothing, normalization, and aggregation. The entire dataset is broken down into two portions. The training data is often used to train the algorithm which provides data points with answers, and the algorithm is used to categories data points as malignant or benign tumor in the testing dataset. In this chapter, four performance metrics are utilized to evaluate several supervised machine learning algorithms: accuracy, recall, precision, and F1-Score.

Rest of the Experiment is split up into nine different sections. The Section 2 covers about breast cancer in both sexes in general. Section 3 delves into the fundamentals of machine learning as well as its various manifestations. Section 4 displays the related work. The methodology of the experiment, as well as the dataset, are detailed in Section 5. The various machine learning techniques utilized in this experiment are explained in Section 6. The simulation findings and interpretations are presented in Section 7. Section 8 concludes the findings and discusses breast cancer.

2 BREAST CANCER

Lobules and ducts make up the breast. The glands that can produce milk are known as lobules. The milk is transported from the lobules to the nipple via the ducts, which are narrow tubes. Fat, connective tissue, lymph nodes, and blood arteries all make up the breast. The tiniest building blocks in the body are cells. Healthy cells that divide only when required by the organism and die when no longer required. Whenever the cells present in the breast develop a malignant tumor, this is referred to as breast cancer. The human body has an enormous cell count. These aberrant cell growths generate a lump, which is commonly referred to as a tumor. The glands that produce breast milk produce these malignant cells. These cancerous cells, which are the main cause of breast cancer, can be classified into many categories based on how they grow and their ability to harm normal cells (Wild et al., 2014, pp 482-494). The ability to effect refers to whether malignant cells can just harm local cells or if they have the potential to spread across the body. Metastasis is the process of malignant cells spreading throughout the patient's entire body. (Wild et al., 2014, pp 482-494

The most common early indicators of breast cancer are a few irregularities that are detected by a mammogram before the patient or a health care practitioner can diagnose it. Patients typically discover a lump or tumor in their breast. Other breast cancer symptoms include discomfort in the breast, which can cause pain, and skin irritation or dimpling, which can make the breast appear red and inflamed. Scaliness, ulceration, or retraction in the breast or around the breast are some of the other symptoms. Chances Breast cancer becomes substantially more common after the age of 40. Women over the age of 50 are more likely to experience it.

Figure 1. Types of cancer

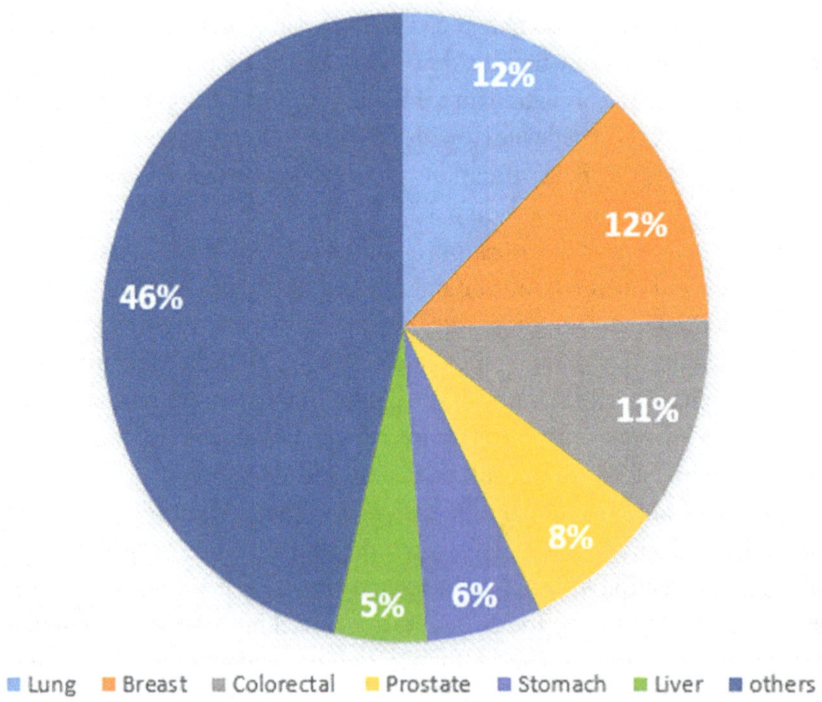

In recent decades, numerous attempts have been made to apply artificial intelligence and other related technologies to aid in the early detection of cancer (Tahmooresi et al., 2018, pp 21-27) Figure 1 graphically displays the prevalence of various cancers in 2018 where Lung and breast cancers were the most common cancers reported globally in 2018, accounting for 12.3% of all new cases diagnosed in both genders. With 1.8 million new cases in 2018, colorectal cancer was the third most common cancer in both genders. Breast cancer was diagnosed in 2,088,849 women worldwide, accounting for 25.4%. One of the most widespread cancers affecting women is breast cancer. (Bray et al., 2018, pp 394-424)

3 MACHINE LEARNING

ML helps in increasing the prediction accuracy without even being specifically designed to do so. The workflow of machine learning employs past data as the input, and using that past data, new output values are forecasted. Major entrepreneurial firms like Facebook, Google, and Uber use machine learning in their technologies. ML has become a critical differentiator for several firms. There are a few machine learning algorithms that are utilized in very particular use-cases, but this paper focuses on three fundamental methods. There are numerous ways to train the model using all of these methods, each with its own set of benefits and drawbacks. These benefits and drawbacks are primarily determined by the type of data being fed to the model. Different types of machine learning classification are depicted in figure 2

A. Supervised Learning

The model is given training data with meaning labels connected to different rows in this type of machine learning. These labels are usually gleaned from a variety of observations. It usually aids the model in learning from labelled training data in order for the model to better predict testing data and enhance accuracy (Han et al., 2011). Usually, data scientists pass attributes and variables they want to look for connections between. Both input and output data are provided to the machine so that it can learn about the data (Sarker et al., 2021, pp 1-18; Sarker, 2021). Supervised learning is concerned with or involves learning from "labelled" data. This means that some information has already been labelled with the correct answer.

Supervised machine learning has two type of algorithms:

1. Classification: In Classification the output variable is divided into Categories, like "Heads" or "tails".
2. Regression: In regression different mathematical techniques are used to forecast few continuous results based predictor variables.

Supervised learning is concerned with or involves learning from "labelled" data. This means that some information has already been labelled with the correct answer.

Types:-

1. Regression
2. Logistic Regression
3. Classification

4. Naive Bayes Classifiers
5. K-NN (k nearest neighbors)
6. Decision Trees
7. Support Vector Machine

B. Unsupervised Learning

The model in unsupervised learning does not have access to the training data's pre-assigned labels or classifications (Mohammed et al., 2016). The model is not supervised in any way in this type of machine learning technique. Because it lacks output data for the input data, unsupervised learning cannot be used in the same way as supervised learning. For instance, clustering is a form of unsupervised learning (Sarker, 2021).

C. Reinforcement Learning

Reinforcement Learning is majorly about taking the right steps to maximize your reward in a given situation (Mohammed et al., 2016). This form of machine learning technology uses no sort of labelled data, and even the outcomes aren't based on the data. The model learns from its own mistakes. The main goal of the agent is to learn in the interactive environment by the process of trial and error, using the remarks from their own experience. By reviewing and testing a variety of possibilities, the model improves its presentation depending on its relationship to the environment and determines how to address its shortcomings and obtain the optimal result (Sarker, 2021).

Figure 2. Types of machine learning

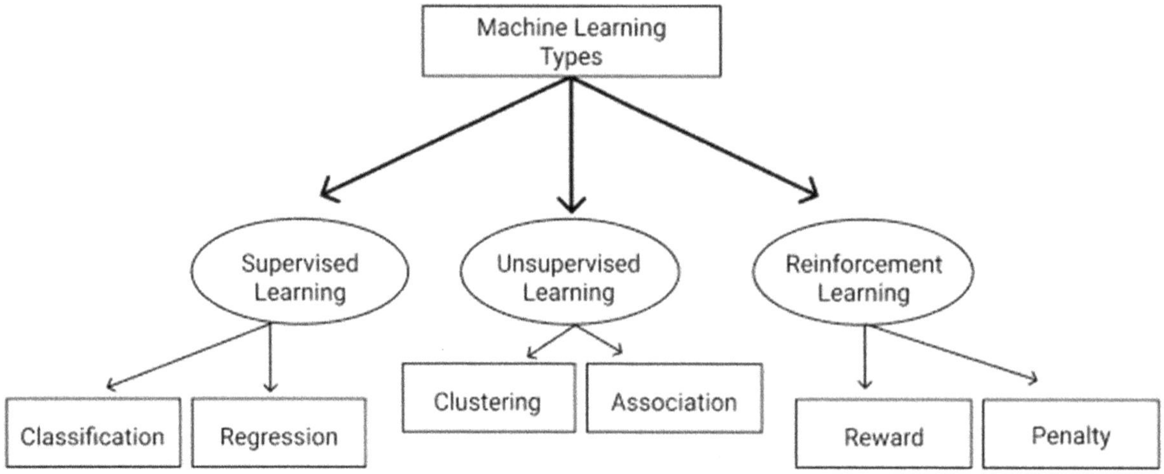

3 LITERATURE SURVEY

Numerous studies have been undertaken on the usage of ML in the detection and treatment of illness, with several approaches or a combination of algorithms being employed to improve accuracy.

Considering the breast cancer dataset, the dataset had a total of 6291 data points and 699 rows and 9 columns. Variable differentiation across several approaches has been demonstrated using various strategies such as Pruned Tree, Bayes theory, and the KNN algorithm with WEKA. The Bayes network is the most accurate, with an accuracy of 89.71% (Bin Othman et al., 2006, pp 520-523). Variance, range, and compactness are all features that are extracted. SVM classification is a method for examining efficiency in an experiment. The outcomes revealed a 95% maximum variance, a 94% range, and an 86% compactness. Based on their findings, SVM can be seen as an acceptable approach for detecting breast cancer. Similarly, (Aruna et al., 2011, pp 37-45) employed naive Bayes, support vector machines, and decision trees to classify a Wisconsin breast cancer dataset, with the highest results coming from the support vector machine (SVM), which had a 96.99% accuracy score (Gc et al., 2015, pp 177-182). Different machine learning methods were applied in different trials on the Wisconsin diagnostic breast cancer dataset (Hazra et al., 2016, pp 39-45), which used three different methodologies. The accuracy of Naive Bayes, Support Vector Machines, and Ensemble was assessed. The highest accuracy was 98.5% for the support vector machine, and 97.3 percent for both Naive Bayes and Ensemble techniques. (Borges et al., 1989, pp 15-19) On the WDBC dataset, two machine learning algorithms, Naive Bayes and J48, were used, with Naive Bayes achieving an accuracy of 97.51% and J48 achieving a 96.5% accuracy (Chaurasia et al., 2014, pp 10-22). The performance classifiers were compared using naive Bayes, SVM, neural networks, and decision tree approaches using the same dataset. With a score of 96.844%, SVM was shown to give the most accurate results in the investigation. A Diffusion-Weighted Magnetic Resonance Image (DWI) was utilized to diagnose breast cancer (Jiang et al., 2017, pp 11-15). They used two types of features on 61 patients' data: the first based on ROI and the second based on ADC. They used the RF technique as well, implementing RF-RFE. The study indicated that the accuracy of RF-RFE and RF and Histogram + GLCM was 77.05%, showing that feature-based texture plays a vital role in improving performance and detection (Delen et al., 2005, pp 113-127). 202,932 patient records were used to study data on breast cancer prediction. The data was divided into two groups: those who survived (93,273) and those who did not (109,659), and the naive Bayes, neural network, and c4.5 decision tree methods were employed to analyse them. According to the findings, the c4.5 decision tree outperformed the other options. Machine that calculates relevance. (Gayathri et al., 2016, pp 1-5) Achieved a 97% accuracy using the WDBC dataset, which contains 699 instances and 11 attributes, while (Kharya et al., 2016, pp 32-37) allotted different weights to different attributes based on their prediction capabilities and achieved a 92% accuracy using the weighted naive Bayes method. (Sivakami et al., 2015, pp 418-429) Used WEKA to create a hybrid classifier using Support Vector Machines and decision trees, which had a 91% accuracy. (Gayathri et al., 2015, pp 1-6) Used Linear Discriminant Analysis for feature selection and trained the dataset with the Mamdani Fuzzy Inference Model, a 93% accurate fuzzy inference method. Wireless cyber mammography images were investigated in a study conducted by (Aminikhanghahi et al., 2015, pp 2252-2256).After selecting and extracting the characteristics, the researcher used two distinct machine learning approaches to verify their accuracy: SVM and GMM. Their findings revealed that if there is no noise or error, SVM is more accurate; otherwise, GMM is better and safer. (Durai et al., 2017, pp 136-139) Choose from many data mining techniques for diagnosing diseases such as breast cancer. They employed LRC and compared it to BFI, ID3, J48, and SVM, as well as four additional approaches. The results demonstrate that LRC is the most precise, with a precision of 99.25 percent. (Ngadi et al., 2016, pp 44-49) Used the NSVC algorithm to compare RBF, Poly, and Linear classification algorithms. They then compared the results against Nave Bayes, DT, K-NN, SVM, RF, and Adaboost, as well as other classification algorithms. RF has the best performance, with a 93 percent accuracy rate. This demonstrates that NSVC is superior to the other approaches. (Asri et al., 2016, pp1064-1069) The same data was used to compare the performance of SVM, decision tree (c4.5), naive Bayes, and KNN machine learning methods. The study compared the accuracy, precision, sensitivity, and specificity of each algorithm in order to classify data in terms of efficiency and effectiveness. SVM received the highest score in the experiment, with an accuracy of 97.13%.

4 METHODOLOGY

4.1 Machine Learning Library

Various machine libraries were used in the experiment's implementation. Numpy (Van der Walt et al., 2011, pp 22-30), scikit-learn (Pedregosa et al., 2011, pp 2825-2830), and Matplotlib (Hunter et al., 2007, pp90-95) are some of the most popular Python libraries used during the course of experiments. NumPy is a package in the Python language that makes it possible to work with different types of arrays. Different functions for matrices, Fourier transformations, and linear algebra functions are also included in Numpy. Scikit-learn is a free-to-use machine learning library. It includes NumPy and SciPy, Python scientific and mathematical libraries. Matplotlib is a Python plotting library for machine learning that is one of the most commonly used and oldest libraries in Python. Machine learning uses numerous visuals to assist in the comprehension of vast amounts of data.

4.2 Dataset

A well-annotated dataset is a prerequisite for developing an innovative and reliable breast cancer detection tool. The lack of samples and the secrecy of the patients' personal information make gathering a dataset extremely difficult. The dataset used was the Wisconsin Diagnostic Breast Cancer (WDBC) dataset (Lichman, 2013) that can be accessed in the UCI ML repository. The dataset includes 569 data points, sorted into 212 malignant (M) and 357 benign (B) categories. The dataset contains 32 attributes overall, although only ten are used for the experiment's clarity. Features derived from a digital image of a breast mass fine needle aspirate (FNA) make up the collection. The mentioned properties describe the characteristics of the cell nuclei in the photograph. Ten real-value features for each nucleus are 1. Radius, [2] texture, [3] perimeter, [4] area, [5] smoothness, [6] compactness, [7] concavity, [8] concave points, [9] symmetry, and [10] fatal dimension. The dataset contains no missing values, making it simple to use and conduct future experiments on.

4.3 Phase of Work

The complete workflow for the experiment is explained in figure 3. The work flow is mainly divided into four parts.

Table 1. Related work on different dataset on breast cancer detection

AUTHOR	APPROACH	DATASET USED	RESULT
Bin Othman et al.	KNN, Bayes Network, and Pruned Tree using WEKA.	There are 6291 number of observations in the Breast Cancer dataset, with 699 row and 9 column.	The Bayes network has the highest accuracy, at 89.71%, followed by the Support Vector Machine (SVM), which has a score of 96.99%.
Aruna et al.	Naive Bayes, SVM, and Decision trees	WDBC	Support vector machine (SVM), which had a 96.99% accuracy score.
Gc et al.	Performance is assessed using SVM classification. Variance, range, and compactness are all features that are extracted.	Breast Cancer dataset	The statistics revealed the maximum variance of 95%, a range of 94%, and compactness of 86%. The highest
Hazra et al.	Ensemble, SVM, and Naive Bayes	WDBC	Accuracy was 98.5% for the support vector machine, and 97.3% for both Naive Bayes and Ensemble techniques.
Borges et al.	Naive Bayes and J48	WDBC	Naive Bayes achieved 97.51% accuracy, while J48 achieved 96.5% accuracy.
Chaurasia et al.	Naive Bayes, SVM, neural networks, and decision tree methods	WDBC	SVM produced the most accurate findings, with a score of 96.84%.
Jiang et al.	The RF-Recursive Feature Elimination (RF-RFE) method	Zhejiang Cancer hospital dataset with Diffusion- Weighted Magnetic Resonance image	The RF-RFE method got an accuracy of 77.05%, a sensitivity of 84.21%, a specificity of 65.21%, and an AUC of 0.76.
Delen et al.	Naive Bayes, neural networks, and decision trees	202,932 patient records were used to study the prediction of breast cancer data	The decision tree performed better than the other strategies.
Gayathri et al.	Machine Learning with Relevance Vectors	WDBC dataset, which contains 699 instances and 11 attributes	Relevance Vector Machine. It achieved a 97% accuracy.
Kharya et al.	Different weights were assigned to different attributes based on their prediction capabilities.	WDBC	92% accuracy using the weighted naive Bayes method.
Sivakami et al.	WEKA was used to develop a hybrid classifier that combined SVMs with decision trees.	Breast cancer dataset	91% accuracy
Gayathri et al.	Linear Discriminant Analysis was used to pick features, and the Mamdani Fuzzy Inference Model was used to train the dataset.	Breast cancer dataset	93% accuracy
Aminikhanghahi et al.	SVM, GMM	DDSM University of South Florida	SVM got a MCC of 78.78%. Sensitivity of 82% and specificity of 96%
Durai et al.	LRC	UCI standard dataset	LRC got a accuracy of 99.25%
Ngadi et al.	NSVC	UCI standard mammography dataset	Accuracy 99%
Asri et al.	SVM, decision tree (c4.5), naive Bayes, and KNN	WDBC	Each algorithm's accuracy, precision, sensitivity, and specificity is measured. SVM received the highest score in the experiment, with an accuracy of 97.13 percent.

Table 2. Description of the dataset

DATASET	NUMBER OF ATTRIBUTES	NUMBER OF INSTANCES	NUMBER OF CLASS
Wisconsin Diagnostic Breast cancer dataset	32	569	2 (Malignant and Benign)

Data File Import: To begin with, the Wisconsin Diagnostic Breast Cancer dataset is downloaded and imported into Python. The dataset contains 569 data points, separated into 212 malignant (M) and 357 benign (B) categories.

Data Preprocessing: There are large clusters of missing and noisy data in real-world datasets. To eliminate these errors and produce confident forecasts, the data is preprocessed. The sequential chart of our proposed model is shown in Figure 3. When cleaning acquired data, noise and missing values are prevalent. To generate an accurate and useful result, the noise in the data must be removed, and missing values must be filled in. Smoothing, standardization, and aggregation are all part of the process.

Splitting of dataset: The entire dataset is broken down into two portions. The training dataset was used to teach the model by providing data points with answers, and the model is then applied to the testing dataset, which contains data points that are classified as benign or malignant tumors. In the experiment, the train and test datasets are split into 60% and 40%, respectively. There are 341 train data points and 228 test data points.

Result: The ultimate goal is to define multiple ML algorithms that can be used to accurately predict the discovery of breast cancer. The main goal is to provide efficient and reliable prediction with a few features and tests. A total of 10 essential attributes are considered in this study, four performance metrics are utilized to evaluate several supervised machine learning algorithms: accuracy, recall, precision, and F1-Score.

5 MACHINE LEARNING ALGORITHMS

5.1 Logistic Regression

Under the supervised learning technique, one of the most popular machine learning algorithms is logistic regression (Pant, 2019). It's a method for predicting a categorical dependent variable from a set of independent variables. Using continuous and discrete datasets, it can generate probabilities and categories fresh data (Ak et al., 2020, pp 111). Using logistic regression, probabilistic values between 0 and 1 are produced. The logistic function's curve represents the possibility of something, such as whether or not the cells are malignant. In logistic regression, an "S" shaped logistic function is fit, which predicts two maximum values (Bassey, 2019). Figure 4 represents logistics regression.

Figure 3. Suggested framework for breast cancer detection

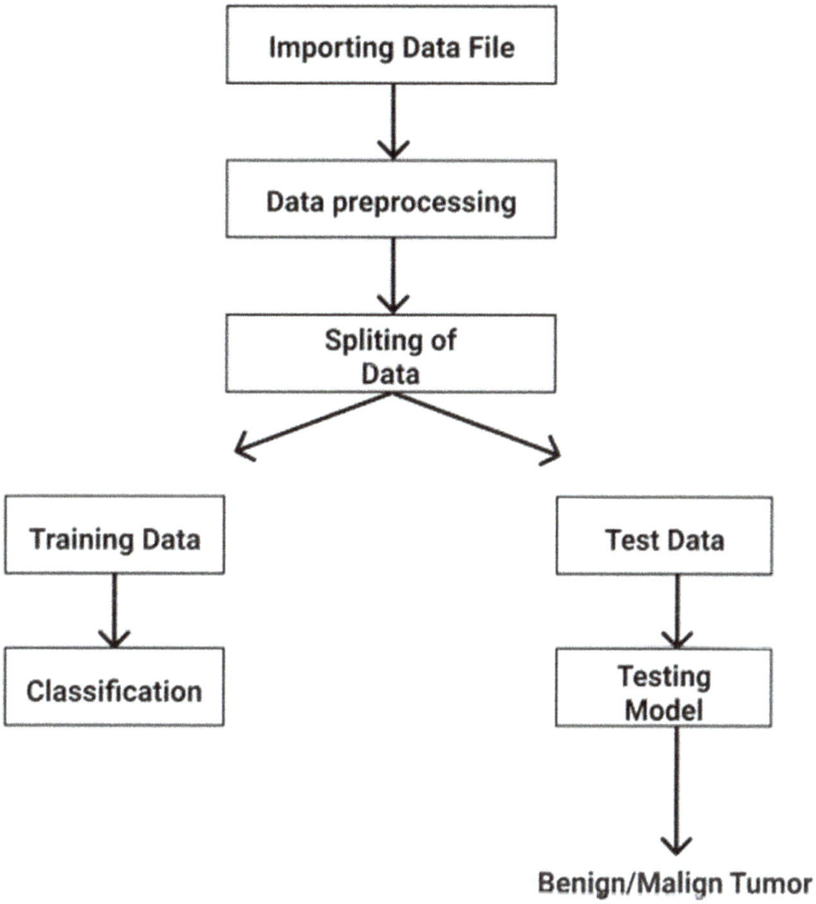

Figure 4. Representation of logistics regression

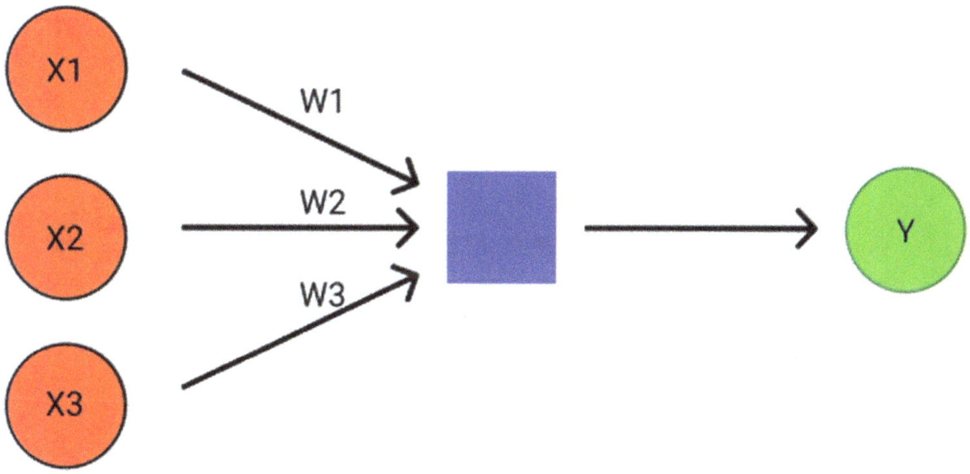

5.2 K-Nearest Neighbor

KNN is a nonparametric classification approach that is one of the most basic and oldest. Based on its neighbors, the KNN method is used to decide where a data set belongs. Regression and classification are examples of supervised learning methods used in this strategy. Before processing a new data point, KNN collects all surrounding data points. A high degree of quality variation is an essential factor in determining the distance (Alarabeyyat et al., 2016, pp 35-39). To make predictions, the Euclidean distance to k-nearest neighbors is used. Because the information already includes categories such as malignant and benign, this method is used to forecast breast cancer. The label is assigned a class depending on its immediate neighbors' class labels (Nechuta et al., 2011, 1319-1331). Figure 5 gives a brief explanation of KNN algorithms working where data points are plotted in the graph and new testing points are classified in any class by comparing the Euclidean distance of new data points to different class.

Figure 5. Representation of KNN algorithm

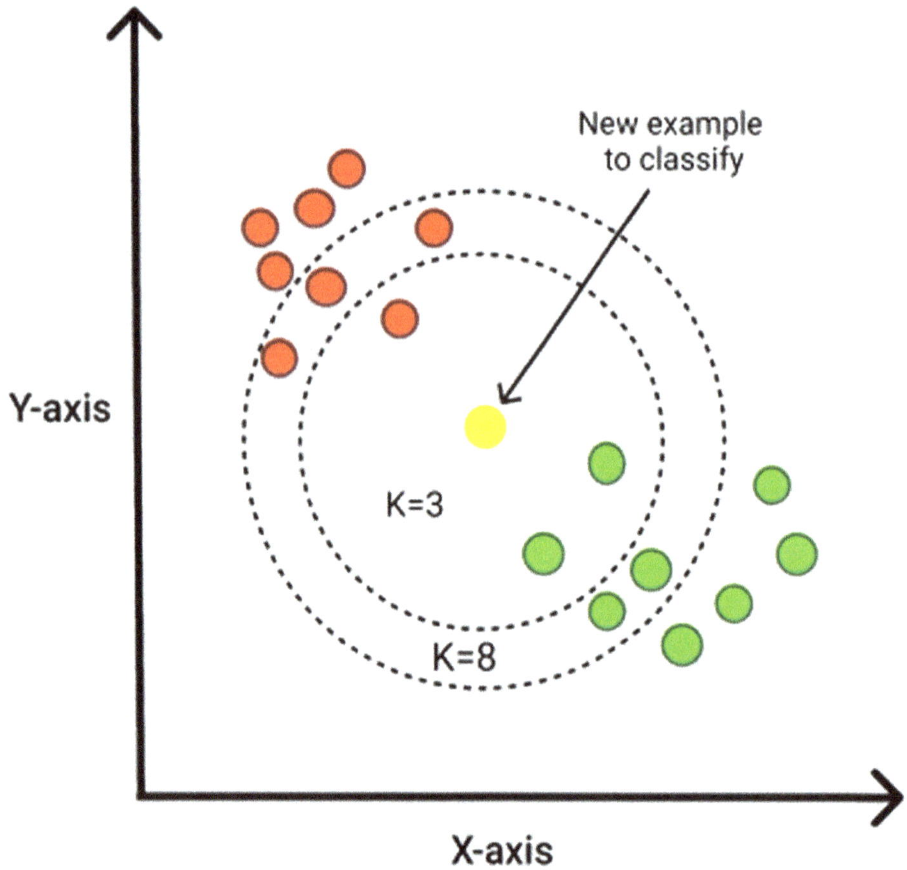

5.3 Decision Tree

The decision tree is the most powerful and extensively used classification and regression approach. The algorithm not only simulates the human mind, but it is also widely used and speedier when analyzing input data, allowing for a better grasp of the issue statement (Olanow et al., 2001). A decision tree is a tree with nodes relating to attributes, nodes pointing to decision rules, and leaf nodes matching the output classes in this technique. The goal is to design a tree-like structure for the input attributes, with each leaf producing a unique output (Pandya et al., 2015, pp 18-21). The complete input training data is accepted as the root when utilizing the decision-tree technique for classification. The depth analysis of the algorithm is taken into account while utilizing the decision-tree approach to solve a classification problem. If the algorithm's depth is increased, the problem of over fitting will arise (Rajaguru, 2019). Figure 6 gives a representation of decision tree.

Figure 6. Representation of decision tree algorithm

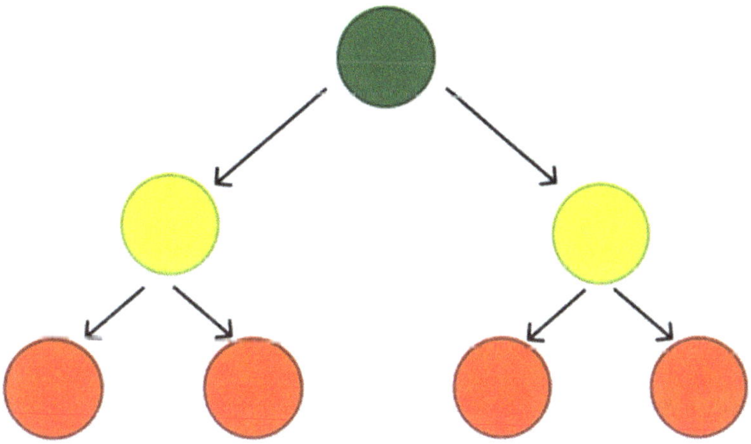

5.4 Random Forest

To solve a classification problem, the random forest technique employs several decision trees. The generic principle of randomized ensembles of decision trees is known as random forest (Bremain 2015, pp 5-32). Recursive partitioning is used in the Random Forest to construct numerous decision trees. A crucial supervised machine learning algorithm is random forest. The bagging method is used to train the system after generating an ensemble of decision trees.

CART is a method in which binary splits recursively partition the tree into homogeneous or near-homogeneous terminal nodes. It is frequently used to construct the Random Forest tree base learner (the tree's endpoints). A successful binary split pushes data from a parent tree node to its two daughter nodes, improving the daughter nodes' homogeneity. Typically, a random forest consists of hundreds to thousands of trees, each of which is generated by bootstrapping the original data. RF trees are constructed using a non-deterministic two-stage randomization technique (Wu &Kumar, 2009; Nguyen et al., 2013) as opposed to CART. Figure 7 gives a detailed description of random forest as different decision trees are created.

Figure 7. Representation of random forest classifier

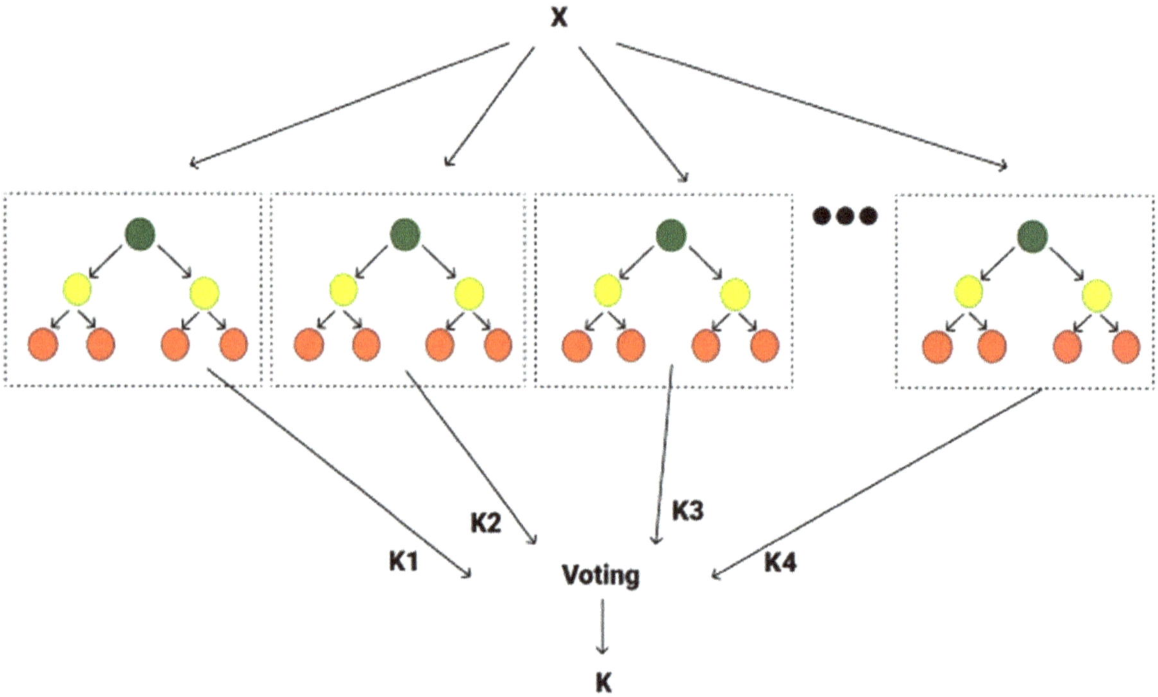

5.5 Support Vector Machine

Support vector machines (SVMs) were invented by Vapnik (Vapnik, 1999) and they have proven to be beneficial in a variety of pattern recognition contexts, outperforming many other categorization algorithms. The purpose of the algorithm is to find an N-dimensional hyper plane that divides the input points into categories. SVM works by selecting critical samples from all classes, known as support vectors, and then utilizing these support vectors to construct a linear function that separates them as broadly as possible. (Byun et al., 2003, pp 459-486)As a result, SVM may be said to be utilized to transfer an input vector to a high-dimensionality space with the goal of determining the optimum hyper plane for classifying the data set. By calculating the best-matched hyper plane, this linear classifier seeks to optimize the distance between the decision hyper plane and the nearest data point, also known as the marginal distance (Williams, 2011; Kourou et al, 2015, 8-17). In Figure 8 two different classes are divided using a hyper plane.

Figure 8. Representation of support vector machine

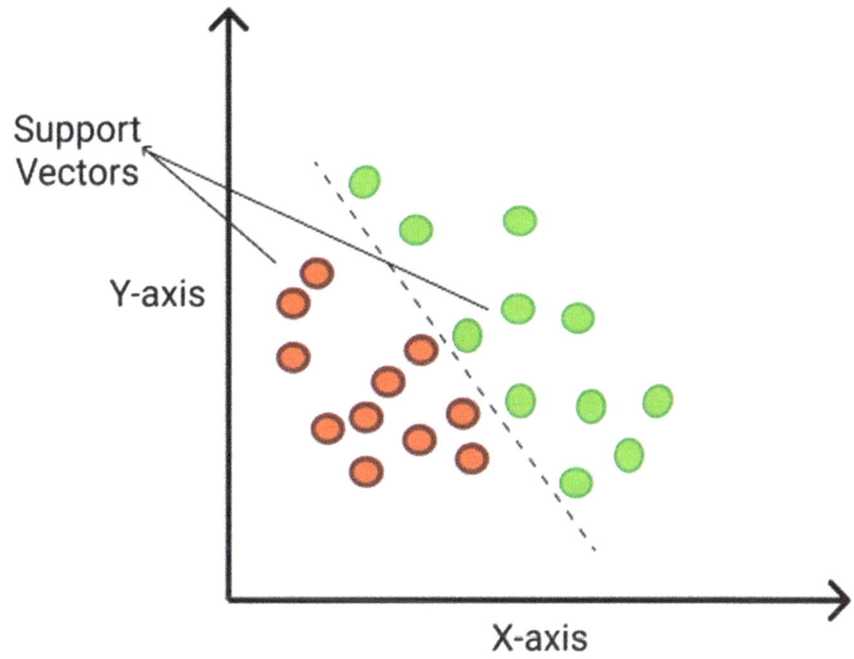

5.6 Artificial Neural Network

Biological neural networks establish the structure of the human brain, and the phrase "artificial neural network" is taken from them. ANN, like the human brain, has numerous layers of neurons that are coupled to one another. Nodes are the names given to these neurons. The goal of an artificial intelligence network is to mimic the network of neurons that make up a human brain so that computers can comprehend how to make human-like judgments. The neural network is made up of layers of artificial neurons called units that are stacked one on top of the other. Figure 9 shows different layers present in artificial neural network. In general, an artificial neural network has three layers:

1. The first layer is the input layer, which receives data from the programmer in a variety of formats.
2. The hidden layer, which sits between the input and output layers, is the second layer. The number of hidden layers can vary depending on the model's requirements. All of the arithmetic that is used to detect hidden features and patterns in the data is done by the hidden layer.
3. The output layer is the third and final layer; in this layer, all of the input data undergoes a series of transformations in order to compute the information that is conveyed through this layer.

5.7 Extreme Gradient Boosting

Tianqi Chen and Carlos Guestrin have proposed a scalable and efficient XGBoost method (Chen et al., 2016, 785-794). Extreme Gradient Boosting (XGBoost) is a new tree-based technique that has lately gained a lot of traction as a powerful data categorization tool (Parashar & Rai, 2020). The XGBoost is a highly scalable end-to-end tree boosting technique for machine learning classification and regression applications (Chen et al., 2015, pp 1-4) .To avoid over fitting, the XGBoost employs a more precise approximation of the learning target as well as a regularization component. It introduces a novel method for estimating leaf nodes and dividing tree nodes.

Figure 9. Representation of artificial neural network

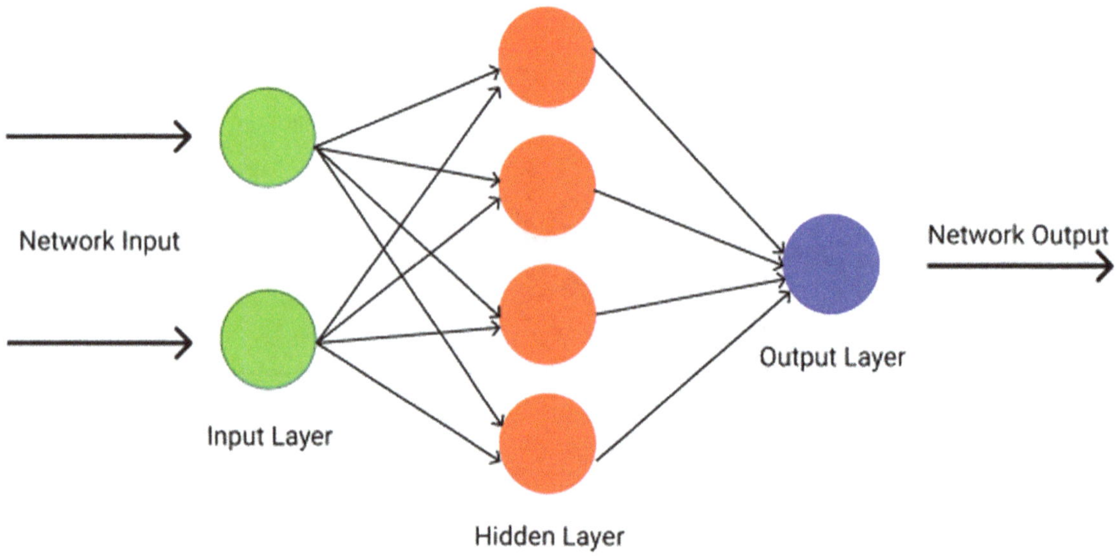

6 RESULT

The results were computed by considering several important characteristics of the dataset. In this study, many different classification and ensemble approaches are applied and used to carry out the results. Python is used to implement all of the algorithms. These are some of the most popular machine learning algorithms for extracting the maximum accuracy from data.

The Confusion Matrix is a matrix that is used to compare the results of several models. The count numbers are used to summarize all of the accurate and wrong predictions, which are then broken down by class. Confusion matrix helps in presenting an extensive picture of performance and types of error shown by all the models separately. The study involves a binary classification problem, so the confusion matrix will be 2 x 2, with four different values. There are two types of classes in the confusion matrix, and they are the positive class and the negative class. The positive class is something we're looking for, whereas the negative class is an alternative. Table 4 shows the True Positive (TP), True Negative (TN), False Positive (FP), and False Negative (FN) values derived using various machine learning techniques.

Table 3. Advantages and disadvantages of all the algorithms used

S. NO	ALGORITHM	ADVANTAGES	DISADVANTAGES
1	Logistic regression	1. Logistic regression is simpler to implement, interpret, and train. 2. It is extendable to multiple classes and provides a natural probabilistic view of class predictions.	1. Complex relationships are difficult to obtain using logistic regression. This algorithm is easily outperformed by more powerful and compact algorithms, such as Neural Networks. 2. Logistic Regression necessitates average or no multi collinearity among independent variables.
2	Decision tree	1. No preprocessing or assumption on distribution of data is needed. 2. Effective to handle correlation	1. Algorithm is not suitable for complicated datasets. 2. Susceptible to have outliners
3	K-nearest neighbor	1. A straightforward machine learning model. 2. There aren't many hyperparameters to tweak.	1. Selection of appropriate K value is important 2. If the sample size is large, the computation cost will be high during runtime.
4	Random forest	1. Model that is accurate and powerful. 2. Overfitting is effectively handled. 3. Supports implicit feature selection and determines the importance of features.	1. When the forest grows in size, the computation becomes more complex and slower. 2. The prediction model is not well described.
5	Support vector machine	1. SVM employs a kernel trick to solve complex problems. 2. SVM employs a convex optimization function, global minima are always achieved. 3. Higher accuracy is provided by hinge loss.	1. For sufficient accuracy, hyper parameters and kernels must be carefully tuned. 2. Larger datasets require more training time.
6	Artificial neural network	1. Artificial neural networks can provide data to be processed in parallel, which means they can handle multiple tasks at the same time. 2. Artificial neural networks have faced opposition. This means that the loss of one or more neurons, or neural networks, has an effect on the performance of Artificial Neural Networks. 3. Artificial neural networks are used to store information on the network so that even in the absence of a data pair, the network does not stop producing results.	1. Large neural networks required a lot of processing time. 2. Due to their structure, artificial neural networks necessitate processors with parallel processing power. As a result, the equipment's realization is dependent. 3. The structure of artificial neural networks is determined by no specific rule. Experience and trial and error are used to determine the best network structure.
7	Extreme gradient boosting	1. XGBoost includes L1 (Lasso Regression) and L2 (Ridge Regression) regularisation to prevent overfitting. 2. XGBoost includes the ability to handle missing values. When XGBoost encounters a missing value at a node, it attempts both the left and right hand split and learns the path that results in a higher loss for each node. 3. XGBoost allows users to perform cross-validation at each iteration of the boosting process, making it simple to obtain the exact number of boosting iterations in a single run.	1. XGBoost performs poorly on sparse and unstructured data. 2. Gradient Boosting is extremely sensitive to outliers because each classifier is forced to correct the errors of the predecessor learners.

A True Positive value (TP) indicates that the value predicted by the classification model corresponds to the actual target value, implying that the actual target value was positive and the model classified it as such. It signifies that the model accurately anticipated the positive class in terms of classes. True Negative (TN) values denote that the value predicted by the classification model matches the actual target value, implying that the actual target value was negative and the model classified it as such. It signifies that the model accurately predicted the negative class in terms of classes. False Positive values (FP), also known as Type 1 errors, indicate that the value predicted by the classification model differs from the actual target value, implying that the real target value was negative and the model categorized it as a positive value. This indicates that the model predicted a positive class wrongly. The False Negative, or Type 2 error, indicates that the value predicted by the classification model differs from the actual target value, implying that the actual target value was positive while the model classified it as negative. This indicates that the model predicted a negative class wrongly.

Table 4. Confusion matrix of multiple ML algorithms

S. NO	ALGORITHM	TP	FN	FP	TN
1	Logistic regression	147	2	4	83
2	Decision tree	144	5	3	76
3	K-nearest neighbor	141	3	6	78
4	Random forest	142	1	10	76
5	Support vector machine	139	2	4	83
6	Artificial neural network	146	0	7	75
7	Extreme gradient boosting	139	1	7	81

The total number of values properly predicted by the model built using the technique is referred to as its accuracy. It generally indicates how much data the model successfully anticipated accurately. The following equation 1 demonstrates how to calculate accuracy mathematically.

$$\text{Accuracy} = \frac{\text{True positive} + \text{True Negative}}{\text{True Positive} + \text{False Positive} + \text{False Negative} + \text{True Negative}} \quad [1]$$

Figure 10. Comparison of different algorithms based on accuracy

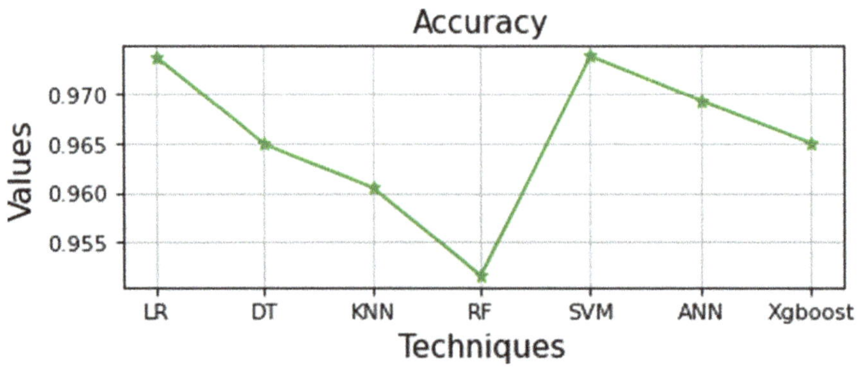

Precision is one statistic used to measure machine learning performance. Precision is determined by dividing true positives by all of the model's positive projected values. The following equation 2 demonstrates how to determine precision in a mathematically accurate manner.

$$\text{Precision} = \frac{\text{True positive}}{\text{True positive} + \text{False Positive}} \qquad [2]$$

Figure 11. Comparison of different algorithms based on precision

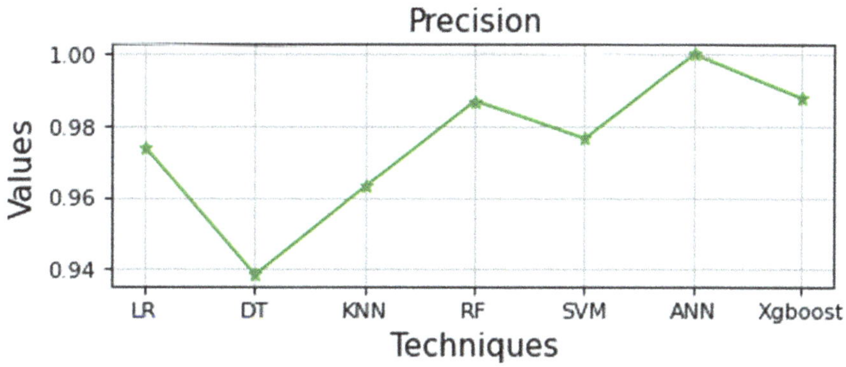

Recall is also known as sensitivity. Recall refers to positive values that are truly positive and are assessed true by the model among all the true or positive set. The recall is calculated by dividing the total number of observations in the actual class by the model's precisely predicted positive observation. . The following equation 3 demonstrates how to determine precision in a mathematically accurate manner.

$$\text{Recall} = \frac{\text{True positive}}{\text{True Positive} + \text{False negaitve}} \qquad [3]$$

Figure 12. Comparison of different algorithms based on recall

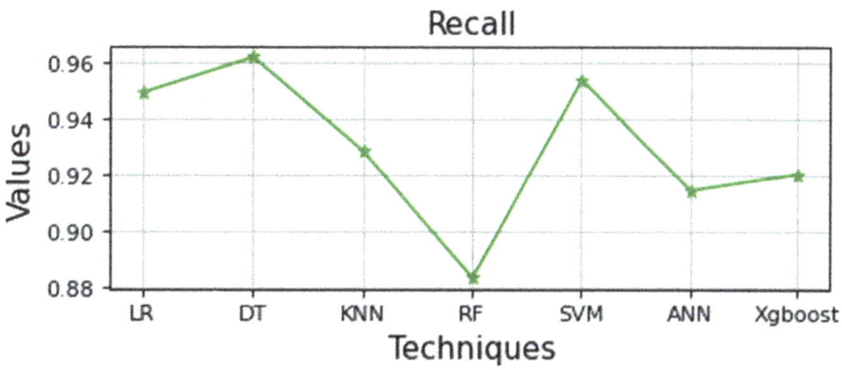

The F1-score is calculated using the precision and accuracy numbers, and it is usually the harmonic mean of both. As a result, both false positives and false negatives are taken into account in this score. The following equation 4 demonstrates how to determine precision in a mathematically accurate manner.

$$\text{F1 Score} = \frac{2*(\text{Recall}*\text{Precision})}{(\text{Recall}+\text{Precision})} \quad [4]$$

Figure 13. Comparison of different algorithms based on F1-score

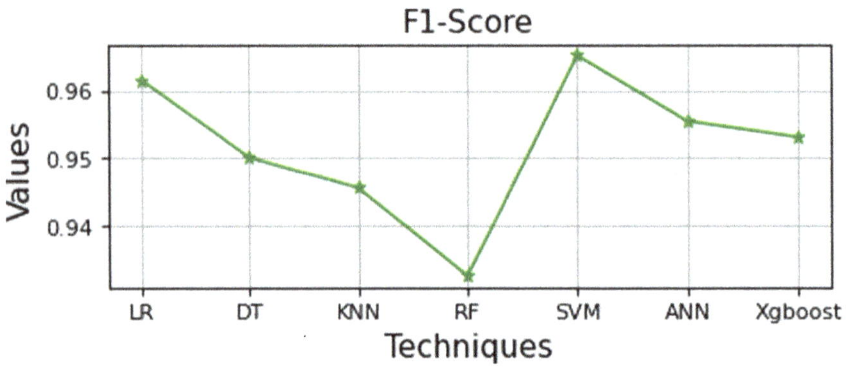

Regarding precision, ANN performed best with a value of 1, and the Decision Tree performed worst with a value of 0.9383. In terms of accuracy, SVM performed best with an accuracy of 97.38% and Random Forest performed worst with an accuracy of 95.16%. In terms of recall, the Decision Tree came out on top with a score of 0.9620, while the Random Forest came in last with a score of 0.8837. In terms of F1 scores, Support Vector Machine came out on top with a score of 0.9651, while Random Forest came in last with a score of 0.9325. Overall, the Support Vector Machine fared the best, scoring the highest on three of the five performance indicators. Random Forest, on the other hand, did poorly, receiving the lowest value in a four-out-of-five metric rating.

Table 5. The outcome of various machine learning methods that were employed

S. NO	ALGORITHM	ACCURACY	PRECISION	RECALL	F1-SCORE
1	Logistic Regression	0.9737	0.9740	0.9494	0.9615
2	Decision tree	0.9649	**0.9383**	**0.9620**	0.95
3	K-nearest neighbor	0.9605	0.9630	0.9286	0.9455
4	Random forest	**0.9516**	0.9870	**0.8837**	**0.9325**
5	Support vector machine	**0.9738**	0.9765	0.9540	**0.9651**
6	Artificial neural network	0.9693	**1.0**	0.9146	0.9554
7	Xgboost	0.9650	0.9878	0.9205	0.9530

8 DISCUSSION

The cause of mortality in women with breast cancer might be linked to a variety of factors depending on the patient's circumstances. Inherited breast cancer, a personal history of breast cancer, radiation exposure, or frequent drinking could all be factors. Aside from these reasons, there should be a proper procedure that may assist people in detecting early breast cancer signs, as there are numerous advantages to early detection. To start, the patient can be provided with a more early prescription to help them overcome the sickness. Second, it can mentally prepare people to battle the disease, according to psychology. To avert fatalities, an early diagnosis approach for patients should be developed.

According to many estimates, the amount of data across the globe is continuously expanding, with unstructured data accounting for more than half of the overall amount of data. To help solve this problem, several researchers are employing different algorithms to assist the healthcare industry and specialists in developing models for early identification and prediction of various diseases, which can greatly benefit individuals. The ultimate goal of the experiment is to establish numerous categorization algorithms that can aid in accurate breast cancer detection.

Non-numerical values were deleted, and each numeric value was standardized in order to prepare the dataset for display. Different machine learning algorithms can be utilized to create tools that aid in the identification and diagnosis of breast cancer, lowering patient mortality rates. The primary goal of these tools is to provide faster analysis of large amounts of data while avoiding potential diagnostic and detection errors. Our findings highlight the importance of accurate early detection in people with breast cancer. Seven different supervised machine learning algorithms are applied to determine if a patient has a malignant tumor or is benign. The amount of missing data should be kept to a minimum or equal to null in order for algorithms to perform perfectly. When the dataset consists of discrete nominal values rather than noisy data, the algorithms learn faster and better. When the noise and missing values were removed, the algorithm achieved a 97.83%, which can be increased further by adding more relevant features and introducing better circumstances for different algorithms.

REFERENCES

Ak, M. F. (2020, June). A comparative analysis of breast cancer detection and diagnosis using data visualization and machine learning applications. In Healthcare (Vol. 8, No. 2, p. 111). Multidisciplinary Digital Publishing Institute. doi:10.3390/healthcare8020111

Alarabeyyat, A., & Alhanahnah, M. (2016, August). Breast cancer detection using k-nearest neighbor machine learning algorithm. In *2016 9th International Conference on Developments in eSystems Engineering (DeSE)* (pp. 35-39). IEEE.

Aminikhanghahi, S., Shin, S., Wang, W., Jeon, S. I., Son, S. H., & Pack, C. (2015, April). Study of wireless mammography image transmission impacts on robust cyber-aided diagnosis systems. In *Proceedings of the 30th Annual ACM Symposium on Applied Computing* (pp. 2252-2256). 10.1145/2695664.2695832

Aruna, S., Rajagopalan, S. P., & Nandakishore, L. V. (2011). Knowledge based analysis of various statistical tools in detecting breast cancer. *Computer Science and Information Technology*, *2*, 37–45.

Asri, H., Mousannif, H., Al Moatassime, H., & Noel, T. (2016). Using machine learning algorithms for breast cancer risk prediction and diagnosis. *Procedia Computer Science*, *83*, 1064–1069. doi:10.1016/j.procs.2016.04.224

Bassey, P. (2019, September 19). Logistic Regression Vs Support Vector Machines (SVM). *Medium.*

Bin Othman, M. F., & Yau, T. M. S. (2007). Comparison of different classification techniques using WEKA for breast cancer. In *3rd Kuala Lumpur international conference on biomedical engineering 2006* (pp. 520-523). Springer. 10.1007/978-3-540-68017-8_131

Borges, L. R. (1989). Analysis of the Wisconsin breast cancer dataset and machine learning for breast cancer detection. *Group*, *1*(369), 15–19.

Bray, F., Ferlay, J., Soerjomataram, I., Siegel, R. L., Torre, L. A., & Jemal, A. (2018). Global cancer statistics 2018: GLOBOCAN estimates of incidence and mortality worldwide for 36 cancers in 185 countries. *CA: a Cancer Journal for Clinicians*, *68*(6), 394–424. doi:10.3322/caac.21492 PMID:30207593

Bray, F., Ren, J. S., Masuyer, E., & Ferlay, J. (2013). *Estimates of global cancer prevalence for 27 sites in the adult*. Academic Press.

Breiman, L. (2001). Random forests. *Machine Learning*, *45*(1), 5–32. doi:10.1023/A:1010933404324

Byun, H., & Lee, S. W. (2003). A survey on pattern recognition applications of support vector machines. *International Journal of Pattern Recognition and Artificial Intelligence*, *17*(03), 459–486. doi:10.1142/S0218001403002460

Chaurasia, V., & Pal, S. (2014). Data mining techniques: To predict and resolve breast cancer survivability. *International Journal of Computer Science and Mobile Computing IJCSMC*, *3*(1), 10–22.

Chen, T., & Guestrin, C. (2016, August). Xgboost: A scalable tree boosting system. In *Proceedings of the 22nd acm sigkdd international conference on knowledge discovery and data mining* (pp. 785-794). 10.1145/2939672.2939785

Chen, T., He, T., Benesty, M., Khotilovich, V., Tang, Y., & Cho, H. (2015). Xgboost: extreme gradient boosting. *R package version 0.4-2, 1*(4), 1-4.

Delen, D., Walker, G., & Kadam, A. (2005). Predicting breast cancer survivability: A comparison of three data mining methods. *Artificial Intelligence in Medicine*, *34*(2), 113–127. doi:10.1016/j.artmed.2004.07.002 PMID:15894176

Durai, S. G., Ganesh, S. H., & Christy, A. J. (2017, February). Novel linear regressive classifier for the diagnosis of breast cancer. In *2017 World Congress on Computing and Communication Technologies (WCCCT)* (pp. 136-139). IEEE. 10.1109/WCCCT.2016.40

Erlay, J., Ervik, M., Dikshit, R., Eser, S., & Mathers, C. (2012). Cancer incidence and mortality worldwide: IARC CancerBase No. 11. *GLOBOCAN*, *1*.

Gayathri, B. M., & Sumathi, C. P. (2015, December). Mamdani fuzzy inference system for breast cancer risk detection. In *2015 IEEE International Conference on Computational Intelligence and Computing Research (ICCIC)* (pp. 1-6). IEEE. 10.1109/ICCIC.2015.7435670

Gayathri, B. M., & Sumathi, C. P. (2016, December). Comparative study of relevance vector machine with various machine learning techniques used for detecting breast cancer. In *2016 IEEE International Conference on Computational Intelligence and Computing Research (ICCIC)* (pp. 1-5). IEEE. 10.1109/ICCIC.2016.7919576

Gc, S., Kasaudhan, R., Heo, T. K., & Choi, H. D. (2015, October). Variability measurement for breast cancer classification of mammographic masses. In *Proceedings of the 2015 Conference on research in adaptive and convergent systems* (pp. 177-182). 10.1145/2811411.2811505

Han, J., Pei, J., & Kamber, M. (2011). *Data mining: concepts and techniques*. Elsevier.

Hazra, A., Mandal, S. K., & Gupta, A. (2016). Study and analysis of breast cancer cell detection using Naïve Bayes, SVM and ensemble algorithms. *International Journal of Computers and Applications, 145*(2), 39–45. doi:10.5120/ijca2016910595

Hunter, J. D. (2007). Matplotlib: A 2D graphics environment. *Computing in Science Engineering, 9*(3), 90-95.

Jiang, Z., Xu, W., & Chen, S. (2017, September). Classification of benign and malignant breast cancer based on DWI texture features. In *Proceedings of the International Conference on Bioinformatics and Computational Intelligence* (pp. 11-15). 10.1145/3135954.3135964

Kharya, S., & Soni, S. (2016). Weighted naive bayes classifier: A predictive model for breast cancer detection. *International Journal of Computers and Applications, 133*(9), 32–37. doi:10.5120/ijca2016908023

Kourou, K., Exarchos, T. P., Exarchos, K. P., Karamouzis, M. V., & Fotiadis, D. I. (2015). Machine learning applications in cancer prognosis and prediction. *Computational and Structural Biotechnology Journal, 13*, 8–17. doi:10.1016/j.csbj.2014.11.005 PMID:25750696

Lichman, M. (2013). *UCI machine learning repository*. http://archive. ics. uci. edu/ml

Moh'd Rasoul, A., Al-Gawagzeh, M. Y., & Alsaaidah, B. A. (2012). Solving mammography problems of breast cancer detection using artificial neural networks and image processing techniques. *Indian Journal of Science and Technology, 5*(4), 2520–2528.

Mohammed, M., Khan, M. B., & Bashier, E. B. M. (2016). *Machine learning: algorithms and applications*. CRC Press. doi:10.1201/9781315371658

Nechuta, S. J., Caan, B. J., Chen, W. Y., Flatt, S. W., Lu, W., Patterson, R. E., Poole, E. M., Kwan, M. L., Chen, Z., Weltzien, E., Pierce, J. P., & Shu, X. O. (2011). The After Breast Cancer Pooling Project: Rationale, methodology, and breast cancer survivor characteristics. *Cancer Causes & Control, 22*(9), 1319–1331. doi:10.100710552-011-9805-9 PMID:21710192

Ngadi, M., Amine, A., & Nassih, B. (2016, November). A robust approach for mammographic image classification using NSVC algorithm. In *Proceedings of the Mediterranean Conference on Pattern Recognition and Artificial Intelligence* (pp. 44-49). 10.1145/3038884.3038892

Nguyen, C., Wang, Y., & Nguyen, H. N. (2013). *Random forest classifier combined with feature selection for breast cancer diagnosis and prognostic*. Academic Press.

Olanow, C. W., Watts, R. L., & Koller, W. C. (2001). An algorithm (decision tree) for the management of Parkinson's disease (2001): Treatment Guidelines. *Neurology, 56*(suppl 5), S1–S88. doi:10.1212/WNL.56.suppl_5.S1 PMID:11402154

Pandya, R., & Pandya, J. (2015). C5. 0 algorithm to improved decision tree with feature selection and reduced error pruning. *International Journal of Computers and Applications, 117*(16), 18–21. doi:10.5120/20639-3318

Pant, A. (2019, January 22). Introduction to Logistic Regression. *Towardsdatascience.*

Parashar, J., & Rai, M. (2020). Breast cancer images classification by clustering of ROI and mapping of features by CNN with XGBOOST learning. *Materials Today: Proceedings*. Advance online publication. doi:10.1016/j.matpr.2020.09.650

Pedregosa, F., Varoquaux, G., Gramfort, A., Michel, V., Thirion, B., Grisel, O., ... Duchesnay, E. (2011). Scikit-learn: Machine learning in Python. *The Journal of Machine Learning Research, 12*, 2825-2830.

Rajaguru, H. (2019). Analysis of decision tree and k-nearest neighbor algorithm in the classification of breast cancer. Asian Pacific journal of cancer prevention. *APJCP, 20*(12), 3777. PMID:31870121

Sarker, I. H. (2021). Machine learning: Algorithms, real-world applications and research directions. *SN Computer Science, 2*(3), 1–21. doi:10.100742979-021-00592-x PMID:33778771

Sarker, I. H., Furhad, M. H., & Nowrozy, R. (2021). Ai-driven cybersecurity: An overview, security intelligence modeling and research directions. *SN Computer Science, 2*(3), 1–18. doi:10.100742979-021-00557-0 PMID:33778771

Sivakami, K., & Saraswathi, N. (2015). Mining big data: Breast cancer prediction using DT-SVM hybrid model. *International Journal of Scientific Engineering and Applied Science, 1*(5), 418–429.

Tahmooresi, M., Afshar, A., Rad, B. B., Nowshath, K. B., & Bamiah, M. A. (2018). Early detection of breast cancer using machine learning techniques. *Journal of Telecommunication, Electronic and Computer Engineering (JTEC), 10*(3-2), 21-27.

Van Der Walt, S., Colbert, S. C., & Varoquaux, G. (2011). The NumPy array: A structure for efficient numerical computation. *Computing in Science & Engineering, 13*(2), 22–30. doi:10.1109/MCSE.2011.37

Vapnik, V. (1999). *The nature of statistical learning theory*. Springer Science & Business Media.

Wild, C. (2014). *World cancer report 2014*. World Health Organization.

Williams, G. (2011). Descriptive and predictive analytics. In *Data Mining with Rattle and R* (pp. 171–177). Springer. doi:10.1007/978-1-4419-9890-3_8

Witten, I. H., & Frank, E. (2002). Data mining: Practical machine learning tools and techniques with Java implementations. *SIGMOD Record, 31*(1), 76–77. doi:10.1145/507338.507355

Wu, X., & Kumar, V. (Eds.). (2009). *The top ten algorithms in data mining*. CRC press. doi:10.1201/9781420089653

Chapter 4
Stress Detection Using Machine Learning Techniques in IoT Environment

Dimple Chehal
J.C. Bose University of Science and Technology, YMCA, India

Parul Gupta
J.C. Bose University of Science and Technology, YMCA, India

Payal Gulati
J.C. Bose University of Science and Technology, YMCA, India

Rosy Madaan
Manav Rachna International Institute of Research and Studies, India

Komal Kumar Bhatia
J.C. Bose University of Science and Technology, YMCA, India

ABSTRACT

Employment of various sensors used in IoT can help create a sustainable urban life. Rapid advancements in IoT have made human existence smarter. Smartness may be associated to office, home, networks, energy consumption, agriculture, education, retail, and even healthcare. Smart health management addresses its populations, such as tracking routine activities, obesity, nutrition intake, heart rate, glucose level, oxygen level, body temperature, or even stress level monitoring. Stress is a condition which is being faced by people irrespective of their age, gender, or profession. But its identification at an early stage can help in preventing the consequences. This work presents nine machine learning techniques for identifying stress using the SWELL dataset. Hence, automated classifiers were utilised to predict working circumstances and stress-related mental states and were compared for accuracy for three stress conditions (no stress, interruption, and time pressure).

DOI: 10.4018/978-1-6684-2508-4.ch004

1. INTRODUCTION

The usage of various Internet of Things (IoT) sensors can lead to a sustainable urban environment, thereby improving the quality of life of citizens of a smart city (Muhammad et al., 2021). Smart healthcare constitutes one of the important aspects of a smart city. Smart Healthcare with IoT applications can be enhanced with the usage of sensors and actuators in patients for monitoring and tracking patients' health and medicines. The data generated by the sensors and actuators in a smart city, upon analysis lead to crucial data insights which can then be utilized to improve any smart city's efficiency and effectiveness. The initial step for the development of any smart city is data analytics. After the collection of a smart city's data through sources such as sensors, smart phones, citizen repositories, city repositories, analytical reasoning can be performed so as to generate the necessary information for good governance and decision making. The integration of IoT and Machine Learning monitoring the patients has drastically improved customised healthcare by enhancing patient care quality while decreasing costs. The Telehealth technologies are seen to be important in resolving substantial challenges for monitoring patients remotely. The key advantages are constant monitoring of a patient's health irrespective of the patient's site, greater accessibility to healthcare, lower healthcare costs, and improved treatment quality. With the advancement of technology, new IoT-based solutions for the collection of data and its analysis have been developed. The data can be collected from different areas within the smart city such as health, education, occupation, energy, weather, pollution, etc. Smart health management tackles both healthy and unhealthy populations, such as monitoring senior or younger people's daily tasks, obesity tracking, nutrition-intake tracking, heart rate, glucose level, oxygen level, body temperature, and even stress level tracking. Stress is a broad phrase that encompasses the psychological and biological activities that occur during emotionally and intellectually challenging situations. It is a disease that affects everyone, regardless of age, gender, or career. Stress leads to the altercation of thermal, acoustic, optical, impedance and electrical signals. As per American Institute of Stress, 80 percent of workers feel stress due to workplace, 50 percent require assistance to learn to handle stress, while 42 percent believe that their colleagues need it. As per the Health and Safety Executive (HSE), stress related to work, anxiety or depression contribute to 44 percent of all sick health cases related to work, further 54 percent of the workforce duration was missed due to illness in 2018-19 (Bobade & Vani, 2020). Stress has been linked to immune system breakdown and an elevated risk of cancer. These figures, as well as the repercussions of stress on humans, need the development of a system capable of recognising stress conditions and treating stress through personalised actions or, if required, medications. The ongoing Covid-19 outbreak has further exacerbated stressful situations across the globe. All people irrespective of their age, gender or profession are facing this condition. It should be dealt on a daily basis lest it endangers our mental sanity and routine work. . But, its identification at an early stage can help in preventing other repercussions that follow. The change in bio signals can help in detection of stress amongst humans. The combined effect of IoT for sustainable healthcare and big data analytics helps to increase medical facilities efficiency by recognising the risk factors, providing diagnosis and the treatment process. It not only meets the hospital management examination index need, but it also achieves superior cost growth between treatment and care services.

This work presents several machine learning techniques for identifying stress in people using the SWELL dataset. Datasets are a crucial tool for training, validating, and testing machine learning-based stress detection systems. The working conditions of 25 workers were modified to collect the dataset. Several features such as facial expressions, computer logging, body postures, heart rate variability and skin conductance were recorded with time pressure and email interruptions as stressor conditions.

Hence, the goal of this article is to create automated classifiers that can predict working circumstances and stress-related mental states from the dataset collected using sensor data that includes computer logs, facial expressions, posture, and physiology. The traditional questionnaire method for stress analysis is fraught with ambiguity and is untrustworthy since it is totally dependent on individual replies, and many respondents might be hesitant to complete the questionnaire.

In recent decades, the machine learning (ML) technique has found several applications in a variety of sectors, including finance, healthcare, energy, networks, materials science and the environment. ML has proven to be quite successful at tackling tough issues in a variety of disciplines. The ML applications are constructed in such a way that they detect and comprehend the incoming data and may make the best judgments based on it on their own. Recommendation, classification, and clustering are three of its most used strategies (Syed, Jabeen, Manimala, & Elsayed, 2019). The two most prevalent ways for implementing ML techniques are classified into supervised and unsupervised approaches. The former uses a predefined dataset for training to understand any function and includes instances such as classifying emails as spam or non-spam, classifying web pages after examining their content as secure or unsecure, and voice recognition, whereas the latter is more commonly used for grouping homogeneous or similar kind of data into integrated clusters with no previously available dataset for training. In the medical area, researchers are utilising the ML algorithms to analyse the neuro-imaging data, comprehend the initial phase of Parkinson's disease using speech data, and many other applications (Fang et al., 2021). We have considered ML algorithms as the tool to forecast the risk of stress, inspired by the results of ML techniques in the medical industry. This prediction is based on characteristics used in the SWELL dataset. The evaluation was conducted on a dataset of over 369289 records.

Artificial neural networks (ANN) have been used in the literature to evaluate the smart city data in order to discover new insights (Dey & Kumar, 2019)(Muhammad et al., 2021)(Manocha, Kumar, Bhatia, & Sharma, 2021). Machine learning and deep learning have been used for data analytics in a smart city, according to the previous literature (Nguyen et al., 2019) (Kadhim, 2019). ML techniques like Random Forest (RF), Extra Trees (ET), Decision Tree (DT), Gradient Boost, K-Nearest Neighbour (KNN), Linear Discriminant Analysis (LDA), Ada Boost, Logistic regression (LR) and Naïve Bayes (NB) were used to evaluate and compare the performance of three-class (no stress vs. interruption vs. time pressure) classifications. Deep learning has received a lot of interest from the academic as well as the professional community because of its ability to process large amounts of data, the need for less manual intervention in data processing (Chen, Hao, Hwang, Wang, & Wang, 2017). It is gaining popularity due to its unique capabilities in dealing with large amounts of data without mandating the need of several algorithms as compared to the usual ML algorithms (Muhammad et al., 2021).

2. RELATED WORK

ML models using physiological feedback towards stressful and emotional conditions have been used to automatically detect stress in the recent years (Bobade & Vani, 2020). WESAD data was collected from fifteen people and physiological data such as acceleration about the three-axis, body temperature, ECG, blood volume pulse,, respiration, electromyogram, and electrodermal activity using wearable devices (Philip Schmidt, A. Reiss, R. Duerichen, 2018). They subjected the individuals to a variety of stress circumstances, including baseline, fun, tension, meditation, and so on. They examined ML methods' performance for detection of stress state: K-Nearest Neighbor (KNN) (Yang & Liu, 1999) (Elmogy, Tariq,

Ibrahim, & Mohammed, 2021)(Mandel J, 2015), Linear Discriminant Analysis (LDA) (Bobade & Vani, 2020), Random Forest (RF) (Sidhu, Kumar, & Rana, 2020), Decision Tree (DT) (Koldijk, Neerincx, & Kraaij, 2018), and AdaBoost (AB) (Barbado, Araque, & Iglesias, 2019). Using common characteristics and standard ML approaches, classiðcation accuracy of up to 80.34 percent and 93.12 percent for the three classes (baseline vs stress vs amusement) and the two classes (non-stress vs. stress) classification issues, respectively was attained.

Wearable sensors were used to assess physiological signals to determine the mental stress. The individuals' ECG, skin conductance, respiration, and EMG and computed a total of 19 physiological characteristics were recorded from them. After studying the correlations and normalising feature values, a subset of nine features were chosen for further analysis, which was subsequently reduced to seven features using the principal component analysis (PCA) technique. Performance-wise, an accuracy of 80 percent was reached between stressful vs non-stressful situations of an individual utilising these variables and other classifiers such as Quadratic Bayes Normal Classifier, Linear Bayes Normal Classifier, K-Nearest Neighbors Classifier, and Fisher's Least Square Linear Classifier (J. Wijsman, B. Grundlehner, H. Liu, 2011).

Saskia Koldijk et al. [6] introduced a new multimodal dataset called SWELL Knowledge Work (SWELL) for stress research and user modelling. The working conditions of 25 workers were altered while they performed their usual routine tasks by introducing two stressor conditions, namely the time constraint and email interruptions to collect the dataset. Body postures, expressions of the face, logging hours on the computer, conductance of skin, and the heart beat rate were all recorded. The dataset was evaluated using validated questionnaires on work load, cognitive effort, and so on. No ML techniques were employed in this benchmark (Koldijk, Sappelli, Verberne, Neerincx, & Kraaij, 2014).

Another important component that might determine a person's stress is facial clues. The framework for identifying followed by assessing emotional responses of stress using face clues that were video-recorded had been created and added to this by Mouth activity, eye events, camera-based photoplethysmographic assessment of heart rate, and head motion parameters were also evaluated. (Giannakakis, G., Pediaditis, M., Manousos, D., Kazantzaki, E., Chiarugi, F., Simos, P.G., Marias, K. and Tsiknakis, 2017) Methods such as Generalized Likelihood Ratio, Naive Bayes classifier, Support Vector Machines, K-nearest neighbours, and AdaBoost classifier were tested. The Adaboost classifier had the highest classification performance in the social exposure procedure, with an accuracy of 91.68 percent.

3. PROPOSED FRAMEWORK

3.1 Dataset

The SWELL -Heart Rate Variability (HRV) dataset for research on user modeling and stress has been considered for this study. It is available through https://www.kaggle.com/qiriro/swell-heart-rate-variability-hrv. The dataset comprises of HRV indices which can be used for user modelling and stress research. Researchers from Radboud University's Institute for Computing and Information Sciences collected the SWELL dataset. It is the result of research done on 25 participants performing routine office tasks (for instance, making work reports, presentations, drafting e-mails and browsing information) The participant experienced standard workplace pressures like unexpected e-mail interruptions with the urge to complete their task on time. As part of this investigation, computer logging, bodily postures, facial expression, skin conductance and the ECG signal were all captured. The researchers also recorded the experience of the individual with mental effort, task load, perceived stress and varying moods. Each participant was subjected to three distinct working circumstances (Cuno, Condori-Fernandez, Mendoza, & Lovon, 2020) (Koldijk et al., 2014):

1. No stress condition: the participants are permitted to perform the activities within 45 minutes, but the participants are unaware of this maximum time limit.
2. Period constraint condition: Under this condition the time given to complete the task was reduced to two-third of the time given during the no stress condition.
3. Interruption condition: As the participants performed their routine duties, they were interrupted by eight mails. Some e-mails were pertinent to their responsibilities (and the participant was asked to take particular actions), while rest were just irrelevant.

The original dataset includes raw ECG signals as well as a feature dataset labelled with the settings under which the data was taken. It also had the heart rate variability (HRV) feature that was calculated once per minute. It skewed the results and concluded that HRV was not a strong predictor of workplace stressors. This is more extensive and enables for 99.25 percent accuracy in predicting the stressor. The details of the dataset used in our study are given in Table 1.

Table 1. Dataset description

Dataset	SWELL HRV
No. of features	36
No. of workers	25
No. of instances	369289
Target attribute	Condition
No. of Conditions	3 (No stress, Time Pressure, Interruption)
Transformed Train Set Instances	258502
Transformed Test Set Instances	110787
Fold Generator	Stratified K Fold
No. of folds	10

3.2 ML Algorithms

ML algorithms are majorly used for:

a. **Classification:** It is a type of supervised learning in which given sample is utilised to decide the allocation of known categories to incoming data (Kou et al., 2020). Alternatively, existing samples of collected classifications determine the classifications of new data. For instance, Gmail, the mail service provider by Google uses this method to identify an email as spam or non-spam by taking into account the emails marked as spam by its user (Syed et al., 2019).

b. **Clustering (also known as segmentation):** It seeks to separate data into distinct clusters. It is also known as unsupervised classification as the output given to the user is uncertain (Rezaimehr & Dadkhah, 2020). The algorithm is not trained on any prior input or output data, but still determines the output for users. Consumer data for example, may be classified into distinct segments or clusters based on criteria such as demographic information or customer purchase behaviour (Lin & Jingtao, 2015). Google uses the clustering algorithms to create linked data groups based on features that are comparable.
c. **Dimensionality reduction:** The process of reducing the number of dimensions or variables in a dataset without losing important information from the data is known as dimensionality reduction. Two well-known variable reduction approaches are Principal Component Analysis (PCA) and Factor Analysis (Jirachanchaisiri, Kitsupapaisan, & Maneeroj, 2019).
d. **Anomaly detection:** Detecting an anomaly entails recognising the things, events, or observations that do not follow the usual anticipated behaviour. It can discover relevant information from the data and is useful in a variety of application sectors. Anomalies are defined as difficulties such as cyber attacks, credit card fraud, a configuration defect, health troubles, or typos in a text. Detecting abnormalities in patient records in healthcare informatics indicates illness epidemics, instrumentation problems, and so on.
e. **Recommender systems:** They provide alternatives to users for their item of interest(s) based on their past purchase history, explicit behaviour such as ratings and reviews and user/item similarity. For instance, Youtube suggests video as recommendation to its users (Chehal, Gupta, & Gulati, 2020).
f. **Ensemble methods:** Some methods are combined to generate strong predictions. For example, decision trees when combined form random forest, the most accurate classification method (Guo et al., 2020).

This study utilised 13 ML algorithms which have been stated below:

1. **Decision Trees classifier:** This classifier is a non-parametric, supervised modelling technique used for regression and classification in machine learning. The classification and regression tree is the traditional name for decision trees (CART) (Hajek & Barushka, 2019). No data processing procedures such as data normalisation is required in it. Moreover it is the binary tree depiction of the given input data. The nodes of the tree denote a variable and the lead node denotes a class label. The leaves represent the class labels which are accepted as input by the target variable in the classification step. The internal nodes, which are made up of tree branches, are employed to make the selections that result in class labels. The purpose is to learn basic decision rules from input data to develop a model which can predict the value of the dependent feature (Raza, Hussain, Hussain, Zhao, & Rehman, 2019).
2. **Random Forest classifier:** It is a variation of decision trees in which stack of decision trees using bagging that uses several random predictors to aggregate predictions (Breiman, 2001). The forecast rule is based on the majority vote or average over all trees. Random forests can produce competitive or even greater prediction strengths (Emmanuel et al., 2021)(Wu, Xindong, 2009).
3. **Extra Trees classifier:** Another meta-estimator or ensemble approach that is based on different sub-sections of a dataset and fits random decision tress on them is known as extra trees classifier.

These randomised decision trees are known as extra trees. The basis for usage of this classifier remains the same as that of random forest (Bhoi & Joshi, 2018).

4. **K Neighbors classifier:** The k closest neighbour (k-NN) technique is often regarded as the most simple non-parametric ML algorithm. This model has no discriminative function with regard to the training instances (Raza et al., 2019). The entire dataset is memorised and represented using the k- NN method. It is also known as the lazy learner as the forecasted values are calculated just-in-time by finding similarity between the input sequence and each training example. The k-NN algorithm is an instance-based learning algorithm that uses raw training cases to produce predictions. Since each sample of the training dataset functions is a case from the issue field, it is referred as learning which is case-based. KNN estimates the proximity among both the new and unknown instance and the training data samples in order to categorise it. The new instance has been turned into a variable or feature vector and is now a component of the variable or feature space. Different distance measures may be used to compute the distance among both the new sample and existing examples in the variable or the feature space.
5. **Gradient Boosting classifier:** Gradient Tree Boosting, also known as Gradient Boosted Decision Trees (GBDT), is a boosting generalisation to arbitrary differentiable loss functions. GBDT is a reliable and efficient off-the-shelf approach that may be applied to regression and classification issues in a range of fields, including Web search ranking and ecology.
6. **Ada Boost classifier:** It is a binary classification boosting algorithm and is also known as adaptive boosting. The goal is to make weak classifiers strong classifiers. It is known to outperform for discrete data (Kumar Gupta & Singh Rana, 2020).
7. **Linear Discriminant Analysis:** This classifier has a linear decision boundary and fits conditional densities of classes to data and uses Bayes' rule. The model assumes that all classes have the same covariance matrix and hence fits a Gaussian density to each class. By projecting the input to the most discriminative directions, the fitted model may be utilised to minimise the dimensionality of the input.
8. **Logistic Regression:** Another name for logistic function is sigmoid function; logistic function is the basis of logistic regression. It is an S-shaped curve that maps any real-valued number between 0 and 1. The logistic function is represented as (Raza et al., 2019):

$$1/_{1+e^{-z}} \tag{1}$$

Where, z is to be mapped between 0 and 1. It uses maximum-likelihood estimation to learn and determine the parameters from the samples of the training data. The purpose of maximum-likelihood estimation is to reduce errors in projected probability during training.

9. **Naïve Bayes:** This method follows the probabilistic paradigm of the Bayes theorem. According to the Bayes theorem's generic notation, for text sample x to be part of class c, the posterior probability is defined as:

$$P(c|x) = \frac{P(c)P(x|c)}{P(x)} \tag{2}$$

P(c| x) is the posterior probability that the sample x belongs to the class
P(c) is the likelihood that the class c (prior probability of class c) is true (regarding the samples).
P(x | c) denotes the likelihood that sample x belongs to class.
P(x) denotes the probability (evidence) of sample x in any class

The probabilistic classifier created utilising the Naïve Bayes technique for text classification (multi-class) leads to categorising text based on word occurrence in every text sample followed by assigning these to distinct classes. Alternatively, Naïve Bayes maintains note of the characteristic that belongs to the class (Hajek & Barushka, 2019) (Trivedi, Dey, & Kumar, 2018).

3.3 Methodology

This section and Figure 1 outline the process followed in this study. The first step involved, collecting of the dataset for detection of stress condition in humans. The dataset was taken from the Kaggle platform. The analysis and details of the dataset and its subset considered have been shown in Table 1. The same has been outlined in sub section 3.1. The dataset was split into 70:30 for performing training and testing of the machine learning algorithms. The data was then inputted to the nine ML algorithms as outlined in sub-section 3.2 and compared for performance across six performance metrics as stated in Section 4 of this study.

Figure 1. Process flow

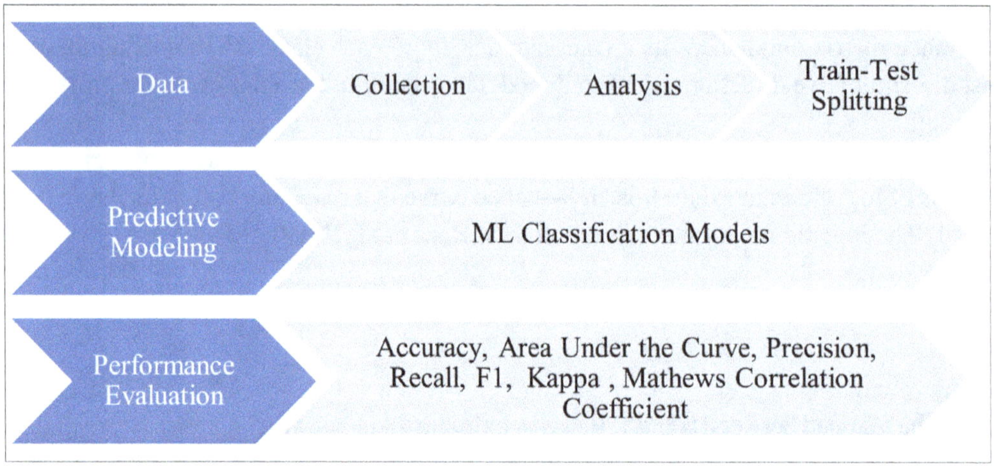

4. RESULT AND DISCUSSION

This study evaluates the performance of various state-of-the-art machine learning models using accuracy, area under the curve (AUC), Recall, Precision, F1 score, Kappa and Mathew's correlation coefficient (MCC) measure as shown in Table 2 and Figure 2 (Cismondi et al., 2013).

Table 2. Performance of ML algorithms

Classifier Model	Accuracy	AUC	Recall	Precision	F1	Kappa	MCC	Time Taken (sec)
Random Forest	**1.0000**	**1.0000**	**1.0000**	**1.0000**	**1.0000**	**1.0000**	**1.0000**	**117.450**
Extra Trees	1.0000	1.0000	1.0000	1.0000	1.0000	1.0000	1.0000	28.822
Decision Trees	0.9999	0.9992	0.9989	0.9990	0.9990	0.9984	0.9984	8.358
K Neighbors	0.9904	0.9987	0.9890	0.9904	0.9904	0.9838	0.9838	3.914
Gradient Boosting	0.9128	0.9854	0.8828	0.9152	0.9117	0.8498	0.8529	710.958
Ada Boost	0.6685	0.7696	0.6012	0.6605	0.6555	0.4129	0.4216	43.081
Linear Discriminant Analysis	0.6251	0.7417	0.5054	0.6098	0.5948	0.3028	0.3229	1.308
Logistic Regression	0.6064	0.7054	0.4867	0.5963	0.5698	0.2553	0.2806	82.827
Naïve Bayes	**0.5525**	**0.6897**	**0.5007**	**0.5509**	**0.5454**	**0.2425**	**0.2454**	**0.239**

Figure 2. Performance of ML algorithms

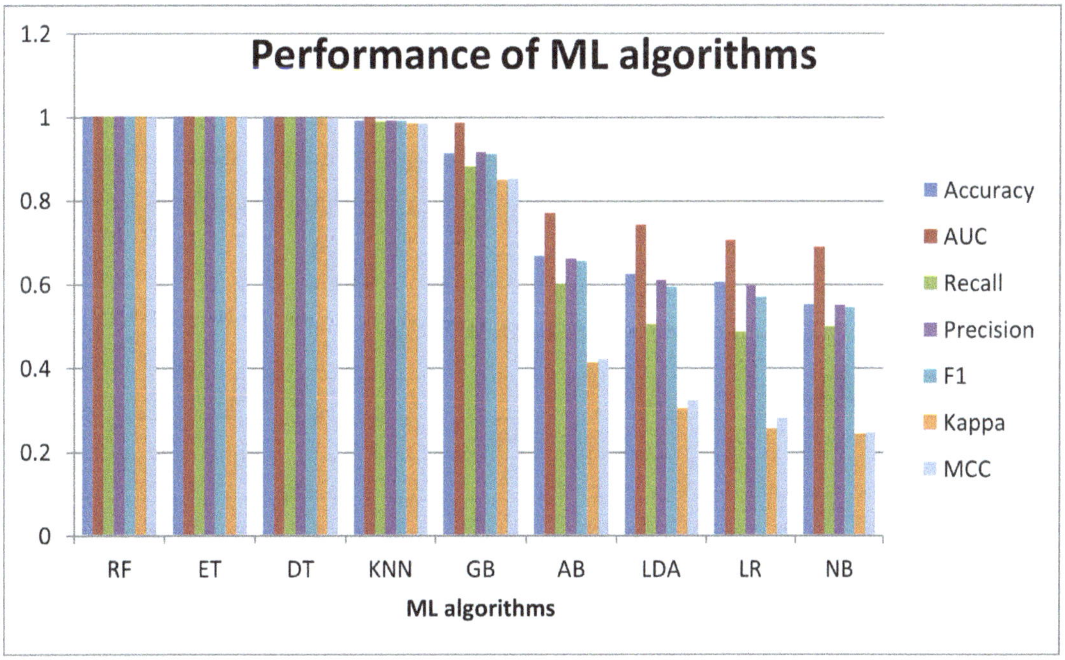

As seen in Table 2, the best classifier model is Random Forest as the accuracy, AUC, recall, precision, F1, Kappa and MCC metric is 100 percent for this model (Kumar, Pannu, & Malhi, 2020) (Kumar Gupta & Singh Rana, 2020). The parameters and their values for the best model are shown in Table 4. The metrics used in table 2 are defined in Table 3.

The metric defined in Table 3 can be explained as follows:

a) TP stands for, True Positive that is, correctly categorised class of interest
b) TN stands for, True Negative that is, correctly categorised as not the class of interest

c) FP stands for, False Positive that is, incorrectly categorised as the class of interest
d) FN stands for, False Negative that is, incorrectly categorised as not the class of interest
e) P' stands for observed agreement and P_e stands for expected agreement

Table 3. Performance metrics

Metric	Definition
Accuracy	$\frac{(TP+TN)}{(TP+TN+FP+FN)}$
Precision	TP/(TP+FP)
Recall	TP/(TP+FN)
F1	(2*Precision*Recall) / (Recall+Precision)
Kappa	$(P'-P_e)/(1-P_e)$
MCC	TP*TN-FP*FN/((TP+FP)(TP+FN)(TN+FP)(TN+FN))$^{1/2}$

As shown in Table 2, the maximum and minimum time taken to classify the stress conditions into three classes is by Gradient Boosting classifier and Quadratic Discriminant Analysis classifier respectively. The worst classifier in terms of performance is Naïve Bayes as its accuracy is 55.25 percent which is very less than the best classifier model.

Table 4. Parameters of the best classifier model (Random Forest)

Parameters	Random Forest
criterion	Gini
max_features	auto
max_leaf_nodes	None
min_samples_leaf	1
min_samples_split	2
n_estimators	100
n_jobs	-1
warm_start	False
bootstrap	True
ccp_alpha	0.0
class_weight	None

5. CONCLUSION

Recent advancements in IoT have changed the way humans exist and interact with each other. The smart existence/interaction may be associated to office, home, networks, energy consumption, agriculture, education, retail and health care. In order to handle both the healthy and unhealthy population of a nation smart health management is indispensable. This should involve tracking routine activities of the elderly or youngsters, obesity, nutrition intake, heart rate, glucose, oxygen level monitoring, body temperature, and even stress level monitoring. This study successfully identified stressful conditions of humans namely, no stress, interruption and time pressure with the help of nine different ML algorithms with the help of SWELL dataset. The study of these classification techniques revealed that RF and ET discriminated between the three working circumstances with 100% accuracy, while DT and KNN discriminated with around 99% accuracy. The results demonstrate that RF, ET, DT, KNN, Gradient Boost models are trustworthy, with accuracy and recall rates of more than 91 percent and 88 percent, respectively. This identification can help in keeping stressful conditions for humans at bay and act as input to recommender systems for generating alternatives of physical activities or medicines or nutrition intake to be undertaken to keep oneself fit and healthy.

REFERENCES

Barbado, R., Araque, O., & Iglesias, C. A. (2019). A framework for fake review detection in online consumer electronics retailers. *Information Processing & Management*, *56*(4), 1234–1244. doi:10.1016/j.ipm.2019.03.002

Bhoi, A., & Joshi, S. (2018). *Various Approaches to Aspect-based Sentiment Analysis*. Retrieved from https://arxiv.org/abs/1805.01984

Bobade, P., & Vani, M. (2020). Stress Detection with Machine Learning and Deep Learning using Multimodal Physiological Data. *Proceedings of the 2nd International Conference on Inventive Research in Computing Applications, ICIRCA 2020*, 51–57. 10.1109/ICIRCA48905.2020.9183244

Breiman, L. (2001). Random Forests. *Machine Learning*, *45*(1), 5–32. doi:10.1023/A:1010933404324

Chehal, D., Gupta, P., & Gulati, P. (2020). Implementation and comparison of topic modeling techniques based on user reviews in e-commerce recommendations. *Journal of Ambient Intelligence and Humanized Computing*, (0123456789). Advance online publication. doi:10.100712652-020-01956-6

Chen, M., Hao, Y., Hwang, K., Wang, L., & Wang, L. (2017). Disease Prediction by Machine Learning over Big Data from Healthcare Communities. *IEEE Access: Practical Innovations, Open Solutions*, *5*, 8869–8879. doi:10.1109/ACCESS.2017.2694446

Cismondi, F., Fialho, A. S., Vieira, S. M., Reti, S. R., Sousa, J. M. C., & Finkelstein, S. N. (2013). Missing data in medical databases: Impute, delete or classify? *Artificial Intelligence in Medicine*, *58*(1), 63–72. doi:10.1016/j.artmed.2013.01.003 PMID:23428358

Cuno, A., Condori-Fernandez, N., Mendoza, A., & Lovon, W. R. (2020). A FAIR evaluation of public datasets for stress detection systems. *Proceedings - International Conference of the Chilean Computer Science Society, SCCC*. 10.1109/SCCC51225.2020.9281274

Dey, D., & Kumar, P. (2019). A novel approach to identify the determinants of online review helpfulness and predict the helpfulness score across product categories. In Lecture Notes in Computer Science (including subseries Lecture Notes in Artificial Intelligence and Lecture Notes in Bioinformatics) (Vol. 11932, pp. 365–388). Springer. doi:10.1007/978-3-030-37188-3_21

Elmogy, A. M., Tariq, U., Ibrahim, A., & Mohammed, A. (2021). Fake Reviews Detection using Supervised Machine Learning. *International Journal of Advanced Computer Science and Applications*, *12*(1), 601–606. doi:10.14569/IJACSA.2021.0120169

Emmanuel, T., Maupong, T., Mpoeleng, D., Semong, T., Mphago, B., & Tabona, O. (2021). A survey on missing data in machine learning. *Journal of Big Data*, *8*(1), 1–37. doi:10.1186/s40537-021-00516-9

Fang, M., Chen, Y., Xue, R., Wang, H., Chakraborty, N., Su, T., & Dai, Y. (2021). A hybrid machine learning approach for hypertension risk prediction. *Neural Computing & Applications*, *0*. Advance online publication. doi:10.100700521-021-06060-0

Giannakakis, G., Pediaditis, M., Manousos, D., Kazantzaki, E., Chiarugi, F., Simos, P. G., Marias, K., & Tsiknakis, M. (2017). Stress and anxiety detection using facial cues from videos. *Biomedical Signal Processing and Control*, *31*, 89–101. doi:10.1016/j.bspc.2016.06.020

Guo, X., Lin, W., Li, Y., Liu, Z., Yang, L., Zhao, S., & Zhu, Z. (2020). DKEN: Deep knowledge-enhanced network for recommender systems. *Information Sciences*, *540*, 263–277. doi:10.1016/j.ins.2020.06.041

Hajek, P., & Barushka, A. (2019). A Comparative Study of Machine Learning Methods for Detection of Fake Online Consumer Reviews. *ACM International Conference Proceeding Series*, 18–22. 10.1145/3383902.3383909

Jirachanchaisiri, P., Kitsupapaisan, J., & Maneeroj, S. (2019). Bayesian flexible mixture model with rating conversion on multi-criteria recommender system. *International Journal of Web Information Systems*, *15*(4), 402–419. doi:10.1108/IJWIS-10-2018-0074

Kadhim, A. I. (2019). Survey on supervised machine learning techniques for automatic text classification. *Artificial Intelligence Review*, *52*(1), 273–292. doi:10.100710462-018-09677-1

Koldijk, S., Neerincx, M. A., & Kraaij, W. (2018). Detecting Work Stress in Offices by Combining Unobtrusive Sensors. *IEEE Transactions on Affective Computing*, *9*(2), 227–239. doi:10.1109/TAFFC.2016.2610975

Koldijk, S., Sappelli, M., Verberne, S., Neerincx, M. A., & Kraaij, W. (2014). The Swell knowledge work dataset for stress and user modeling research. *ICMI 2014 - Proceedings of the 2014 International Conference on Multimodal Interaction*, 291–298. 10.1145/2663204.2663257

Kou, G., Yang, P., Peng, Y., Xiao, F., Chen, Y., & Alsaadi, F. E. (2020). Evaluation of feature selection methods for text classification with small datasets using multiple criteria decision-making methods. *Applied Soft Computing*, *86*, 105836. doi:10.1016/j.asoc.2019.105836

Kumar, R., Pannu, H. S., & Malhi, A. K. (2020). Aspect-based sentiment analysis using deep networks and stochastic optimization. *Neural Computing & Applications*, *32*(8), 3221–3235. doi:10.100700521-019-04105-z

Kumar Gupta, V., & Singh Rana, P. (2020). Ensemble Technique for Toxicity Prediction of Small Drug Molecules of the Antioxidant Response Element Signalling Pathway. *The Computer Journal*, *00*(0). Advance online publication. doi:10.1093/comjnl/bxaa001

Lin, D., & Jingtao, S. (2015). A recommender system based on contextual information of click and purchase data to items for e-commerce. *Third International Conference on Cyberspace Technology (CCT 2015)*, 1–6. 10.1049/cp.2015.0823

Mandel, J. S. P. (2015). A Comparison of Six Methods for Missing Data Imputation. *Journal of Biometrics & Biostatistics*, *06*(01), 1–6. doi:10.4172/2155-6180.1000224

Manocha, A., Kumar, G., Bhatia, M., & Sharma, A. (2021). IoT-inspired machine learning-assisted sedentary behavior analysis in smart healthcare industry. *Journal of Ambient Intelligence and Humanized Computing*, (0123456789). Advance online publication. doi:10.100712652-021-03371-x

Muhammad, A. N., Aseere, A. M., Chiroma, H., Shah, H., Gital, A. Y., & Hashem, I. A. T. (2021). Deep learning application in smart cities: Recent development, taxonomy, challenges and research prospects. In *Neural Computing and Applications* (Vol. 33). Springer London. doi:10.1007/s00521-020-05151-8

Nguyen, G., Dlugolinsky, S., Bobák, M., Tran, V., López García, Á., Heredia, I., Malík, P., & Hluchý, L. (2019). Machine Learning and Deep Learning frameworks and libraries for large-scale data mining: A survey. *Artificial Intelligence Review*, *52*(1), 77–124. doi:10.100710462-018-09679-z

Philip Schmidt, A., Reiss, R., & Duerichen, K. V. L. (2018). Introducing WESAD, a multimodal dataset for wearable Stress and Affect Detection. *International Conference on Multimodal Interaction 2018.*

Raza, M., Hussain, F. K., Hussain, O. K., Zhao, M., & Rehman, Z. (2019). A comparative analysis of machine learning models for quality pillar assessment of SaaS services by multi-class text classification of users' reviews. *Future Generation Computer Systems*, *101*, 341–371. doi:10.1016/j.future.2019.06.022

Rezaimehr, F., & Dadkhah, C. (2020). *A survey of attack detection approaches in collaborative filtering recommender systems. Artificial Intelligence Review*. Springer Netherlands. doi:10.100710462-020-09898-3

Sidhu, R. K., Kumar, R., & Rana, P. S. (2020). Machine learning based crop water demand forecasting using minimum climatological data. *Multimedia Tools and Applications*, *79*(19–20), 13109–13124. doi:10.100711042-019-08533-w

Syed, L., Jabeen, S., Manimala, S., & Elsayed, H. A. (2019). Data science algorithms and techniques for smart healthcare using iot and big data analytics. In *Studies in Fuzziness and Soft Computing* (Vol. 374). doi:10.1007/978-3-030-03131-2_11

Trivedi, S. K., Dey, S., & Kumar, A. (2018). Capturing user sentiments for online Indian movie reviews: A comparative analysis of different machine-learning models. *The Electronic Library*, *36*(4), 677–695. doi:10.1108/EL-04-2017-0075

Wijsman, J., Grundlehner, B., & Liu, H., H. H. and J. P. (2011). Towards mental stress detection using wearable physiological sensors. In *2011 Annual International Conference of the IEEE Engineering in Medicine and Biology Society* (pp. 1798–1801). 10.1109/IEMBS.2011.6090512

Wu, X., & V. K. (2009). *The top ten algorithms in data mining.* CRC Press.

Yang, Y., & Liu, X. (1999). A re-examination of text categorization methods. *Proceedings of the 22nd Annual International ACM SIGIR Conference on Research and Development in Information Retrieval, SIGIR 1999*, 42–49. 10.1145/312624.312647

Chapter 5
Smart Prediction of Pulmonary Diseases Using Artificial Intelligence and Deep Learning

Tanvi Gupta
Manav Rachna International Institute of Research and Studies, India

Supriya P. P.
https://orcid.org/0000-0001-8054-8567
Manav Rachna International Institute of Research and Studies, Faridabad, India

ABSTRACT

As a result of global urbanization and the drive for more sustainable and livable cities, smart cities are becoming increasingly significant. It is widely known that air pollution exists all around us as a result of numerous automobiles on the road, stubble burning, and industrial air pollution, all of which impair our health, particularly our lungs. Chronic diseases are growing more common as our society ages. Chronic respiratory problems such as asthma and chronic obstructive pulmonary disease (COPD) impact millions of people globally, and the number is growing every day. COPD, for example, afflicted roughly 251 million individuals worldwide in 2016, and claimed the lives of 3.17 million people (i.e., 5% of the population). There are many distinct sorts of the pulmonary diseases: COPD, pulmonary fibrosis, asthma, and lung cancer, to name a few. This chapter explains the three machine learning algorithms that helped to diagnose pulmonary diseases based on the dataset.

The lung is a vital organ in the human body that is prone to damage under several circumstances (Sheffield, 2017). Airborne particles, environmental pollutants, occupational pollutants, and industrial pollution are varied possible causes. These harm human health. As a result, several lung disorders such as COPD, Asthma, Pulmonary Fibrosis, and Lung Cancer have emerged. Because the lungs are an interior bodily organ, detecting such disorders was previously challenging. However, technology will play an increasingly important role in medical science over time. Technologies such as the Internet of Things (IoT), Artificial intelligence (AI), and Deep Learning (DL) have played an important role in improving

DOI: 10.4018/978-1-6684-2508-4.ch005

disease detection without causing pain to patients. Diagnosing an internal organ is quite tough, but sensors, Machine Learning(ML), and the prediction of images through AI have made it easier and painless.

When compared to those with diagnosed Asthma (Alan Kaplan et al., 2021), underdiagnosis can result in decreased quality of life, increased number of general practitioner visits, absence from school or work, and increased hospitalizations, as well as failure to prescribe appropriate medication(s). Indeed, failure to deliver inhaled corticosteroids to those with Asthma (whether or not they have COPD) shows an increase in hospitalizations. As a result, the purpose of this chapter is to examine prediction models for pulmonary ailment diagnoses, such as Deep Learning and AI. Various predictive models aid in the prediction of disease depending on the symptoms provided.

Respiratory disease (Sheffield, 2017) has a significant impact on people's health. As demonstrated in Table 1, the most common diseases are Asthma, COPD, Sleep-Disordered Breathing, Tuberculosis (TB), Pulmonary Hypertension, and Pulmonary Fibrosis. To be more specific, 235 million people(Devi Prasad Shetty,2010) have Asthma, 200 million people have COPD, 65 million people have moderate-to-severe COPD, 1–6% of the adult population (more than 100 million) has sleep-disordered breathing, 9.6 million people develop tuberculosis (TB) each year, millions have pulmonary hypertension, and millions have pulmonary fibrosis worldwide.

At least two billion people are affected by the negative effects of biomass fuels, one billion by outdoor air pollution, and one billion by cigarette smoke. Every year, four million people die due to chronic respiratory disease. To examine pulmonary problems, the data is acquired from the local health department in Albuquerque, New Mexico. Table 2 shows many attributes in the data that can be used to identify the disease and its types.

Table 1. Statistics of respiratory diseases of the year 2019

Respiratory Diseases	Population affected(Total=7.7 billion in the world)	Percentage
Asthma	235 million	3.05%
COPD	200 million	2.59%
COPD(moderate-to-severe)	65 million	0.844%
Sleep-disordered breathing	100million (approx.)	1.29%
Tuberculosis	9.6 million	0.124%

Table 2. Statistics of the respiratory disease based on pollution of the year 2019

Respiratory Disease from	Population affected (Total=7.7 in the world)	Percentage
Biomass Fuels	2 billion	25.97%
Outdoor Air Pollution	1 billion	12.98%
Cigarette Smoke	1 billion	12.98%

Certain Machine Learning(ML) Algorithms used to predict the disease using the symptoms are discussed here:

1. **Naïve Bayes Classifier Algorithm:** Based on the Bayes theorem (SonooJaiswal, 2021), it is a "supervised learning strategy" for dealing with classification problems. It's most typically employed in text categorization with a big training dataset. This is a simple and effective classification algorithm that aids in the construction of fast ML models capable of making quick predictions. It's a probabilistic classifier, which means it makes predictions based on an object's probability. Spam filtration, sentiment analysis, and article classification are all common uses for the same.

Bayes' Theorem

a. This is also known as "Bayes' Rule" or "Bayes' law," and it is a conditional probability method for determining the likelihood of a hypothesis with previous knowledge.
b. The formula for Bayes' theorem is given by eq.1, where A is hypothesis and B is observed event:

$$P\left(\frac{A}{B}\right)=P\left(\frac{B}{A}\right)P(A)/P(B) \quad (1)$$

Where,

P(A|B) is Posterior probability: Probability of hypothesis A on the observed event B.

P(B|A) is Likelihood probability: Probability of the evidence given that the probability of a hypothesis is true.

P(A) is Prior Probability: Probability of the hypothesis before observing the evidence.

P(B) is Marginal Probability: Probability of Evidence.

Consider the workings of the Naive Bayes' Classifier as an example. Assume there is a weather dataset and a variable called "Play" as an objective variable. As a result, based on the weather conditions, it is required to select whether or not to play on a specific day using this dataset. To resolve this problem, one must follow the steps below:

1. Create frequency tables from the given dataset.
2. Create a Likelihood table by calculating the probability of the provided attributes.
3. Apply the Bayes' theorem to determine the posterior probability.

There are three types of Naive Bayes' Model, which are given below:

- **Gaussian:** This model assumes that attributes are regularly distributed. If predictors take continuous values rather than discrete values, the model assumes these values come from a Gaussian distribution.
- **Multi-nomial:** This Naive Bayes classifier is used when the data is multi-nominally distributed. It is typically used to tackle document classification problems, such as determining whether the document belongs to the Sports, Politics, or Education category. The predictors of the classifier are based on the frequency of words.

- **Bernoulli**: This classifier functions similar to the Multi-nomial classifier, with the exception that the predictor variables are independent Booleans variables. Determine whether a given word appears in a document, for example, this paradigm is also well-known in document categorization jobs.

SUPPORT VECTOR MACHINE

These introduced in the 1960s and improved in the 1990s are supervised ML techniques that can be used for classification as well as regression (ElearningProviders, 2006),. They are, nevertheless, most typically used in categorization problems. SVMs have a distinct implementation strategy when compared to other ML algorithms. Because of their ability to handle both continuous and categorical variables, they've recently garnered a lot of traction. This model is essentially a representation of separate classes in a hyperplane in a multidimensional space. To minimize the error, SVM will iteratively construct the hyperplane. The goal of SVM is to divide datasets into classes to find the "Maximum Marginal Hyperplane (MMH)".

The following concepts are important in SVM:

- Support Vectors: These are the data points that are closest to the hyperplane, and between them, a dividing line will be drawn.
- A "hyperplane" is a decision plane or space that divides a collection of things into discrete classes.
- Margin is defined as the distance between two lines on a set of data points from different classifications. It is possible to compute the perpendicular distance between the line and the support vectors. A wide margin is considered a good margin, whereas a tiny margin is considered a bad margin.

The main goal of SVM is to divide the datasets into classes to find a "Maximum Marginal Hyperplane (MMH)".

K-NEAREST NEIGHBOR (K-NN) ALGORITHM FOR MACHINE LEARNING

The Supervised Learning Technique is used in K-Nearest Neighbor, a simple ML methodology. It assumes that the new case/data and previous cases are comparable, and it assigns the new case to the category that is closest to the existing categories It saves all available data and groups fresh data points into categories based on their similarity. As new data is generated, the K-NN algorithm can quickly classify it into the appropriate category. This method can be applied to both Regression and Classification problems, but it is more commonly employed for Classification. It's a non-parametric method, which means no assumptions about the underlying data are made. It's also known as a lazy learner algorithm because it doesn't learn from the training set right away, instead of storing the data and acting on it later during classification. During the training phase, this method simply saves the dataset, and when new data is received, it is categorized into a group that is quite similar to the new data.

Consider the following scenario: there is a snapshot of an animal that could be a cat or a dog, and we want to know if it is a cat or a dog. The K-NN technique can be used for this identification because it is based on a similarity metric. It will compare the new data set to photos of cats and dogs and divide it into two groups based on the most similar qualities.

Need for K-NN Algorithm

Assume there are two categories, A and B, and we have a new data point X1 to which we wish to assign it. This type of challenge necessitates the use of a K-NN algorithm. K-NN is used to determine the category or class of a dataset. Consider Figures 1 and 2:

Figure 1. Before K-NN

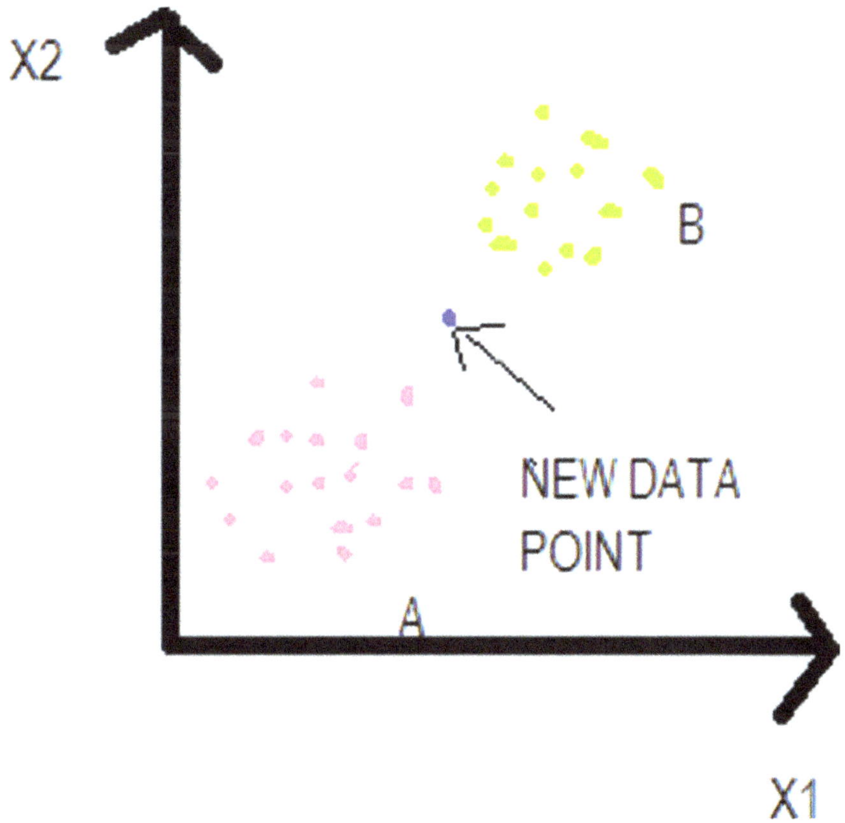

Figure 2. After K-NN

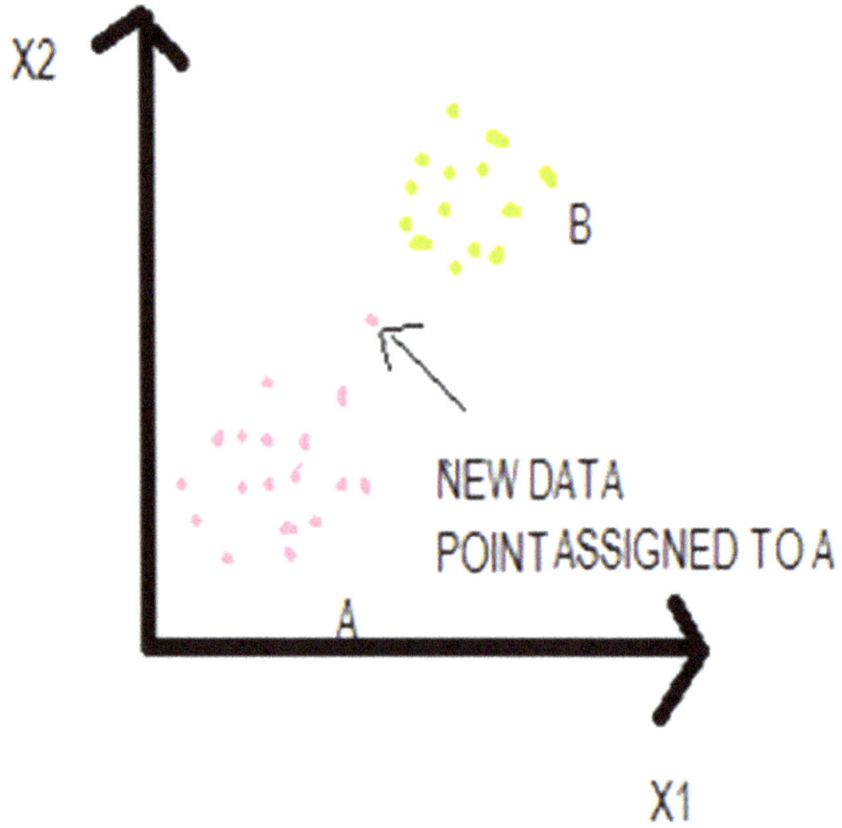

Working of K-NN

The K-NN working can be explained based on the below algorithm:

Step 1: Decide on the number of neighbors (K).
Step 2: Determine the Euclidean distance between K neighbors.
Step 3: Using the calculated Euclidean distance, find the K- closest neighbors.
Step 4: Count the number of data points in each category among these K- neighbors.
Step 5: Assign the new data points to the category with the greatest number of neighbors.
Step 6: The model is now complete.

Suppose, a new data point is there and it is needed to put it in the required category. Consider Figure3:

Figure 3. Categorizing A and B before K-NN

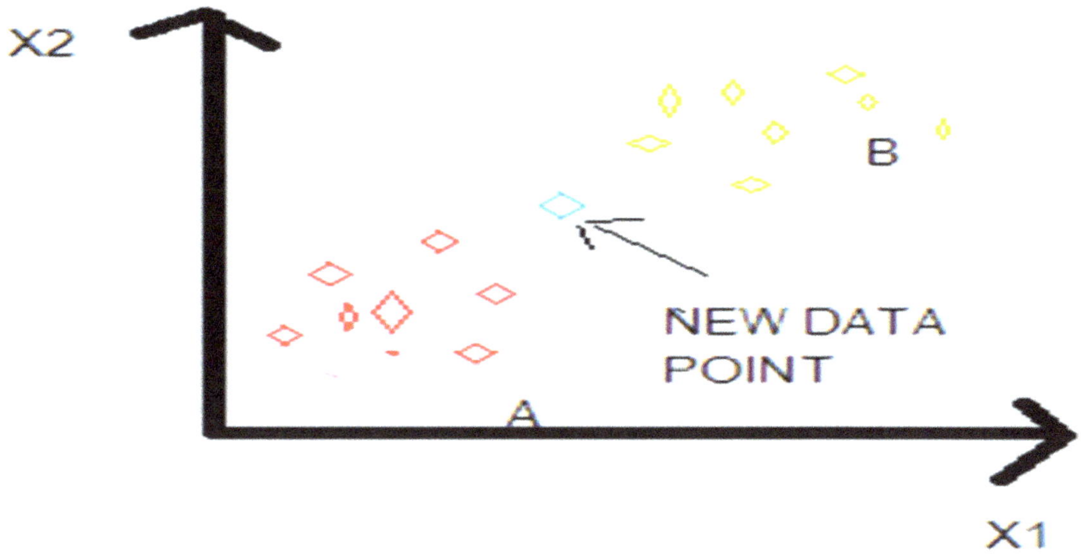

1) Firstly, the number of neighbors was chosen, So, Consider the K=5.
2) Next, as in Figure 4, the **Euclidean distance** between the data points is calculated. The Euclidean distance is the distance between two points. It can be calculated as:

Figure 4. Euclidean distance $\left(\left|\sqrt{(X2-X1)^2+(Y2-Y1)^2}\right|\right)$

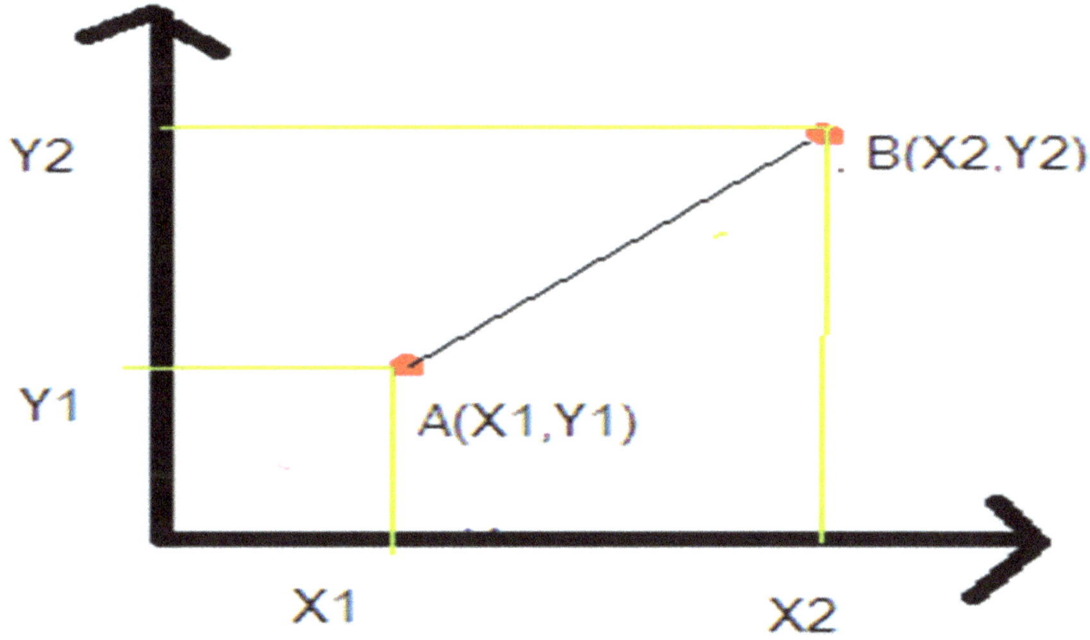

3) By Calculating the Euclidean distance the nearest neighbors are getting, as three nearest neighbors in Category A and two nearest neighbors in Category B. Consider Figure 5:

Figure 5. New data point must belong to category A

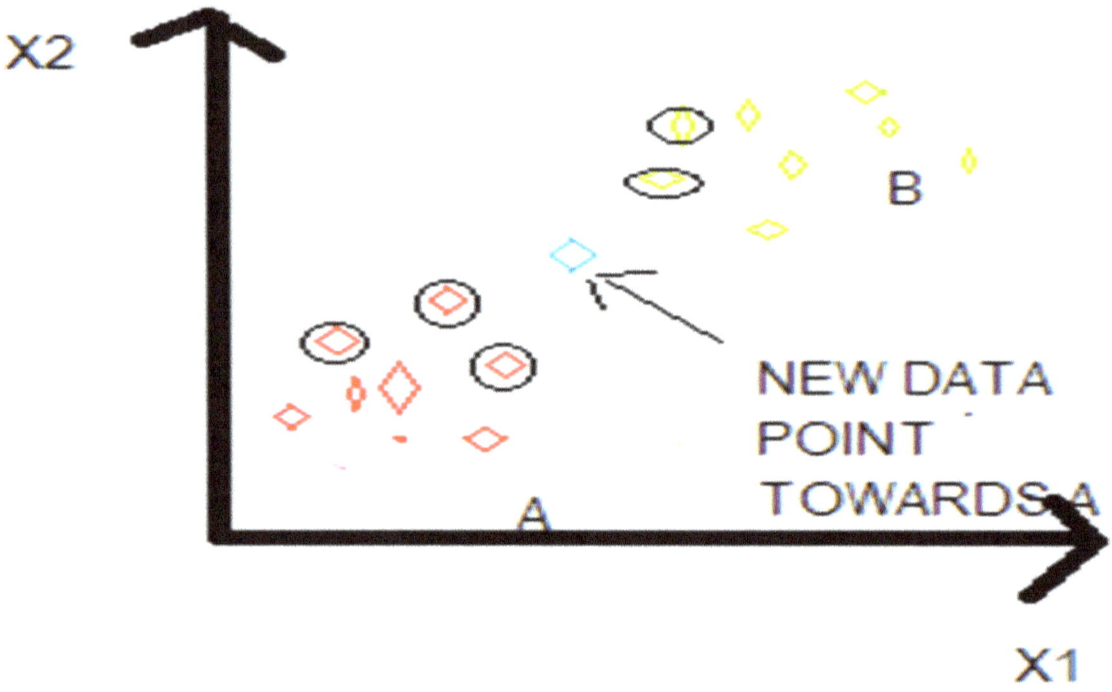

4) As, the three nearest neighbors are from Category A is seen, hence this new data point must belong to Category A.

Selection of the value of K in the K-NN Algorithm

Here are some things to keep in mind while deciding on a value for K in the K-NN algorithm:

1) Because, there is no single approach to identify the best value for K, several values to find the best one has experimented with. The most popular K value is 5.
2) A very low value for K, such as “K=1” or “K=2”, can be noisy and cause outlier effects in the model.
3) Large values of K are preferred, but they may cause problems.

The K-NN Algorithm has the following advantages:

1) It is straightforward to implement.
2) It can handle noisy training data.
3) It may be more successful if the training data is large.

Consequences of K-NN Algorithm:

1) It is always needed to determine the value of K, which might be difficult at times.
2) The Computation Cost is considerable since the distance between data points for all training samples is calculated.

Literature Survey

According to S Vijayarani et al.(2015), advances in sequencing technology have resulted in an exponential increase in the number of protein sequences in public databases. "Sequential information" has successfully been used to show structures, functions, evolutionary linkages, and so on. Based on sequence information, a variety of computer algorithms have been developed to classify protein sequences and forecast diseases. The classification of biological sequences is an important topic in bioinformatics, genomics, and proteomics. The existence of enormous amounts of this sequence data, their indistinctness, and, most importantly, the exorbitant costs of laboratory investigations demand the use of data mining in sickness prediction algorithms that are utilized in place of laboratory trials. Protein sequence analysis has recently attracted a lot of attention because proteins and their sequences are involved in a lot of disorders. The use of data mining techniques in protein sequence analysis provides an efficient tool for examining proteins to learn about their properties, as well as a method for developing better medications. In this study, the Naive Bayes classifier is used to predict hemoglobin protein-based diseases. This classifier's performance is measured by its classification accuracy and execution time.

According to Nida Khateeb et al.(2017) the healthcare industry creates huge amounts of healthcare data, which can be transformed into valuable information by utilizing various data mining techniques. This knowledge can subsequently be employed in a range of decision-making scenarios, such as finance, marketing, and the healthcare business. Cardiovascular disease is one of the most important yet difficult activities in the health care sector that must be handled swiftly, efficiently, and with proper automation. Various Heart Disease Prediction systems have been investigated in this area, and previous work has combined several medical features and risk indicators utilizing various data mining methodologies. The number of parameters and data mining techniques utilized define the degree of accuracy stated in each of those articles. The number of parameters and datasets employed in the experiments, however, was insufficient to claim high accuracy. We utilized the K-nearest neighbor classifier with 14 attributes to achieve an accuracy of roughly 80%. Furthermore, the superiority of K-NN classifier-based heart disease prediction systems has been demonstrated using several dominant classifiers.

To forecast COVID-19 recovered and dead patients, P Theerthagiri et al.(2021) applied multiple ML classification approaches. The Prediction Model is validated using the k-fold cross-validation resampling technique. Performance criteria such as prediction accuracy, precision, recall, mean square error, confusion matrix, and kappa score are used to evaluate each algorithm's prediction scores. Based on the prediction results of multiple machine learning classification methods on the COVID-19 dataset, this study reveals that the K-NN algorithm predicts COVID-19 possibilities better than other algorithms for the smaller (730 record) dataset. For the preprocessed dataset, the K-Nearest Neighbor (K-NN) classification technique achieves 80.4 percent prediction accuracy and 1.5 to 3.3 percent higher accuracy than other algorithms. The K-NN system correctly predicts 92 percent of the dead cases (true positive rate), with a misclassification rate of 0.077 percent. Furthermore, with an error rate of 0.19, the K-NN method exceeds the other technique in terms of accurate COVID-19 prediction. It also produces the receiver operator characteristic curve, which has an output value of 82%. This study shows that the K-NN algorithm predicts COVID-19 possibilities better than other algorithms for the smaller (730 record) dataset based on the prediction results of multiple ML classification methods on the COVID-19 dataset.

According to KetutAgungEnriko, Muhammad Suryanegara, DadangGunawan et al.(2016), heart disease is now the major cause of death. The treatment of heart disease patients has developed, for example, through the use of Machine-To-Machine (M2M) technology, which allows for remote patient monitoring. To use M2M to care for a remote heart disease patient, his or her medical state should be checked regularly at home. As a result, administering complex tests that necessitate the expertise of specialists is difficult. Meanwhile, certain aspects of the patient's health can be used to predict heart illness. The application of data mining methods can improve the prediction of heart disease. Some algorithms used for this purpose include Naive Bayes, Decision Trees, and K-Nearest Neighbor (K-NN). This research will employ data mining techniques to predict cardiac disease and to simplify parameters for usage in M2M remote patient monitoring. To boost accuracy, K-NN is used with a parameter weighting approach.

According to S. Durga, Kasturi Karuppiah, et al.(2017), data mining is defined as the process of analyzing enormous amounts of data to extract relevant information. Data mining techniques such as association rule mining, classification, and clustering are used to research the various types of diseases. In data mining, classification is a key issue. A classifier creates a short and unambiguous definition for each class that may be used to classify successive entries given a database with a collection of records, each with a single class label. In medical systems, data mining is critical. It extracts information from data and presents it in a human-readable fashion. It is the result of a collaborative effort between humans and computers. The two primary goals of data mining are prediction and description. Prediction is forecasting unknown or future values of other variables of interest using some variables or fields in the data set. The goal of description is to discover patterns in data that humans can comprehend. It's quite good for predicting ailments like heart disease and lung disease. Lung cancer is one of the world's most hazardous diseases. If detected early enough, lung cancer can be treated by applying Naive Bayes and Artificial Neural Networks to massive amounts of healthcare data. Massive amounts of data are generated in the healthcare industry, but they are not mined to uncover hidden information. The Naive Bayes algorithm aims to deliver accurate classifications even when working with little or incomplete data sets. The study's goal is to detect and diagnose lung problems as early as possible, allowing doctors to preserve the patient's life. This article shows how lung cancer was predicted and controlled using data mining techniques.

According to Dr.T.Christopher et al.(2016),Lung cancer is still the top cause of cancer-related mortality in both men and women, and its prevalence is increasing globally. Lung cancer is defined as the uncontrolled proliferation of abnormal cells that begin in one or both lungs. Cancer detection is not an easy process, but if it is identified early, it is treatable. We used classification algorithms such as Naive Bayes, Bayesian networks, and the J48 algorithm to predict lung cancer. Initially, data from one hundred cancer and non-cancer patients were collected, preprocessed, and evaluated using a classification algorithm for lung cancer prediction. There are one hundred instances and twenty-five attributes in the collection. The primary goal of this work is to give customers an earlier warning as well as a performance analysis of the categorization methods.

The Comparison of different Machine Learning Algorithms with Implementation

1) Dataset

Kaggle was used to collect the dataset. This data was acquired from the public health department to detect many chronic respiratory illnesses in the state of New Mexico, The United States (Temporal coverage: 2019-03-31 to 2021-04-01). This data has many attributes, including Name, Age, Sex, Diseases, Treatments, and Nature, where Name, Sex, Diseases, Treatments, and Nature are string values. This data set currently contains over 37000 records and is updated quarterly.

Figure 6. Sample dataset having parameters: symptoms, age, sex, treatment, nature, disease; Note: 0-male,1-female, 2-cannot says

Symptoms	Age	Sex	Treatment	Nature	Disease
shortness of breath	56	0	Omalizumab	medium	Asthma
shortness of breath	58	0	Omalizumab	medium	Asthma
shortness of breath	67	0	Omalizumab	high	Asthma
coughing	87	1	Omalizumab	high	Asthma
shortness of breath	65	1	Mepolizumab	high	Asthma
tight feeling in the chest	54	0	Mepolizumab	medium	Asthma
shortness of breath	78	0	itraconazole	high	Asthma
fever	67	0	inhaler	high	Asthma
cold	56	0	inhaler	medium	Asthma
cold	59	0	Omalizumab	medium	Asthma
fever	60	0	Omalizumab	high	Asthma
fever	50	0	Mepolizumab	medium	Asthma
cold	56	0	inhaler	medium	Asthma
shortness of breath	78	1	inhaler	high	Asthma
Fatigue, feeling run-down or tired	56	2	antibiotics	high	Bronchiectasis
Fatigue, feeling run-down or tired	78	2	antibiotics	high	Bronchiectasis
Coughing up yellow or green mucus daily	70	1	hypertonic saline	high	Bronchiectasis
fever	65	1	hypertonic saline	high	Bronchiectasis
whistling sound while you breathe	55	0	hypertonic saline	medium	Bronchiectasis
whistling sound while you breathe	56	0	hypertonic saline	medium	Bronchiectasis
Chest pain	71	0	hypertonic saline	high	Bronchiectasis
Chest pain	78	1	hypertonic saline	high	Bronchiectasis
Chest pain	74	1	hypertonic saline	high	Bronchiectasis
Chest pain	67	1	hypertonic saline	high	Bronchiectasis
Shortness of breath that gets worse durin	65	1	hypertonic saline	high	Bronchiectasis
Chest pain	57	1	hypertonic saline	high	Bronchiectasis
Chest pain	76	1	hypertonic saline	high	Bronchiectasis

2) Implementation (Psuedo Codes)

i) Naive Bayes Algorithm for prediction of disease based on the symptoms (finding accuracy) pseudo codes:

1. import libraries
2. read dataset ("respiratory symptoms and treatment1.csv")
3. find X = dataset.iloc[:, [0, 1,2]].values and y = dataset.iloc[:, 5].values

4. import library LabelEncoder
5. find X[:,0] = le.fit_transform(X[:,0])
6. Import library train_test_split
7. X_train, X_test, y_train, y_test = train_test_split(X, y, test_size = 0.10, random_state = 0)
8. import library StandardScaler
9. sc = StandardScaler()
10. X_train = sc.fit_transform(X_train)
11. X_test = sc.transform(X_test)
12. import library GaussianNB
13. classifier.fit(X_train, y_train)
14. y_pred = classifier.predict(X_test)
15. display y_pred
16. import confusion_matrix,accuracy_score
17. find cm = confusion_matrix(y_test, y_pred)
18. find ac = accuracy_score(y_test,y_pred)
19. display cm
20. display ac

Confusion matrix:

```
[ 0 0 0 0 0 9 0 14 5 0 2 0 0 0 0 0 0]
[ 0 0 0 0 0 0 0 0 0 0 0 0 0 0 0 15 0]
[ 0 0 0 0 2 5 0 5 0 0 0 6 0 0 4 0 0]
[ 0 0 0 0 4 6 0 12 8 0 0 0 0 0 0 5 0]
[ 0 0 0 0 25 0 0 2 3 0 0 0 9 5 0 10 0]
[ 0 0 0 0 0 36 0 16 0 0 0 0 0 0 0 0 0]
[ 0 0 0 0 0 9 0 19 6 0 0 0 8 0 0 0 0]
[ 0 0 0 0 0 6 0 94 24 0 4 0 0 0 0 31 0]
[ 0 0 0 0 5 28 0 50 35 0 17 0 16 0 12 52 9]
[ 0 0 0 0 12 23 0 23 0 0 10 0 18 4 0 37 0]
[ 0 0 0 0 0 0 0 17 0 0 17 0 0 0 0 6 0]
[ 0 0 0 0 0 16 0 15 14 0 0 0 0 0 0 0 0]
[ 0 0 0 0 14 0 0 0 0 0 0 0 26 0 0 12 0]
[ 0 0 0 0 0 10 0 29 14 0 3 0 0 0 0 2 0]
[ 0 0 0 0 22 16 0 4 16 0 0 0 0 0 26 16 0]
[ 0 0 0 0 0 14 0 64 8 0 0 0 51 0 0 39 0]
[ 0 0 0 0 0 0 0 2 0 0 0 0 19 0 0 26 0]]
```

Accuracy:

0.23317683881064163

ii) Support Vector Machine(SVM) Machine Learning Algorithm

1. import libraries
2. find X = dataset.iloc[:, [0,1,2]].values and y = dataset.iloc[:, 5].values
3. import library train_test_split
4. X_train, X_test, y_train, y_test = train_test_split(X, y, test_size = 0.20, random_state = 0)
5. import LabelEncoder
6. le = LabelEncoder()
7. X[:,0] = le.fit_transform(X[:,0])
8. import library svm
9. clf=svm.SVC(kernel='linear')
10. clf.fit(X_train, y_train)
11. y_pred = clf.predict(X_test)
12. import metrics
13. display ("Accuracy:",metrics.accuracy_score(y_test, y_pred))

Accuracy: 0.221665623043206

iii) K-Nearest Neighbor(K-NN) Machine Learning Algorithm

1. read dataset ("respiratory symptoms and treatment1.csv")
2. import libraries KNeighborsClassifier
3. find X = dataset.iloc[:, [0,1,2]].values and Y = dataset.iloc[:, 5].values
4. X_train, X_test, Y_train, Y_test = train_test_split(X, Y, test_size = 0.2, random_state=42)
5. import LabelEncoder
6. le = LabelEncoder()
7. find X[:,0] = le.fit_transform(X[:,0])
8. find K-NN = KNeighborsClassifier(n_neighbors=17)
9. find K-NN.fit(X, Y)
10. display(K-NN.predict(X_test))
11. import numpy as np
12. find neighbors = np.arange(1, 9)
13. calculatetrain_accuracy = np.empty(len(neighbors))andtest_accuracy = np.empty(len(neighbors))
14. for loop-> i, k in enumerate(neighbors):
    K-NN = KNeighborsClassifier(n_neighbors=k)
    K-NN.fit(X, Y)
15. Compute training and test data accuracy
    train_accuracy[i] = K-NN.score(X, Y)
    test_accuracy[i] = K-NN.score(X, Y)
16. import matplotlib.pyplot as plt
17. plot -> (neighbors, test_accuracy, label = 'Testing dataset Accuracy')
    Plot->(neighbors, train_accuracy, label = 'Training dataset Accuracy')

Figure 7. Accuracy for K-NN algorithm

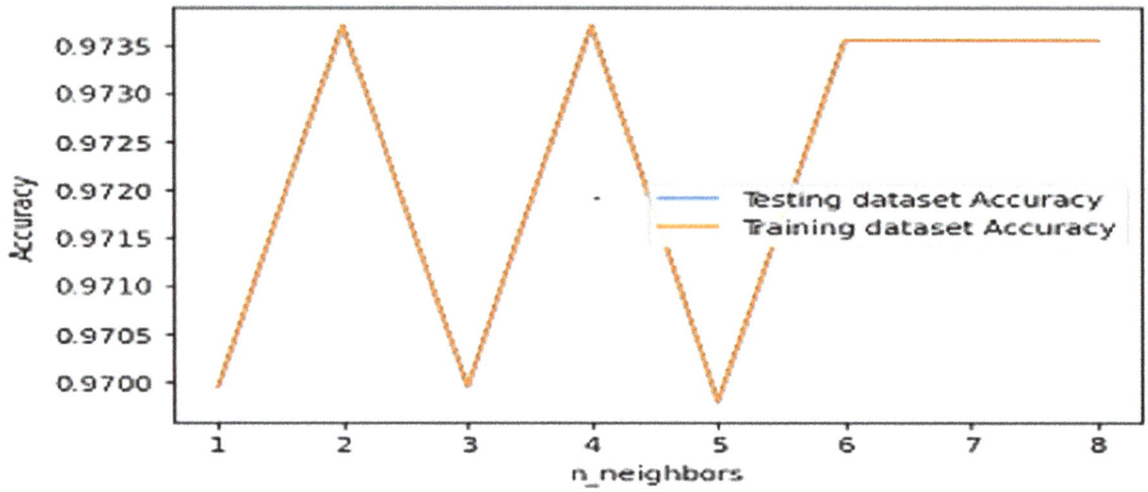

Accuracy above 6 clusters=0.9735
Accuracy percentage= 97.35%

Table 3. Comparison table of ML algorithms for predicting pulmonary disease

Machine Learning Algorithms	Accuracy	ACCURACY PERCENTAGE
NAÏVE BAYES ALGORITHM	0.23317683881064163	23%
SUPPORT VECTOR MACHINE ALGORITHM	0.221665623043206	22%
K-NN(K-NEAREST NEIGHBOUR) ALGORITHM	0.9735(K>=6)	97%

Basically, Naïve Bayes algorithm use conditional probability to predict the disease, whereas support vector machine helps to sort the two data group using hyperplane in multidimensional area and K-NN algorithm use the concept of feature similarity, where a new point is assigned according to how similar the point is to other points in neighbor in the training datasets.

But, from the above Table3, it can be said that out of the three Machine Learning Algorithms, KNN(K-Nearest Neighbor) Algorithm can be considered to be better algorithm for prediction of Pulmonary diseases. Here, Accuracy Percentage is a parameter that is considered.

CONCLUSION AND FUTURE SCOPE

Based on the dataset, this chapter discusses that K-NN outperforms the other two machine learning algorithms for lung disease diagnosis. In terms of accuracy, K-Nearest Neighbor (K-NN) outperforms the Support Vector Method (SVM) and Naive Bayes. Furthermore, several new technologies and algorithms may be created in the future to aid in the detection of lung problems, thereby saving lives.

REFERENCES

Christopher, T., & Jamera Banu, J. (2016). Study of Classification Algorithm for Lung Cancer Prediction. *International Journal of Innovative Science, Engineering & Technology, 3*(2), 42–49.

Durga & Karuppiah. (2017). Lung disease prediction system using data mining techniques. *Journal of Advanced Research in Dynamical and Control Systems, 9*(5), 62-66.

Elearning Providers. (2006). https://www.tutorialspoint.com/machine_learning_with_python/machine_learning_with_python_classification_algorithms_support_vector_machine.htm

Enriko, Suryanegara, & Gunawan. (2016). Heart Disease Prediction System using k-Nearest Neighbor Algorithm with Simplified Patient's Health Parameters. *Journal of Telecommunication, Electronic and Computer Engineering, 8*(12).

Jaiswal. (2021). https://www.javatpoint.com/machine-learning-naive-bayes-classifier

Kaplan, A., Cao, H., FitzGerald, J. M., Vogelmeier, C. F., Pfister, P., & Mastoridis, P. (2021). Artificial Intelligence/Machine Learning in Respiratory Medicine and Potential Role in Asthma and COPD Diagnosis. *The Journal of Allergy and Clinical Immunology, 9*(6), 2255–2261. PMID:33618053

Khateeb & Usman. (2017). Efficient Heart Disease Prediction System using K-Nearest Neighbor Classification Technique. *Proceedings of the International Conference on Big Data and Internet of Thing*. 10.1145/3175684.3175703

Sheffield. (2017). The Global Impact of Respiratory Disease. In *Forum of International Respiratory Societies* (2nd ed.). European Respiratory Society.

Shetty. (2010). https://www.narayanahealth.org/blog/respiratory-diseases-causes-symptoms-preventive-measures/

Theerthagiri, Jacob, Ruby, & Yendapalli. (2021). Prediction of COVID-19 Possibilities using K-NN Classification Algorithm. *International Journal of Current Research and Review, 13*(6).

Vijayarani & Deepa. (2015). Naïve Bayes Classification for Predicting Diseases in Haemoglobin Protein Sequences. *International Journal of Computational Intelligence and Informatics, 3*(4).

Chapter 6
A Computational Model Approach for a Lifestyle Disorder:
Hypertension

Komal Arora
Manav Rachna International Institute of Research and Studies, India

Deepak Kumar
https://orcid.org/0000-0001-9419-8895
Manav Rachna International Institute of Research and Studies, India

Pooja Khurana
Manav Rachna International Institute of Research and Studies, India

ABSTRACT

Hypertension is known to be one of the most common medical and lifestyle disorders, signalized by the elevated levels of blood pressure, that is systolic and diastolic blood pressures more than 140 mm/Hg and 90 mm/Hg, respectively, associated with the various risk factors for cardiovascular diseases, chronic kidney disease, and some of the neurodegenerative diseases. Major lifestyle parameters such as lack of physical activity, high concentration of salt in diet, alcohol consumption, smoking, stress, and high weight are significantly related to this disease. Computational models of physiological frameworks can significantly help with our comprehension of the frameworks under study and can likewise be utilized in educating and examination apparatuses. Computational models can supplement exploratory and clinical investigations, yet additionally challenge flow standards, reclassify our comprehension of systems driving lifestyle, and shape future research.

DOI: 10.4018/978-1-6684-2508-4.ch006

INTRODUCTION

In the modern world of competition where advancement in technology has reached its height to a level that is also affecting the habits of many individuals to a great extent. Lifestyle (the way of life one lives) greatly influenced the behavior, habits, interests, opinions, and attitude. The bad quality of lifestyle is one of the main reasons for developing many health-related issues that are primarily based on the individual's habit that cause them to shift from the activity to a sedentary lifestyle. Hypertension, one of the very common lifestyle diseases, refers to the increased blood pressure, which is a third leading disease contributing about 10.8% of all the total deaths in India (Rajkumar and Romate 2020). It's a diverse disease where blood pressure levels mainly depend upon the lifestyle factors such as obesity, lack physical of physical activity, the salt concentration in diet, alcohol consumption, stress, smoking, weight, the quality of life one lives, forming a direct link between the increased blood pressure levels and cardiovascular risks, also causing the increased risk for kidney, diseases, thyroid problems and sleep apnea. Many anti-hypertensive drugs are available in the market, but due to their cost, side-effects and resistance, effective treatment is restricted. However, modifiable lifestyle such as better stress management, good intake of diet (diet full with fruits as well as vegetables that are low in sodium content but high in potassium value, no drinking and smoking) can help to manage the Hypertension. The objective of this paper is to design a mathematical model that depicts the change in blood pressure levels in consideration to different controlled lifestyle factors like salt consumption, physical exercise, stress and to optimize the mathematical model using Genetic Algorithm, the approach that is highly effective in diagnosing medical conditions.

Background

Hypertension, a heterogeneous disorder, characterized by the level of systolic and diastolic blood pressure more than 140/mm Hg and 90 mm Hg respectively (Kokubo et al. 2015). The process of circulating the blood throughout the body is carried out by the Heart. When heart beats, it results in the formation of peaks and troughs in blood pressure referred to as systolic and diastolic, considering normal blood pressure as 120/80 mm Hg. The blood pressure above 140/90 mm Hg termed as Hypertension, usually measured by an instrument sphygmomanometer (David et al. 2018).

Epidemiology

Hypertension, a multifactorial disorder, revealed to be the most significant risk factor for those who have affected lifestyle. Reports from WHO, GBD and Non- Communicable Risk Factor Collaboration showed the high pervasiveness of high BP in India as well as reported greater than 1 million people that are suffering from this disease (Foex and. Sear 2004). Hypertension has become the third leading rank in terms of causing death, contributing to about 10.8% of all deaths in India (Rajkumar and Romate 2020). 29% of stroke and 24% of all heart attacks is directly associated with Hypertension (Gupta et al. 2018).

Table 1. "Classification of blood pressure parameters" Range in mm Hg

Normal range	Pre-Hypertension stage	Hypertension Stage 1	Hypertension Stage 2
Systolic- less than 120. Diastolic- less than 80.	120-139 80-89	150-159 90-99	Greater than or equal to 160. Greater than or equal to 100.

Pathophysiology

Different physiological mechanisms play a key role in maintaining optimum blood pressure levels. Any change in the system or mechanism results in the development of essential hypertension. Arteries constrict and dilate due to the stimulation caused by a Sympathetic Nervous System and thus are involved in the maintenance of blood pressure levels. Interaction of Sympathetic nervous system with the renin-angiotensin system causes increased absorption of sodium resulting in sodium retention in the body and hence is known to be related to hypertension. Renin converts angiotensinogen to angiotensin 1 (inactive substance) which gets converted to angiotensin 2 by angiotensin converting enzyme. Blood pressure rises due to angiotensin 2 (a potent vasoconstrictor) and results in hypertension. Release of aldosterone is also stimulated by Renin that causes the further increase in the levels of blood pressure related to water and sodium retention (Beevers 2001).

Regulation of blood pressure levels: Maintaining optimum levels of blood pressure is essential to live a quality life. However, it's not as easy to restore the normal levels once disturbed. There are normal regulatory mechanisms that our body does in order to ensure the maintenance of blood pressure levels.

Autonomic nervous system (ANS): ANS acts as the important factor in regulating BP for short span of time. There are baroreceptors present in the aortic arch and in carotid sinus that detects or senses the change in BP levels in response to tension caused by the walls of the arteries. Elevated pressure in the walls of arteries constricts the blood vessels resulting in baroreceptors trigger which sends feedback to the ANS (Autonomic Nervous System) that lower down blood pressure by reducing cardiac output and heart rate via parasympathetic fibers. Similarly, baroreceptors also detect decreased blood pressure and sends feedback for the stimulation of sympathetic response that increase cardiac output and heart rate, thus rises the blood pressure levels (Beevers et al. 2001, Joyner et al. 2008, Wallin et al. 2007, Charkoudian et al.2009 and Joyner et al. 2010).

Renin- Angiotensin-Aldosterone System (RAAS): It is one of the system responsible for maintaining long-term optimum blood pressure levels. Granular cells of kidney released renin, a peptide hormone, which converts angiotensinogen to angiotensin I followed by conversion by angiotensin-converting enzyme, which converts angiotensin I to angiotensin II (a potent vasoconstrictor). Angiotensin II directly acts on the kidney leading to the increased reabsorption of the sodium. Aldosterone release is also promoted by Angiotensin II. Bradykinin, a potent vasodilator, degraded by the enzyme Angiotensin converting enzyme. Breakdown of Bradykinin facilitates the overall process of constriction. The role of aldosterone is to regulate the sodium expression by promoting the retention ability of salt and water. It also increases the mobility of sodium ions by increasing the Na-K ATPase activity. As a result of more sodium ions in the kidney, the process of excretion of water decreased, resulting in the more blood volume and hence high blood pressure (Souza et al. 2018, Niarchos et al. 1979)

Anti-Diuretic Hormone (ADH): ADH, a kind of Nano-peptide, whose synthesis takes place in hypothalamus region of brain, regulates the blood pressure levels by being secreted in response to volume contraction. After being released, reabsorption of sodium stimulated by ADH, which then promotes reabsorption of water in the kidneys. ADH also cause vasoconstriction when its concentration rises and these two phenomena (increased water reabsorption and vasoconstriction) increase the blood volume in arteries and hence levels of blood pressure. Conversely, increased blood volume inhibited the secretion of ADH and thus reduced secretion of ADH will be there. This is how the blood pressure levels are regulated by vasopressin (ADH) (Cuzzo et al. 2020)

Natriuretic peptides: Salt and water balance are also regulated by heart in addition to kidney, where atrial natriuretic peptide, a cardiac hormone, mediates this function. Natriuretic and vasodilatory actions of these peptides regulate homoeostasis of blood volume and hence blood pressure levels. Increase in the levels of sodium and blood pressure resulting in the secretion of Atrial Natriuretic Peptide (ANP) from human's heart, which fixes to receptor as a ligand and receptor is present in the blood vessels and kidney. The binding of ANP to its receptor promotes the excretion of salt that lowers down the volume of blood and hence causes blood vessel relaxation. Conversely, decrease in the blood pressure levels slows down the secretion of ANP. Prostaglandins tends to be local vasodilators that reduces the reabsorbtion of sodium and thus extreme vasoconstriction is prevented. It has been reported in a study that deficiency of ANP results in hypertension whereas its overexpression causes hypotension in mice. BNP, Brain Natriuretic Peptide and CNP i.e. C-type natriuretic peptide are also the members of Natriuretic peptide family. BNP and CNP have similar chemical structure and share common pathways of biosynthesis, despite the fact that they both are encodes by different sets of genes. proANP and proBNP are the precursors of ANP and BNP respectively, which becomes active by the action of Corin, meaning corin plays a key role in process of biosynthesis and action of natriuretic peptide in the regulation (Potter et al. 2006, John et al. 1995, Steinhelper et al. 1990, Zhou et al. 2009, Armaly 2013, and Beevers et al. 2001).

Short term chemical control: Chemically control of blood pressure levels takes place by the vasodilators and vasoconstrictors that cause the dilation or constriction of the blood vessels, which results in the vascular resistance, thus increases or lowers down the levels of blood pressure respectively. There is a rise in systemic blood pressure by the process of vasoconstriction whereas, dilation of blood vessels causes the increase in blood flow and decrease the levels of systemic blood pressure. Vasoconstriction is the effect resulting from the mechanism that possess calcium ions in high quantity and the presence of phosphorylated myosin in the smooth muscle cells of vasculatory system. ATP, angiotensin II, epinephrine are some of the examples of endogenous vasoconstrictors. Vasodilation happens when myosin light- chain phosphatase dephosphorylates the myosin present within the smooth muscle cells of vasculatory system and when calcium ions pump out of the intracellular compartment via symporters and antiporters of calcium. Lactic acid and arginine are endogenous vasodilators.

Hypertension and Lifestyle

Many lifestyle, physical factors around us influence the levels of blood pressure to a great extent. These factors may include lack of physical activity, high concentration of salt in diet, alcohol consumption, smoking, stress, high weight, excessive intake of drugs, other diseases, the quality of life one lives, forming a direct link between the increased blood pressure levels and cardiovascular risks. However, blood pressure levels are autoregulated by the different mechanisms or pathways undergo in the body that are mentioned above, but still the responses are varied or slow due to the reasons like getting a split-second or slow response from the autonomic or sympathetic nervous system.

Figure 1. Physiological mechanism expressing change in functional areas due to hypertension

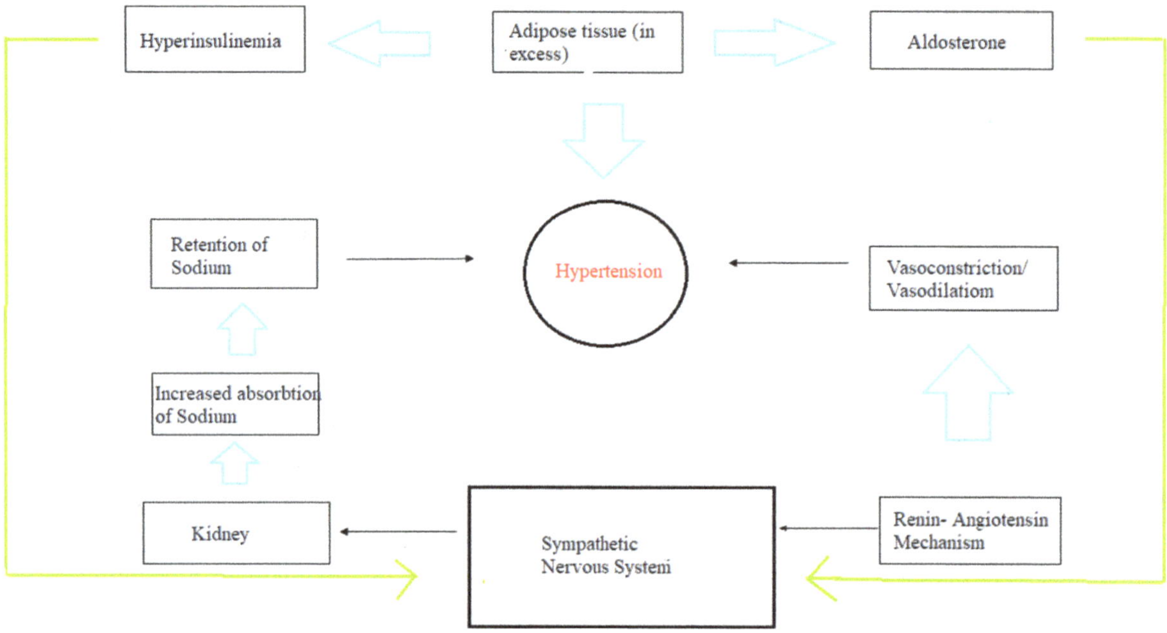

Important lifestyle parameters along with their relationship with blood pressure levels are described herein to show how and to what extent these factors associated with Hypertension.

Essential/ Primary Hypertension: When the specific cause of the rise in the level of blood pressure is not known, it referred to as Essential Hypertension and it takes into account 90% of all the cases associated with Hypertension (Bolívar 2013). However, some lifestyle factors are responsible for the rise of Essential Hypertension.

Controlled Factors

Obesity- Many metabolic syndromes such as insulin sensitivity impairment, intolerance to glucose, dyslipidemia associated with obesity which also increases the level of blood pressure and hence increases the risk of cardiovascular disease (Pouliot et al. 1994)

Physical activity- Physical activity follows an inverse relationship with blood pressure levels. The more the physical activity, the lower the levels of blood pressure and vice versa (Blair et al. 1984). Meta-analysis studies showed the lowering of systolic blood pressure of around 7-11 mm Hg on doing various physical activities (Fagard 1995).

Dietary Interventions- Diet greatly affects the levels of blood pressure in the body.

Na: K ratio- With age, the consumption of salt in the diet of an individual increases. Consuming salt more than 10mg/ml per day disturbs the normal balance causing the problem for the kidneys in water removal. The excess of fluid causes an additional strain on delicate blood vessels leading to higher blood pressure. Thus, high consumption of salt is positively correlated with hypertension and hence showing its linear dependency on high blood pressure. Data from several studies showed the strong association of Na: K ratio with blood pressures (Perez and Chang 2014). Studies from RCT suggests that potassium intake in high amount and sodium intake in low amount decrease mean blood pressure levels (Sacks

2001). Reduced sodium intake (100 mill moles reduction) resulted in decrement in the levels of blood pressure for about 6 mm Hg systolic in hypertensive and around 2 to 3 mm Hg systolic in normotensives (Kumanyika, and Cutler 1997).

Fruit, vegetables, fats, and fiber- Consumption of diet which includes fruits, vegetables, fiber with the lower amount of total and saturated fat keeps the population with lower blood pressure as compared to the normal population (Rouse et al.1983).

Protein- Intake of protein follows an inverse relationship with blood pressure levels. It has been showed in Inter salt study that higher protein consumption reduced blood pressure levels with an average difference of about 3.0/2.5 mm Hg between subjects whose protein intake was 1/3rd below the population mean (Stamler et al.1996).

Alcohol- Studies from controlled trials showed that drinking heavily can cause potentially reversible Hypertension. (Puddey et al.1987).

Stress- Hypertension results from stress by causing elevation in the levels of blood pressure. Nervous system stimulation causes stress which produce vasoconstriction hormones in high quantity that are responsible for causing increase in the blood pressure levels (Kulkarni et al. 1998).

Uncontrolled Factors

The following two uncontrolled factors are:

Age- Outcomes of various studies considering various parameters with age showed that increasing age increase the hypertension's prevalence and particularly systolic blood pressure after 60 years of age. (Anderson 1999, and Pinto 2007).

Gender Men younger than 65 reliably have more elevated blood pressure levels compared to ladies of a similar age group. One study reported that white adults of age group 18-29 years, only 1.5% of females and 5% of males are suffering from Hypertension (Everett and Zajacova 2015, and Cutler et al. 2008).

Mathematical Modeling

By the use of a mathematical model, Averina et al. developed a new conceptual paradigm for the haemodynamics of salt-sensitive hypertension, demonstrating that excretion of sodium is not dependent on BP & neuronal stimulation resulting in hypertension. Data was also reproduced to the previous models' solutions supporting the relation between release of sodium and variations in BP. They contrasted the conventional version of their novel model to a simplified Guyton–Coleman model in which natriuresis is regulated by the whole-bovine procedures and the resistance in arteries are regulated by the pressure–natriuresis procedures. They demonstrated the changes in salt inputs and Angiotemsion II in response to renal excretion using reduced GC model. Their findings demonstrated that the model can offer a theoretically novel substitution for Guyton's theory (Averina et al., 2012). The compliance of a vessel for every compartment has been supposed as constant considering usual blood pressure range and they assumed it as linear.

They have described their model as:

$$V_j = V_{j,U} + C_j P_j,\ j=a,s,r,v.$$

Table 2. Summarized studies depicting the change in blood levels based on different controlled/uncontrolled factors

Sources	Factors	Results
Pouliot et al., 1994.	Obesity	Insulin sensitivity impairment, intolerance to glucose, dyslipidemia associated with obesity which also increases the level of blood pressure.
Fagard, 1995.	Physical exercise	Lowering of systolic blood pressure of around 7-11 mm Hg.
Sacks et al., 2001; Cutler et al., 1997; Rouse et al., 1983; Stamler et al., 1996; Puddey et al., 1987.	Dietary interventions	Potassium and sodium intake in high and low amount respectively decrease mean blood pressure levels. Reduced sodium intake (100 mill moles reduction) rresulted in decrement in the levels of blood pressure for about 6 mm Hg systolic in hypertensive. Fiber with lower amount of total and saturated fat keeps the population with lower blood pressure as compared to the normal population. Higher consumption of protein in diet reduced blood pressure with an estimated difference of about 3.0/2.5 mm Hg in individuals. Drinking heavily can cause potentially reversible Hypertension.
Kulkarni et al., 1998.	Stress	Nervous system stimulation causes stress which produce vasoconstriction hormones in high quantity that are responsible for causing increase in the blood pressure levels
Gunnar, 1999; Pinto, 2007.	Age	With increasing age, hypertension's prevalence increased significantly, especially after 60 years of age risk of systolic hypertension increased dramatically.
Everett and Zajacova, 2015; Cutler et al., 2008.	Gender	Males younger than 65 reliably have more elevated blood pressure levels compared to females of a similar age group
Yang M.H. et. Al., 2017	Lifestyle	Weight gain, physical inactivity, and high salt intake were associated with inadequate blood pressure control.

Where,

Vj represents the total volume of the blood restricted in section j
Vj,v represents the volume of blood in section j
Pi represents the blood pressure in section j
Ci represents the adherence of section j

Aterial section, splanchic and extra splanchic compartments, venous compartment have been represented as a,s,r and v.

Tiffin et al. published Computational Analysis of Candidate Disease Genes and Variants for Salt-Sensitive Hypertension in Indigenous Southern Africans in 2010. They selected and prioritised putative aetiological genes for salt-sensitive hypertension using computational approaches such as text- and data-mining.

Furthermore, they differentiated gene recurrence and SNPs copy number of target genes in the populations residing in Africa. They were trying to find out the potential gene having potent changeability/variability within two different groups of population. This identification of gene variability in different groups of population can help in determine the prevalence of a disease and thus in finding potent gene. The two potent genes they determined were Type 1 receptor of Angiotensin II and the precursor of Parathyroid hormone. Morever, they added that these genes could be investigated further to find out the genes responsible for the etiology of hypertension. (Tiffin et al., 2010).

Because the relationship between macrostructural mechanical loading, microstructural cellular changes, and macrostructural adaptation is unclear, and because chronic arterial hypertension initiates a series of events known to collectively initiate arterial wall thickening, Sáez et al presented a Computational modelling of hypertensive growth in the human carotid artery in which they described a microstructurally motivated computational model for chronic arrhythmia. They used a traditional idea based on the multiplicative decomposition of the deformation gradient into an elastic and a growth portion to simulate growth. They hypothesised, based on clinical data, that the driving factor for development is the strain experienced by smooth muscle cells. They built their model on top of a finite element framework, where growth is recorded locally as an internal variable. To begin, they explored the impact of hypertension expansion in a genuine human carotid artery to highlight the properties of their model. Both subjectively and numerically, their findings corresponded well with experimental data presented in the literature (Saez et al., 2014).

HumMod, a large physiological model, was used by John et al to explore hypotheses of blood pressure (BP) salt sensitivity. In the normal functioning of renal system, they studied various factors including levels of Angiotemsion II, activity of sympathetic nervous system, decrease number of nephrons, the hemodynamics of systemic circulation, renal artery sternosis, consequences of changes in salt intake on neuro- hormonal levels. For four weeks, they performed simulations with salt consumption ranging from "30-1000 milli mol per day". Redponsiveness to salt was raised when functional renal mass was reduced or ANG II was repaired. Salt sensitivity was related with lower variations in renal blood flow but larger changes in glomerular filtration rate, renal sodium reabsorption, and total peripheral resistance, which was caused by the failure of ANG II to adapt to changes in salt consumption (TPR). They found no significant effect on salt sensitivity after clamping TPR at normal or high levels. There were no discernible links between BP salt sensitivity and renal vascular resistance or extracellular fluid volume. Their rigorous mathematical model of cardiovascular, renal, endocrine, and sympathetic nervous system physiology supports the concept that certain kinds of kidney failure, such as poor ANG II regulation or enhanced tubular sodium reabsorption, contribute to BP salt sensitivity. Higher preglomerular resistance, increased RSNA, or failures to lower TPR, on the other hand, do not appear to affect salt sensitivity. Their model provides a venue for evaluating competing long-term BP control approaches during salt consumption variations (John et al., 2017).

Until recently, the only mathematical model for long-term management of arterial pressure was the G-C model developed by Guyton and Coleman. The notion that sodium excretion is governed by renal perfusion pressure, or the so-called'renal function curve,' lies at the heart of this model. Thus, according to the G-C model, all kinds of hypertension are caused by a fundamental shift of the renal function curve to a higher operating pressure. However, some recent experimental findings in the AngII–salt model of hypertension, which is caused by a high salt consumption combined with angiotensin II treatment, are inconsistent with the G-C model. They created a novel mathematical model that does not confine the causation of salt-sensitive hypertension to basic renal failure. Their model is the first known mathematical counter-example to the assumption that all salt-sensitive forms of hypertension require a fundamental shift in renal function: they demonstrated that the requirement is not required in at least one salt-sensitive type of hypertension. This computational model was dubbed the "neurogenic model" by the researchers. They explained how, despite basic differences in processes governing sodium excretion and vascular resistance between the G-C model and the neurogenic model, they produce identical haemo-dynamic profiles of AngII–salt hypertension. Furthermore, the steady-state connections between arterial pressure and sodium excretion, which is commonly referred to as the renal function curve,' were identical in both models. Their findings revealed that salt-sensitive hypertension is caused by neurogenic dysfunction as well as renal failure, as anticipated by the G-C model (Viktoria, 2015).

BP = CO. T P R

A mathematical research is carried out to determine how & why arterial pressure volume (P-V) relationship, systolic and diastolic pulse amplitude, and structure influence outcomes of non-invasive osci/lometric finger mean blood pressure estimate using maximum oscillation criterion (MOC). Several exponential simulations of a relaxed finger artery as well as a partially constricted artery have been investigated. A novel version of error equation is being proposed (Raamat, 1999).

P_{pulse} is calculated as:

$$P_{pulse} = P_{syst} - P_{diast}$$

Also P_0 defined as

$$P_0 = P_{mean} - P_{diast}$$

And $k_{pulse} = \frac{P_0}{P_{pulse}}$.

Trans-mural pressure P_{transm} is represented as:

$$P_{transm} = P_a - P_{cuff}$$

Based on the selected model, the relationship between blood pressure and volume:

$$V = \begin{cases} V_0 . e^{\frac{C_{max}}{V_0} P_{transm}} & for\ P_{transm} \leq 0 \\ V_{max} - (V_{max} - V_0) . e^{-\frac{C_{max}}{V_{max} - V_0} P_{transm}} & for\ P_{transm} \geq 0 \end{cases}$$

Where,

P_{transm} represents "transmural pressure"
V represents volume of blood in arteries at particular P_{transm},
V0 represents volume of blood in arteries at 0 transmural pressure
V_{max} represents the full expansion of arteries
C_{max} *represents* maximum slope.

Secondary/ Non- Essential Hypertension

In the remaining 10% of cases, elevated blood pressure is associated with some another disease, called Secondary Hypertension. It can be reduced if the main determinant/ cause is treated well. The causes may include sleep apnea, alcohol addiction, adrenal gland diseases, dysfunctional thyroid gland, and coarctation of aorta and may be more (Charles et al., 2007).

Description the of Genetic Algorithm: Genetic Algorithm was developed by John Holland (also known as father of Genetic Algorithm) in early 1970's. It is the evolutionary computing methods that are based on the population models. Working of GA is described in brief steps as (J. McCall, 2005):

1. Initialization. Random selection/creation of initial population (set of solution) results in the commencement of the algorithm.
2. Selection: Identify the good solutions in a population.
3. Fitness evaluation. In this, each solution is assigned with the fitness value depending upon the actual degree of closeness with the optimal solution of the problem.
4. Crossover: This operation involves the exchange of genetic information in the mating pool between the set of solutions.
5. Mutation: Generating new offspring from single parent. In addition to crossover, mutation also has a role in searching the optimal solution.
6. Elitism: Elitism is the preservation of few best solutions.

Figure 2. Mechanism of genetic algorithm

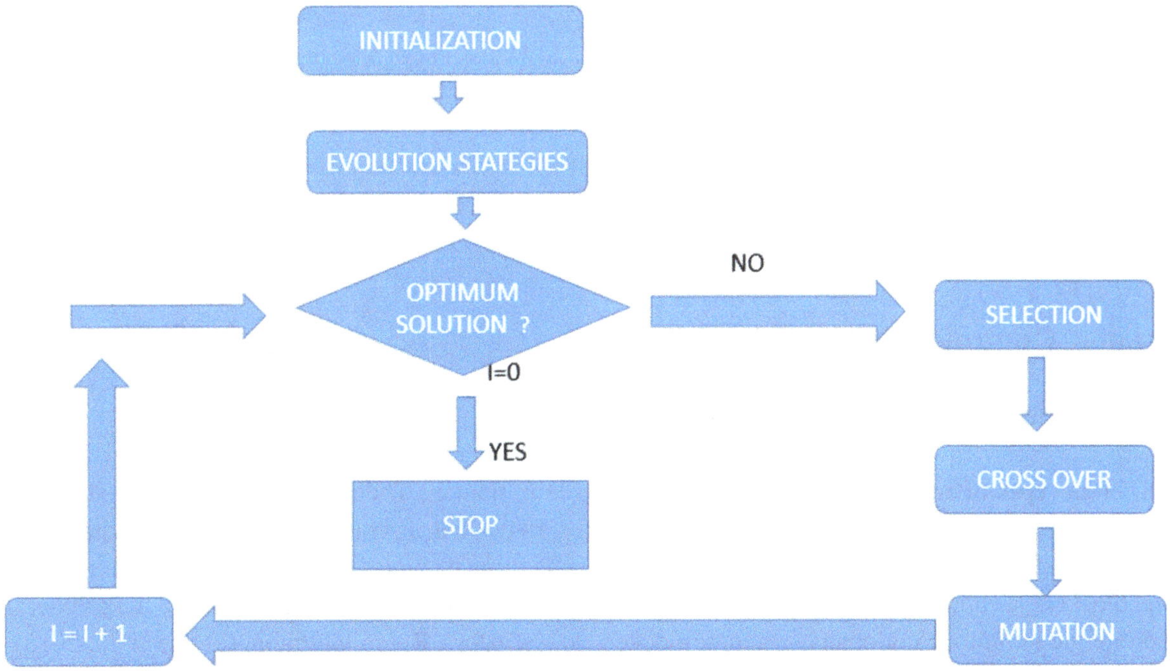

Achieving the maximum number of generations or satisfactory level of fitness results in the termination of algorithm and the solutions of the new generation is used in the next iteration of the algorithm.

Table 3. Terminology of genetic algorithm

Nature	Computation	Additional information
Population	Set of solutions	the number of chromosomes available to test
Individual	Solution to a problem	Single solution
Fitness	Quality of a solution	Fitness is computed for each individual.
Chromosome	Encoding for a solution (strings)	1 1 0 1
Gene	Part of the encoding solution	1 or 0

General solution of problem using Genetic Algorithm: The solutions to the problem can be solved using Genetic Algorithm tool i.e. GUI (Graphical User Interface). It allows to use GA without working at the command line. Genetic Algorithm tool can be opened by entering 'Gatool' in the command prompt of MATLAB. This example shows how to solve a problem using the Genetic Algorithm (GA) solver in Global Optimization Toolbox.

$$\begin{array}{l} Min.\ \sum f(x_1, x_2, x_3 \ldots x_n) = B \\ subject\ to\ \sum a_{ij} x_j \leq b_i \end{array} \quad \text{for } i,j = 1,2,\ldots,n$$

The bounds on the variables are given lower bound to upper bound as: $l_i £ x_i £ u_i$

MAIN FOCUS OF THE ARTICLE

The focus of the article is to design a mathematical model considering various lifestyle factors and its optimization using genetic algorithm.

Issues, Controversies, Problems

1. Treatment

Different types of antihypertensive drugs are available in market. Their classification is based on the mechanism of action and side effects. Class of antihypertensive drugs include diuretics, including thiazides, chlorthalidone, and indapamide, Angiotensin-converting enzyme (ACE) in blocker, calcium channel blockers, Central agonists, Alpha-adrenergic receptor, Beta-blockers and alpha-blockers, Peripheral adrenergic inhibitor, Angiotensin receptor blockers, vasodilators, Renin inhibitors (Moise et al., 2015). These drugs can decrease the vascular resistance and cardiac output or both, but their cost, developing resistance against these drugs are the great disadvantages that the individuals having hypertension suffering from. Therefore, modifiable lifestyle such as better stress management, good intake of diet can help to manage the Hypertension to a great extent along with an appropriate concentration of drug.

Hypertension is a metabolic disorder signalized by elevated levels of blood pressure i.e. more than 140 mm/Hg and 90 mm/Hg respectively. Can this disease be influenced by the way of life one lives? Do lifestyle parameters raise the risk of developing hypertension? What type of treatments available for curing Hypertension? Are these treatments efficacious or have any side effects reported? Can improved lifestyle factors manage hypertension? Many studies reported the correlation of various controlled and uncontrolled lifestyle factors with the development of hypertension. Also, genetic algorithm being used in the estimation, diagnosis and optimization of high levels of blood pressures. Based on that we have developed a mathematical model considering some of the lifestyle parameters showing interdependence on hypertension and tried to optimize the same using Genetic Algorithm.

SOLUTIONS AND RECOMMENDATIONS

The importance of Mathematical modeling in treating Hypertension is to determine how levels of blood pressure affect or change by different lifestyle factors including age, diet, stress and also upon the concentration of the drug.

Blood Pressure vs. Salt and Age

With age, activities like sodium regulation and water retention becomes less efficient. Consuming salt more than 2.3 mg/ml per day disturbs the normal balance of kidneys to remove water and electrolytes. The excess of fluid causes an additional strain on delicate blood vessels leading to higher blood pressure. Thus, high consumption of salt is positively correlated with hypertension and hence showing its linear dependency on high blood pressure.

$$BP \; \alpha \; SA$$

$$BP = k_1 SA \tag{1}$$

k_1= Coefficient of salt effects

Blood Pressure vs. Drug Intake and Physical Exercise

$$BP\alpha(D + P)$$

$$BP = k_2 D + k_3 P \tag{2}$$

k_2= Coefficient of drug intake, k_3= Coefficient of physical exercise

Blood Pressure vs. Stress

During stress conditions, stimulation of nervous system produces large amount of vasoconstricting hormones like adrenaline, Cortisol, Norepinephrine which have been reported to elevate the levels of blood pressure. Stress is one of the reasons that indirectly leads to hypertension by elevating the repeated cycles of blood pressure and thus showing the direct relation with high blood pressure.

$BP\ \alpha\ \mathrm{k}4_{\mathrm{H}}$

$$BP = k_4 H \tag{3}$$

k_4= Coefficient of stress {0-1}

Formation of Mathematical Model and Parameter Relationship

Adding all the above equations we get

$$3BP = k_1 SA + k_2 D + k_3 P + k_4 H$$

$$BP = k'_1 SA + k'_2 D + k'_3 P + k'_4 H \tag{4}$$

Where,

$$k'_1 = {}^{k_1}\!/_3,\quad k'_2 = {}^{k_2}\!/_3,\quad k'_3 = {}^{k_3}\!/_3,\quad k'_4 = {}^{k_4}\!/_3$$

$$BP = a_1 SA + z_1$$

where z_1 is a constant

$$BP = b_1 D + b_2 P + z_2$$

where z_2 is a constant

$$BP = c_1 H + z_3$$

where z_3 is a constant

Adding all these above equations we get,

$$3BP = a_1 SA + b_1 D + b_2 P + c_1 H + z_1 + z_2 + z_3$$

$$BP = a'_1 SA + b'_1 D + b'_2 P + c'_1 H + Z \tag{5}$$

$$a_1^{'} = {a_1}/{3},\quad b_1^{'} = {b_1}/{3},\quad b_2^{'} = {b_2}/{3},\quad c_1^{'} = {c_1}/{3},\quad Z = \frac{z_1 + z_2 + z_3}{3}$$

Adding (4) and (5)

$$2BP = (a_1^{'} + k_1^{'})SA + (b_1^{'} + k_2^{'})D + (b_2^{'} + k_3^{'})P + (c_1^{'} + k_4^{'})H + Z$$

$$BP = \alpha SA + \beta D + \gamma P + \lambda H + \delta \tag{6}$$

Optimization of the Problem using Genetic Algorithm

Since many studies reported the role of genetics in the development of hypertension, the future generation of hypertensive patients are high prone to hypertension as compared to normal ones. This genetic algorithm is a proof that improved lifestyle parameters not only prevents or manage hypertension in the current generation but also in the future generations.

In this work we use genetic algorithms to solve linear equation problem (eq. 6).

Table 4. Parametric values for Systolic BP

Salt (S) gm/day	Age (A) years	Drug (D)	Physical Activity (P)	Hypertension (H)	Blood Pressure (BP)
2	30	1	200	0.1	120
4	33	1.4	250	0.3	140
5	40	1.6	350	0.4	160
7	37	2	500	0.8	200

Source: (McLoone 2014, Beevers 2001, Joyner 2008, and Yang 2017)

Evaluation of the constants using the above table for Systolic Blood pressure. From equation (6), we get

$$120 = 60\alpha + \beta + 200\gamma + 0.1\lambda + \delta$$

$$140 = 132\alpha + 1.4\beta + 250\gamma + 0.3\lambda + \delta$$

$$160 = 200\alpha + 1.6\beta + 350\gamma + 0.4\lambda + \delta$$

$$200 = 259\alpha + 2\beta + 500\gamma + 0.8\lambda + \delta$$

Hence solving the above simultaneous equations system, we get

α= -0.27848, β=90.6962, γ=0.252152, λ=--44.1772 and δ=22

Now from equation (6), we get the objective function

Min.BP = -0.27848 * SA + 90.6962 * D + 0.252152 * P – 44.1772 * H + 22 (7)

Where Systolic Blood pressure (BP=[120,200]), salt and age multiplication (SA=[60,259]), Drug (D=[1,2]) Physical activity (P=[200, 500]), and Hypertension (H=[0.1,0.8]).

MATLAB code for optimize function of Systolic Blood pressure:

```
function y = systolicbp(x)
    char x;
    y=(-0.0278*x(1)+90.696*x(2)+0.2522*x(3)-44.18*x(4))+22;
end
```

use the genetic algorithm tool box and Lower bound [60 1 200 0.1 22]; and upper bound [259 2 500 0.8 22];

Systolic **Blood pressure function (Objective function value) returned by ga = 120.591**85963660019

Figure 3 shows the plot of the best value for diastolic blood pressure is 120.719 mmHg and mean value is 120.725 mmHg and over the 163 iterations. Best fitness values have been represented by the bottom points of the plot and the average fitness values have been represented by the points present above the bottom points in the plot. The best and mean value in the current generation displayed numerically at the top of the plot.

Figure 3. Plots of the best fitness value over the 163 iterations (Generations)

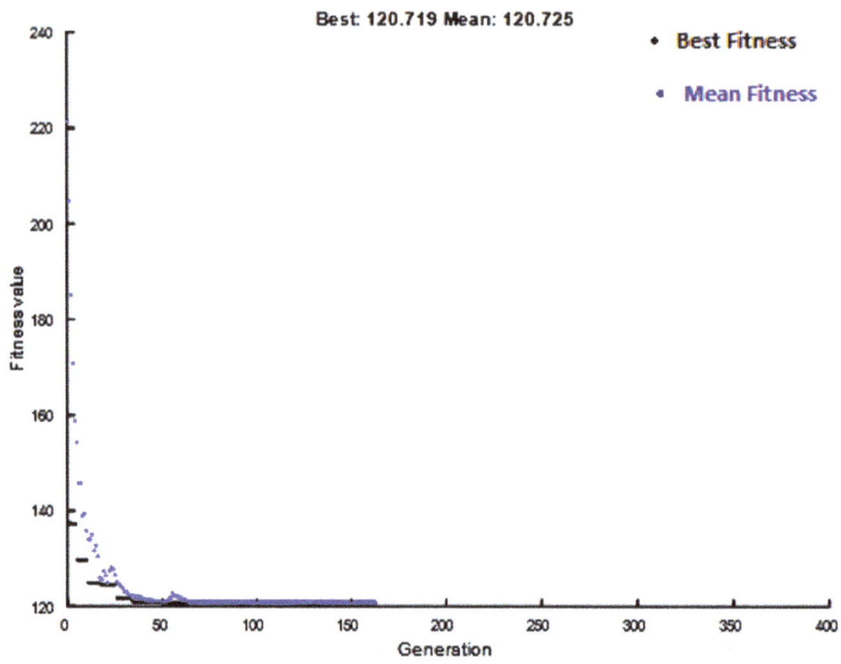

Figure 4 shows the plots of the Current best individuals variables over the 209 iterations which represents the variable 1 (Salt and age) and variable 3 (Physical activities) are important. From the plot it is clear that best individual is corresponding to variable 1.

Figure 4. Plots of the current best individuals' variables over the 209 iterations (Generations)

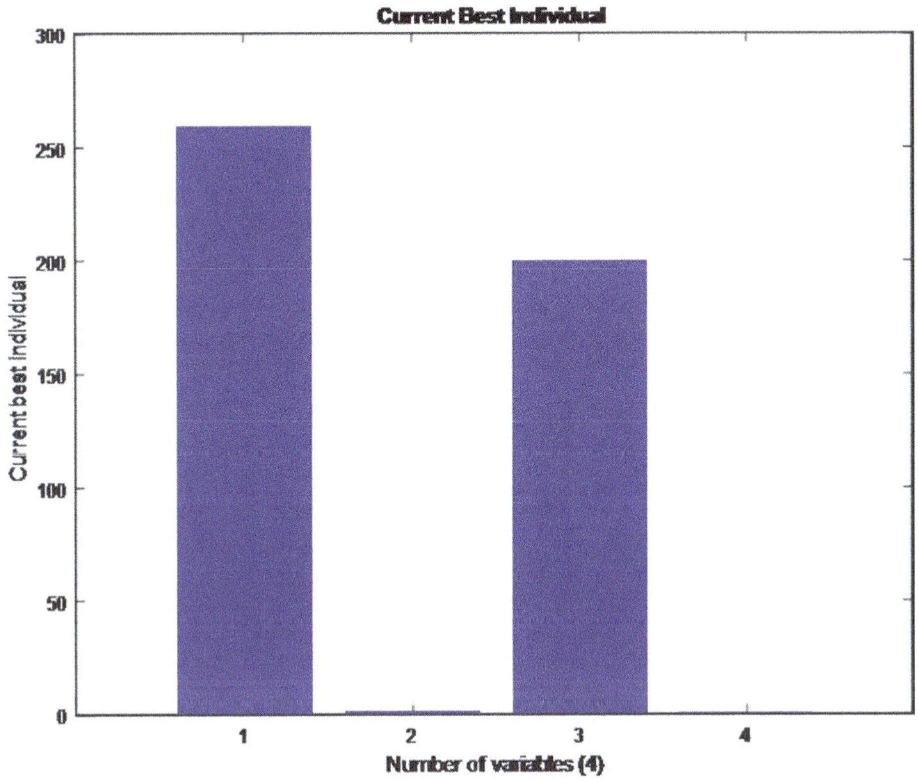

Figure 5 shows the plots of the fitness function value i.e. 120.719 over the 98 iterations. Scaled fitness (expectation) of the best-found solutions in the Genetic Algorithm.

Figure 6 shows the plots of the mean scores of values of Fitness function over the 104 iterations. Note that all individuals lie between 120 and 280.

Evaluation of the constants using the above table for Diastolic Blood pressure. From equation (6), we get

$$80 = 60\alpha + \beta + 200\gamma + 0.1\lambda + \delta$$

$$100 = 132\alpha + 1.4\beta + 250\gamma + 3.0\lambda + \delta$$

$$110 = 200\alpha + 1.6\beta + 350\gamma + 0.4\lambda + \delta$$

$$130 = 259\alpha + 2\beta + 500\gamma + 0.8\lambda + \delta$$

Figure 5. Plots of the fitness function value over the 98 iterations (Generations)

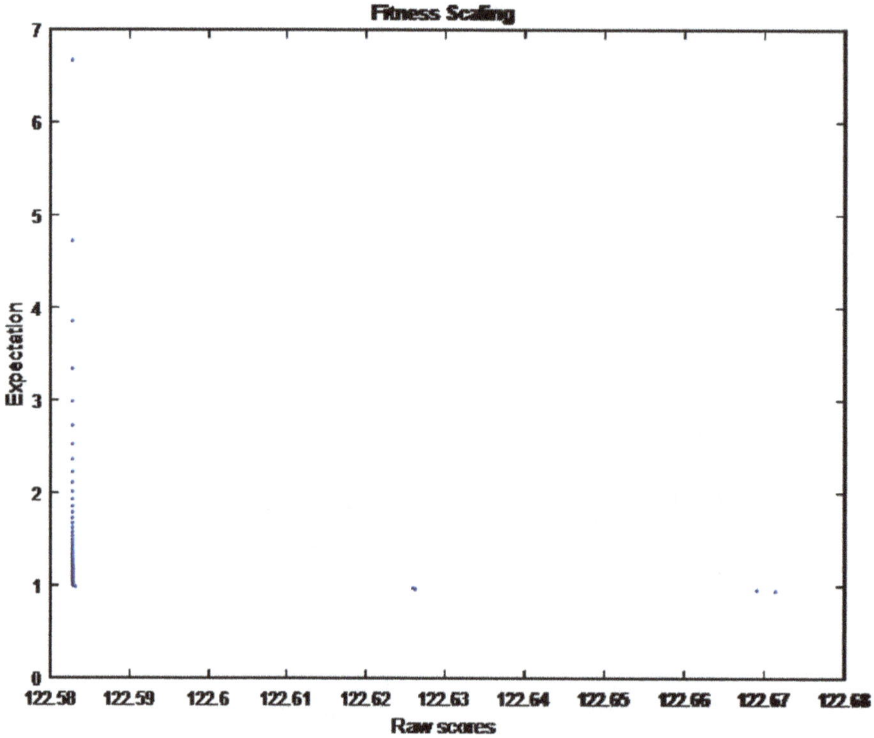

Figure 6. Plots of the mean scores of values of fitness function over the 104 iterations (Generations)

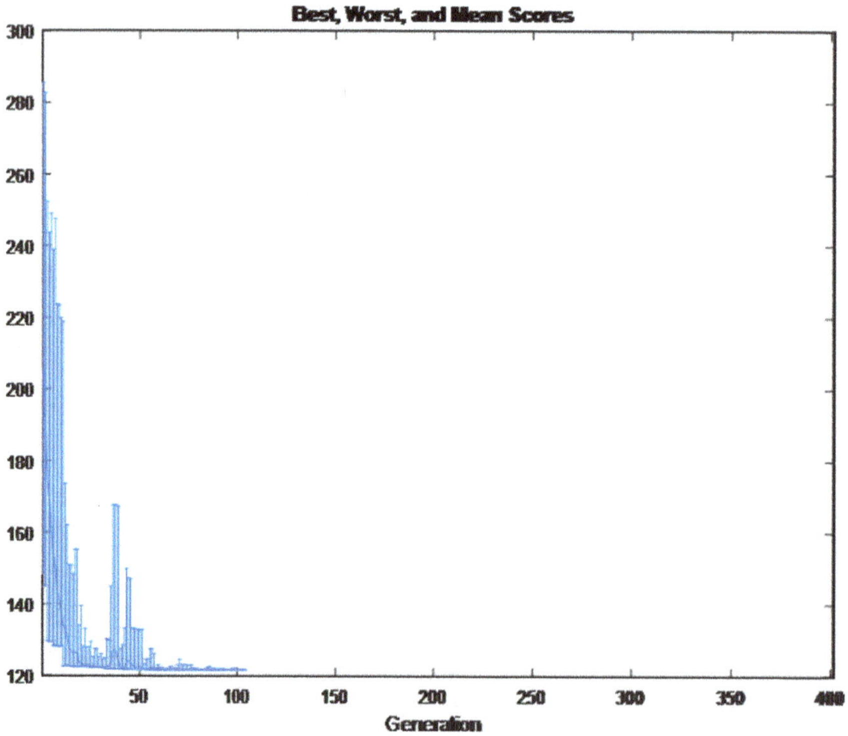

Hence solving the above simultaneous equations system, we get

α= -0.11392, β=80.28481, γ=0.048608, λ=-31.7089 and δ=44

Now from equation (6), we get

$$\text{Min.BP} = -0.11392 * SA + 80.28481 * D + 0.048608 * P - 31.7089 * H + 44 \quad (8)$$

Where *D*iastolic Blood pressure (BP=[80,130]), salt and age multiplication (SA=[60,259]), Drug (D=[1,2]) Physical activity (P=[200, 500]), and Hypertension (H=[0.1,0.8]).

MATLAB code for optimize function of Diastolic Blood pressure:

```
function y = diastolicbp(x)
    char x;
    y=(-0.114*x(1)+80.285*x(2)+0.0486*x(3)-31.71*x(4))+44;
end
```

use the genetic algorithm tool box and Lower bound [60 1 200 0.1 44]; and upper bound [259 2 500 0.8 44];.

Diastolic **Blood pressure (Objective function valuc) returned by ga = 79.7502**8909597836

Table 5. Parametric values for diastolic BP

Salt (S) gm/ day	Age (A) years	Drug (D)	Physical Activity (P)	Hypertension (H)	Blood Pressure (BP)
2	30	1	200	0.1	80
4	33	1.4	250	0.3	100
5	40	1.6	350	0.4	110
7	37	2	500	0.8	130

Source: (McLoone 2014, Beevers 2001, Joyner 2008, and Yang 2017)

Figure 7 shows the plot of the best value for diastolic blood pressure is 79.1148 mmHg and mean value is 79.1228 mmHg and over the 322 iterations. Best fitness values have been represented by the bottom points of the plot and the average fitness values have been represented by the points present above the bottom points in the plot. The best and mean value in the current generation displayed numerically at the top of the plot.

Figure 8 shows the plots of the Current best individuals variables over the 292 iterations which represents the variable 1 (Salt and age) and variable 3(Physical activities) are important. From the plot it is clear that best individual is corresponding to variable 1.

Figure 9 shows the plots of the fitness function value is 79.1148 over the 343 iterations. Scaled fitness (expectation) of the best-found solutions in the Genetic algorithm

Figure 10 shows the plots of the mean scores of values of Fitness function over the 214 iterations. It has to be noted that all the individuals' range between 79 and 200.

Figure 7. Plots of the best fitness value over the 322 iterations (Generations)

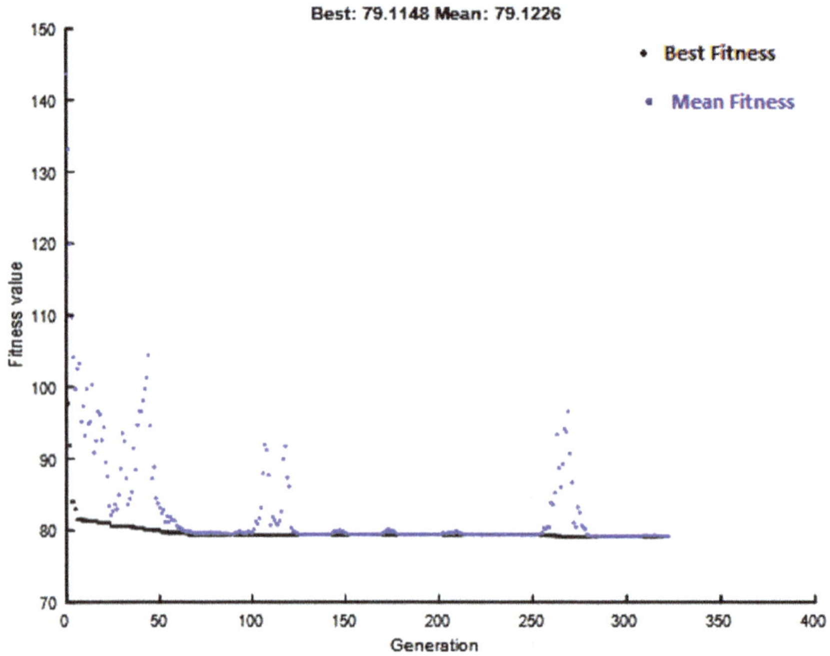

Figure 8. Plots of the current best individuals' variables over the 292 iterations (Generations)

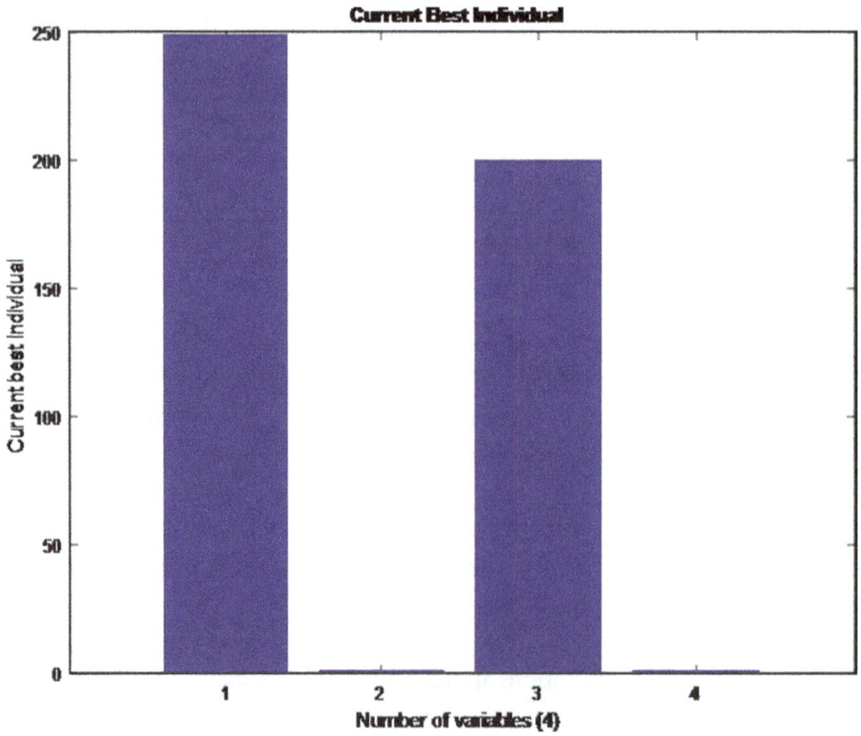

Figure 9. Plots of the fitness function value over the 343 iterations (Generations)

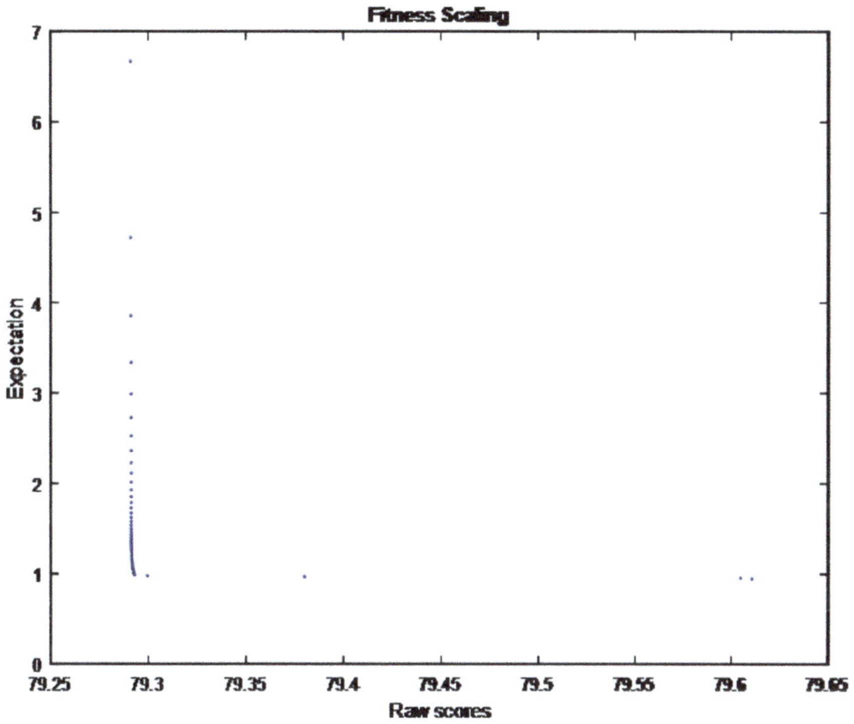

Figure 10. Plots of the mean scores of values of fitness function over the 214 iterations (Generations)

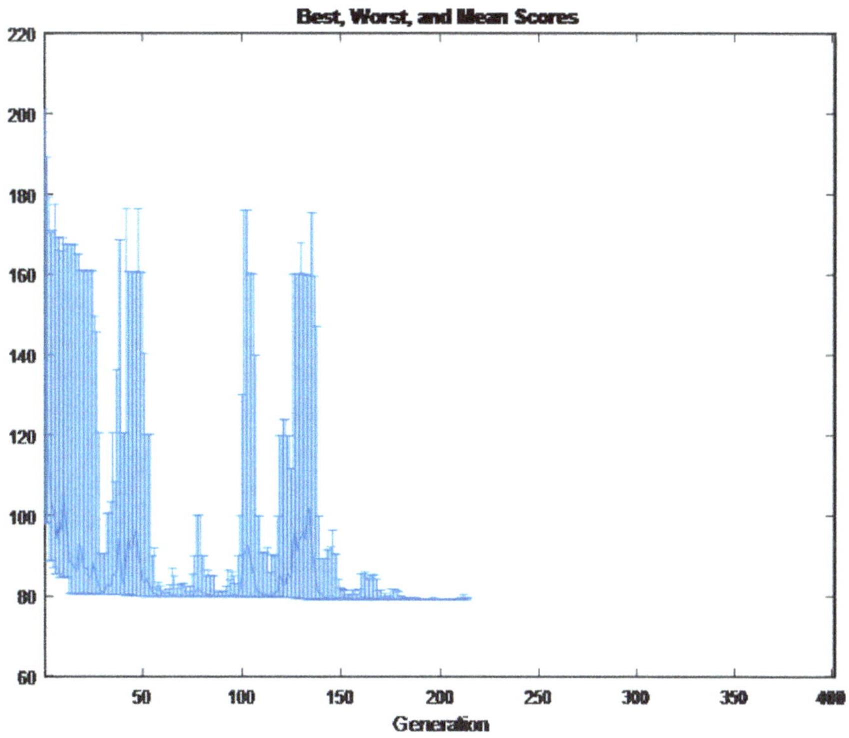

CONCLUSION

Major lifestyle parameters such as lack of physical activity, high concentration of salt in diet, alcohol consumption, smoking, stress, and high weight significantly related to this disease. Genetics also play an important role in the development of hypertension. The complexity of disease is appropriate to quantitative methodologies as it gives difficulties and chances to new turns of events. This work generalized a mathematical model of hypertension considering the lifestyle parameters including stress, physical activity, consumption of salt (concerning age) in which we have shown how the concentration of drug and lifestyle factors affect the rate of change of blood pressure. This mathematical model acts as a parental template for deciding the appropriate concentration of drug for proper medication along with the lifestyle parameters. The genetic algorithm has presented an optimized system that attains high classification performance, with simple interpretation. Hypertension, characterized by a rise in blood pressure levels, more than 140 mm/Hg and 90 mm/Hg in case of systolic and diastolic blood pressure. 29% of stroke and 24% of all heart attacks are directly associated with Hypertension. The unhealthy quality of lifestyle is one of the main reasons for developing many health-related issues that are primarily based on the individual's habit that cause them to shift from the activity to a sedentary lifestyle. The lifestyle is major factor of Hypertension and as the epidemic rates of hypertension are too high due to bad lifestyle, the significance of this research is to ensure that how modifiable lifestyle parameters can restore the elevated blood pressure levels with the help of Mathematical Model. Novelty, being analyzing and comparing the controlled lifestyle parameters with the blood pressure levels by designing a Mathematical Model and optimizing the same using Genetic Algorithm (evolutionary algorithm) approach. A computational model wherein sodium discharge has been autonomous of pulse as well as neural actuation has triggered vasculature hypertension. Our model duplicates the arrangements of prior models, yet still shows the experimentally grounded connection between progressions in sodium discharge and blood pressure. Cardiac levels being carefully controlled inside body by a variety of interrelated mechanisms on an intermediate-, middle-, and long-term scale. In pathologic situations, pulse rate may be persistently elevated above normal values, resulting in progression of cardiovascular disease and increased mortality. Building a total image of the mechanisms associated with circulatory strain control is crucial for the turn of events of a superior comprehension of the cycles that might prompt hypertension.

The multi factorial disorder- Hypertension depends greatly upon the lifestyle factors which an individual enrolls in his life. Bad lifestyle measures such as excess fat consumption, smoking, drinking, no physical activity, stress tends to increase the cause of developing many diseases and ultimately affect the blood pressure leading to a condition called Hypertension. Using Mathematics, we have generalized a mathematical model which shows the inter dependence of different lifestyle factors on the change in blood pressure levels. The model also determines a concentration of drug (dosage) to be intake corresponding to that blood pressure level. This work is a measure of how controlled lifestyle parameters and appropriate concentration of drug helps in the management of Hypertension. In this work, we applied a genetic algorithm to optimize the systolic and diastolic blood pressure of human being. Our results suggest that the genetic algorithm approach is highly effective on medical diagnosis problems which shows the optimized systolic blood pressure (120.719 mmHg) and diastolic blood pressure (79.1148 mmHg). This work demonstrates a prime advantage mathematical model, which is the ability to find an output.

ACKNOWLEDGMENT

The authors thank to Department of Biotechnology, MRIIRS LAB to provide data sets on lifestyle-disorder to provide facts which motivates authors to do research work.

FUNDING

This research received no specific grant from any funding agency in the public, commercial, or not-for-profit sectors.

REFERENCES

Anderson, G. H. (1999). Effect of age on hypertension: Analysis of over 4,800 referred hypertensive patients. *Saudi Journal of Kidney Diseases and Transplantation, 10*(3), 286. PMID:18212439

Armaly, Z., Assady, S., & Abassi, Z. (2013). Corin: A new player in the regulation of salt–water balance and blood pressure. *Current Opinion in Nephrology and Hypertension, 22*(6), 713–722. doi:10.1097/01.mnh.0000435609.35789.32 PMID:24100222

Averina, V. A., Othmer, H. G., Fink, G. D., & Osborn, J. W. (2012). A new conceptual paradigm for the haemodynamics of salt-sensitive hypertension: A mathematical modelling approach. *The Journal of Physiology, 590*(23), 5975–5992. doi:10.1113/jphysiol.2012.228619 PMID:22890716

Averina, V. A., Othmer, H. G., Fink, G. D., & Osborn, J. W. (2012). A new conceptual paradigm for the haemodynamics of salt-sensitive hypertension: A mathematical modelling approach. *The Journal of Physiology, 590*(23), 5975–5992. doi:10.1113/jphysiol.2012.228619 PMID:22890716

Bashir, L. Z. (2015). Solve simple linear equation using evolutionary algorithm. *World Scientific News, 19*, 148–167.

Beevers, G., Lip, G. Y., & O'Brien, E. (2001, April 14). The pathophysiology of hypertension. *British Medical Journal, 322*(7291), 912–916. doi:10.1136/bmj.322.7291.912 PMID:11302910

Blair, S. N. (1984). Physical fitness and incidence of hypertension in healthy normotensive men and women. *Journal of the American Medical Association, 252*(4), 487–490. doi:10.1001/jama.1984.03350040017014 PMID:6737638

Bolívar, J. J. (2013). Essential Hypertension: An approach to its etiology and neurogenic pathophysiology. *International Journal of Hypertension, 2013*, 1–11. doi:10.1155/2013/547809 PMID:24386559

Charkoudian, N., & Rabbitts, J. A. (2009). Sympathetic neural mechanisms in human cardiovascular health and disease. *Mayo Clinic Proceedings, 84*(9), 822–830. doi:10.4065/84.9.822

Charles, L., Triscott, J., & Dobbs, B. (2017). Secondary hypertension: Discovering the underlying cause. *American Family Physician, 96*(7), 453–461. PMID:29094913

Chatterjee, A. N., & Roy, P. K. (2020). *Smoking habit: A bio mathematical study*. Communications in Mathematical Biology and Neuroscience. doi:10.28919/cmbn/4319

Clemmer, J. S., Pruett, W. A., Coleman, T. G., Hall, J. E., & Hester, R. L. (2017). Mechanisms of blood pressure salt sensitivity: New insights from mathematical modeling. *American Journal of Physiology. Regulatory, Integrative and Comparative Physiology*, *312*(4), R451–R466.

Cuzzo, B., Padala, S. A., & Lappin, S. L. (2020). *Vasopressin (Antidiuretic Hormone, ADH)*. StatPearls.

De Souza, A. M. A., West, C. A., de Abreu, A. R. R., Pai, A. V., Mesquita, L. B. T., Ji, H., & Sandberg, K. (2018). Role of the renin angiotensin system in blood pressure allostasis-induced by severe food restriction in female fischer rats. *Scientific Reports*, *8*(1), 10327. Advance online publication. doi:10.103841598-018-28593-6 PMID:29985423

Elliott, W. J. (2009). Trends in hypertension prevalence, awareness, treatment, and control rates in United States adults between 1988–1994 and 1999–2004. *Yearbook of Cardiology*, *5-7*, 5–7. Advance online publication. doi:10.1016/S0145-4145(08)79400-0

Everett, B., & Zajacova, A. (2015). Gender differences in hypertension and hypertension awareness among young adults. *Biodemography and Social Biology*, *61*(1), 1–17. doi:10.1080/19485565.2014.929488 PMID:25879259

Fagard, R. H. (1995). The role of exercise in blood pressure control: Supportive evidence. *Journal of Hypertension*, *13*(11), 1223–1227. doi:10.1097/00004872-199511000-00001 PMID:8984117

Foëx, P., & Sear, J. W. (2004). Hypertension: Pathophysiology and treatment. *Continuing Education in Anaesthesia, Critical Care & Pain*, *4*(3), 71–75. doi:10.1093/bjaceaccp/mkh020

Gerage, A. M., Benedetti, T. R. B., Farah, B. Q., Santana, F. da S., Ohara, D., Andersen, L. B., & Ritti-Dias, R. M. (2015). Sedentary behavior and light physical activity are associated with brachial and central blood pressure in hypertensive patients. *PLoS One*, *10*(12), e0146078. doi:10.1371/journal.pone.0146078 PMID:26717310

Gupta, R., Gaur, K., & Ram, C. V. (2018). Emerging trends in hypertension epidemiology in India. *Journal of Human Hypertension*, *33*(8), 575–587. doi:10.103841371-018-0117-3 PMID:30254382

John, S., Krege, J., Oliver, P., Hagaman, J. R., Hodgin, J. B., Pang, S. C., Flynn, T. G., & Smithies, O. (1995). Genetic decreases in atrial natriuretic peptide and salt-sensitive hypertension. *Science*, *267*(5198), 679–681. doi:10.1126cience.7839143 PMID:7839143

Joyner, M. J., Charkoudian, N., & Wallin, B. G. (2008). A sympathetic view of the sympathetic nervous system and human blood pressure regulation. *Experimental Physiology*, *93*(6), 715–724. doi:10.1113/expphysiol.2007.039545 PMID:18326553

Joyner, M. J., Charkoudian, N., & Wallin, B. G. (2010). Sympathetic nnervous ssystem and blood pressure in humans. *Hypertension*, *56*(1), 10–16. doi:10.1161/HYPERTENSIONAHA.109.140186 PMID:20497993

Kojuri, J., Boostani, R., Dehghani, P., Nowroozipour, F., & Saki, N. (2015). Prediction of acute myocardial infarction with artificial neural networks in patients with non-diagnostic electrocardiogram. *Journal of Cardiovascular Disease Research*, *6*(2), 51-19.

Kokubo, Y., Iwashima, Y., & Kamide, K. (2015). Hypertension: Introduction, Types, Causes, and Complications. *Pathophysiology and Pharmacotherapy of Cardiovascular Disease*, 635–653. doi:10.1007/978-3-319-15961-4_30

Kulkarni, S., O'Farrell, I., Erasi, M., & Kochar, M. S. (1998). Stress and hypertension. *WMJ: Official Publication of the State Medical Society of Wisconsin*, *97*(11), 34. PMID:9894438

Kumanyika, S. K., & Cutler, J. A. (1997). Dietary sodium reduction: Is there cause for concern? *Journal of the American College of Nutrition*, *16*(3), 192–203. doi:10.1080/07315724.1997.10718674 PMID:9176824

Lee, C. Y. W., & Burnett, J. C. Jr. (2007). Natriuretic peptides and therapeutic applications. *Heart Failure Reviews*, *12*(2), 131. Advance online publication. doi:10.100710741-007-9016-3 PMID:17440808

McCall, J. (2005). Genetic algorithms for modelling and optimisation. *Journal of Computational and Applied Mathematics*, *184*(1), 205–222. doi:10.1016/j.cam.2004.07.034

McGrath, M. F., de Bold, M. L. K., & Adolfo, J. (2005). The endocrine function of the heart. *Trends in Endocrinology and Metabolism*, *16*(10), 469–477. doi:10.1016/j.tem.2005.10.007 PMID:16269246

McLoone, V. (2014). *Modelling of Long and Short Term Blood Pressure Control Systems* (Doctoral dissertation). National University of Ireland, Maynooth, Ireland.

McLoone, V. I. (2014). *Modelling of long and short term blood pressure control systems* (Doctoral dissertation). National University of Ireland Maynooth.

Meelab, S., Bunupuradah, I., Suttiruang, J., Sakulrojanawong, S., Thongkua, N., Chantawiboonchai, C., & Sakboonyarat, B. (2019). Prevalence and associated factors of uncontrolled blood pressure among hypertensive patients in the rural communities in the central areas in Thailand: A cross-sectional study. *PLoS One*, *14*(2), e0212572. doi:10.1371/journal.pone.0212572 PMID:30779818

Moise, N., Schwartz, J., Bring, R., Shimbo, D., & Kronish, I. M. (2014). Antihypertensive drug class and adherence: An electronic monitoring study. *American Journal of Hypertension*, *28*(6), 717–721. doi:10.1093/ajh/hpu199 PMID:25344354

Niarchos, A. P., Pickering, T. G., Case, D. B., Sullivan, P., & Laragh, J. H. (1979). Role of the renin-angiotensin system in blood pressure regulation. The cardiovascular effects of converting enzyme inhibition in normotensive subjects. *Circulation Research*, *45*(6), 829–837. doi:10.1161/01.RES.45.6.829 PMID:498446

Ogwumu, O., Amoo, S., Eguda, F., Adeyefa, E., & Abubakar, S. (2015). A mathematical model for estimating the weight of human beings using some anthropometric parameters (A Case Study of Taraba State of Nigerias Community). *British Journal of Mathematics and Computer Science*, *8*(2), 147–158. doi:10.9734/BJMCS/2015/10987

Parlikar, A. S., & Dahe, P. D. (2019). Application of linear programming-genetic algorithm combination for Urmodi reservoir operation. In *International Conference on Reliability, Risk Maintenance and Engineering Management* (pp. 98-103). Springer.

Perez, V., & Chang, E. T. (2014). Sodium-to-potassium ratio and blood pressure, hypertension, and related factors. *Advances in Nutrition*, *5*(6), 712–741. doi:10.3945/an.114.006783 PMID:25398734

Pinto, E. (2007). Blood pressure and ageing. *Postgraduate Medical Journal*, *83*(976), 109–114. doi:10.1136/pgmj.2006.048371 PMID:17308214

Potter, L. R., Abbey-Hosch, S., & Dickey, D. M. (2006). Natriuretic peptides, their receptors, and cyclic guanosine monophosphate-dependent signaling functions. *Endocrine Reviews*, *27*(1), 47–72. doi:10.1210/er.2005-0014 PMID:16291870

Pouliot, M.-C., Després, J.-P., Lemieux, S., Moorjani, S., Bouchard, C., Tremblay, A., & Lupien, P. J. (1994). Waist circumference and abdominal sagittal diameter: Best simple anthropometric indexes of abdominal visceral adipose tissue accumulation and related cardiovascular risk in men and women. *The American Journal of Cardiology*, *73*(7), 460–468. doi:10.1016/0002-9149(94)90676-9

Puddey, I. B., Beilin, L. J., & Vandongen, R. (1987). Regular alcohol use raises blood pressure in treated hypertensive subjects. *Lancet*, *329*(8534), 647–651. doi:10.1016/S0140-6736(87)90413-2 PMID:2882082

Raamat, R., Talts, J., Jagomägi, K., & Länsimies, E. (1999). Mathematical modelling of non-invasive oscillometric finger mean blood pressure measurement by maximum oscillation criterion. *Medical & Biological Engineering & Computing*, *37*(6), 784–788.

Rajkumar, E., & Romate, J. (2020). Behavioural Risk Factors, Hypertension Knowledge, and Hypertension in Rural India. *International Journal of Hypertension*, *2020*, 1–7. doi:10.1155/2020/8108202 PMID:32231796

Rouse, I. L., Armstrong, B. K., & Beilin, L. J. (1983). The relationship of blood pressure to diet and lifestyle in two religious populations. *Journal of Hypertension*, *1*(1), 65–72. doi:10.1097/00004872-198306000-00011 PMID:6681026

Sacks, F. M., Svetkey, L. P., Vollmer, W. M., Appel, L. J., Bray, G. A., Harsha, D., ... Karanja, N. (2001). Effects on blood pressure of reduced dietary sodium and the dietary approaches to stop hypertension (DASH) diet. *The New England Journal of Medicine*, *344*(1), 3–10. doi:10.1056/NEJM200101043440101 PMID:11136953

Saez, P., Peña, E., Martínez, M. A., & Kuhl, E. (2014). Computational modeling of hypertensive growth in the human carotid artery. *Computational Mechanics*, *53*(6), 1183–1196. doi:10.100700466-013-0959-z PMID:25342868

Stamler, J., Elliott, P., Kesteloot, H., Nichols, R., Claeys, G., Dyer, A. R., & Stamler, R. (1996). Inverse relation of dietary protein markers with blood pressure. *Circulation*, *94*(7), 1629–1634. doi:10.1161/01.CIR.94.7.1629 PMID:8840854

Steinhelper, M. E., Cochrane, K. L., & Field, L. J. (1990). Hypotension in transgenic mice expressing atrial natriuretic factor fusion genes. *Hypertension*, *16*(3), 301–307. doi:10.1161/01.HYP.16.3.301 PMID:2144261

Tiffin, N., Meintjes, A., Ramesar, R., Bajic, V. B., & Rayner, B. (2010). Computational analysis of candidate disease genes and variants for salt-sensitive hypertension in indigenous Southern Africans. *PLoS One*, *5*(9), e12989. doi:10.1371/journal.pone.0012989 PMID:20886000

Wallin, B. G., & Charkoudian, N. (2007). Sympathetic neural control of integrated cardiovascular function: Insights from measurement of human sympathetic nerve activity. *Muscle & Nerve*, *36*(5), 595–614. doi:10.1002/mus.20831 PMID:17623856

Yang, M. H., Kang, S. Y., Lee, J. A., Kim, Y. S., Sung, E. J., Lee, K. Y., Kim, J.-S., Oh, H. J., Kang, H. C., & Lee, S. Y. (2017). The effect of lifestyle changes on blood pressure control among hypertensive patients. *Korean Journal of Family Medicine*, *38*(4), 173. doi:10.4082/kjfm.2017.38.4.173 PMID:28775806

Zhou, Y., Jiang, J., Cui, Y., & Wu, Q. (2009). Corin, atrial natriuretic peptide and hypertension. *Nephrology, Dialysis, Transplantation*, *24*(4), 1071–1073. doi:10.1093/ndt/gfn727 PMID:19131349

Chapter 7
Recent Developments of Smart Hospitals and Challenges

Kannadhasan S.
https://orcid.org/0000-0001-6443-9993
Cheran College of Engineering, India

Nagarajan R.
Gnanamani College of Technology, India

Jisha Chandra C.
Gnanamani College of Technology, India

Manjushree Kumari J.
Gnanamani College of Technology, India

ABSTRACT

Remote monitoring is a healthcare tool that enables physicians to stay connected to their patients from afar and offer treatment anytime it is needed. The sensing devices may be worn, implanted, or sensors in the surrounding environment can be linked to the internet, allowing physicians and caregivers to deliver patients with effective and timely medicine. This application is used to remotely monitor the patient's vital parameters using sensors, gadgets, and items in their environment. The patient's essential data is transferred and exchanged in real time between the patient and the caretakers. Its primary use is in the treatment of chronic diseases such as diabetes, heart disease monitoring, asthma, and so on. In many sectors, recent technological advancements and connectivity have resulted in the rise of internet of things (IoT) and artificial intelligence (AI) applications.

DOI: 10.4018/978-1-6684-2508-4.ch007

INTRODUCTION

One area where IoT and AI, alone or in combination, are having a huge impact is the healthcare industry, which is always under pressure to decrease costs while serving a rapidly growing ill population. These technologies might help healthcare organisations reap the advantages of a more connected and responsive world. Patients, physicians, payers, and drug developers would all benefit if the industry can achieve "greater interconnectedness in a single ecosystem." Smart pills, wearable monitors, and sensors enable healthcare providers to collect data in real time, and AI systems can help analyse that data to detect changes in a patient's condition, suggest treatment options, and identify trends, boosting patient adherence, improving patient outcomes, and speeding the discovery and access to new treatments. The internet of things (IoT) is a growing network of smart gadgets connected to each other over the internet. The Internet of Things has contributed significantly to improving people's quality of life. Smart healthcare, smart cities, industrial automation, agriculture, and transportation are just a few of the internet of things' diverse uses. Sensing devices and objects detect and collect essential data in the Internet of Things, which can subsequently be processed and analysed for better decision making.

As a consequence, physical devices in the actual world may be linked to give computation-based performance. As a consequence, the Internet of Items (IoT) is a developing network of smart devices, actuators, smart phones, and things with low-memory processors that are connected to the internet in order to collect and exchange data and perform requested services. In this research, the internet of things is leveraged to deliver smart healthcare. The Internet of Things allows for machine-to-machine, sensor-to-device, patient-to-device, patient-to-doctor, and device-to-doctor interactions. Remote monitoring, early detection, chronic disease management, elder care, medical treatment for institutionalised patients, and other healthcare IoT applications are only some of the possibilities. It allows us to link intelligently, resulting in a more efficient healthcare system. However, even with the advantages, there remain security and privacy vulnerabilities that are key problems for IoT applications (B. G. Ahn et.al, 2015; A. Dwivedi.et.al,2003).

This software makes use of mobile technology to provide users remote access to current healthcare systems or organisations that offer care. Automation of e-health systems has become easier because to the broad availability of smart mobile apps, portals, and websites. In healthcare, smart devices are utilised to record and monitor critical care parameters as well as sickness data. They're primarily used to give fitness solutions by monitoring target activities and storing data from the gadgets. They're usually used as fitness trackers for patients, as well as smart diagnostic devices like blood pressure monitors, pedometers, and Google Glass, which collect data from sensors for later examination by physicians.

This programme allows for virtual care consultations, medicine distribution, and teaching, among other things, via remote connection and effective solutions. The notion of providing remote medical assistance, such as teleconsultations and mobile video solutions, has grown immensely popular in a few countries and areas. This initiative monitors the elderly in order to assist them in becoming more self-sufficient. Wearable and implanted sensors are two examples of technology that might be used to monitor elderly individuals without involving humans. The monitoring gadgets track the elderly's vital signs and relay them to a regular smartphone, which works as a node for transmitting real-time data to doctors. The data collected may be used to provide medical assistance to the elderly, and local hospitals could be contacted in the case of an emergency.

Smartphone apps might be used to provide care to individuals who are in need. Several open source programmes for offering healthcare solutions have been developed in order to provide efficient healthcare facilities. Among them are diagnose apps (Diagnose, 5MCC, Prognosis, 5-minute infectious disease consult), drug reference apps (Medical doctor: reference tool, Epocrates, FDA drugs, Lab values), calculator apps (MedCalc, caddy medical calculator, uBurn lite), and clinical communication apps (Voalte one, mVisum, Vocera). The processing capabilities of smart IoT devices are limited by low-speed CPUs. These devices are designed for use in limited contexts where inefficient procedures are carried out, and a security solution that minimises resource consumption while maximising security is necessary to increase their efficacy. Because these devices have limited on-device memory and can only execute lightweight protocols or programmes, the same is true for memory computation. Smart devices used in IoT healthcare, such as blood pressure monitors and temperature sensors, go into sleep mode when no readings need to be recorded to preserve battery life.

As a consequence, a design solution to deal with the energy, power, and processing limits of these devices should be devised. Other security risks linked to mobility and scalability must be addressed. This article gives a quick summary of smart healthcare as an Internet of Things (IoT) application that has transformed the conventional medical system. Smart healthcare systems have reduced the complexity and problems associated with the use of IoT settings. The IoT devices that have been deployed gather critical data regarding the patient's health, enabling for speedy decision-making. This article discusses the many ways in which healthcare may be provided to a needed patient through remote monitoring, senior care management, virtual consultation, and other approaches. In order to improve everyone's quality of life, it's also necessary to secure the security and privacy of healthcare data. This study (M. S. D. Gupta, et.al,2015; N. Pereira,et.al, 2007) highlights existing security issues as well as open areas that pose hazards to researchers.

As a consequence, a standardised design should be proposed to reduce security concerns while also addressing issues such restricted settings, cost-effectiveness, scalability, and interoperability of healthcare apps. The Internet of Things (IoT) is a network that enables physical equipment, humans, animals, and other items with sensors and software to communicate with one another. One of the most important areas of future technology is usually viewed as this. Cloud computing and IoT will become more intertwined as technology improves. Cloud computing gives you access to almost unlimited storage and processing power. Medical science and the smart hospital system are discussed in this article. There are areas in underdeveloped countries where people do not have enough access to a good healthcare system.

According to a recent study, patients in Australia, Canada, Germany, New Zealand, the United Kingdom, and the United States lacked comprehensive health records. This made identifying symptoms and diagnosing sickness more challenging. Furthermore, there was no system in place to ensure that the doctor was contacted once the patient was released. Health is an important aspect of life, and with each new day comes a new ailment. Physicians and medical institutions are in greater demand as the world's population expands. It's also vital that we provide a high-quality, error-free healthcare system that is accessible to patients, physicians, and caregivers.

The growing elderly population, together with the rise in chronic illness that has followed it, has put a pressure on the healthcare system. Hospital beds are at a premium, and there aren't enough doctors or resources to care for such a large number of patients. The Internet of Things (IoT) has emerged as a means of alleviating the current healthcare system's pressure. The Internet of Things (IoT) enables remote patient sensing via the use of various hardware and software components. Patients, physicians, and caregivers may access patient information at any time and from any place, and they can be contacted in an emergency. The kidney is one of the most important organs in the human body. It is a bean-shaped organ that helps the human body remove waste and excess fluids via urine. When kidney function is lost, waste piles up in the body, potentially harming other organs and triggering a heart attack. According to a research conducted by the American Kidney Fund, kidney disease is the ninth leading cause of death in the United States. In the United States, roughly 31 million people suffer from chronic renal disease.

Renal failure is most often caused by diabetes and high blood pressure. The Internet of Things (IoT) is envisioned as a network of billions of linked items that can detect, communicate, and exchange data. This data can then be analysed to give a wealth of data for planning, management, and decision-making. The Internet of Things will have a significant impact on healthcare, industry, agriculture, telecommunications, and transportation. Despite the popularity of the IoT idea and its promised benefits, its adoption has been slower than expected (K. Kakousis.,et.al, 2010; C. He.,et.al,2013).

SMART HOSPITAL TECHNOLOGIES

We may never return to our prior condition since COVID-19 has had such tremendous impact on individuals from all areas of life. COVID-19 is proven to be a catalyst for digital transformation since it has produced or expanded digital technology applications and use cases. It has also forced governments, businesses, and individuals to rethink their objectives, viewpoints on societal/ethical issues, and commercial practises. As a consequence, many of the above-mentioned reasons for IoT adoption being slower than predicted in various areas have been fixed or decreased. Governments have spent a lot of money on IoT and other technology to combat COVID-19, for example.

COVID-19-induced lifestyle changes, such as working/studying from home, have spawned new IoT use cases with clear ROI, such as remote asset control, workforce monitoring, and remote employee collaboration. As a consequence, many businesses have increased their IoT spending and the pace with which they adopt IoT programmes. Furthermore, the fight against COVID-19 has resulted in a softer stance on privacy issues, improved technical confidence, and accelerated approval procedures. This also opens the way for a more rapid adoption of IoT across many businesses. In addition, regulatory advancements such as corporate cleaning and monitoring rules are hastening the use of IoT in smart buildings.

This article discusses COVID-19's possible impact on IoT adoption in a variety of fields, including healthcare, smart homes, smart buildings, smart cities, transportation, and industrial IoT. To that end, we looked at recent studies from Gartner, Yole, McKinsey, and other consulting firms, as well as relevant research literature over the last several years. COVID-19 does not seem to have aided IoT adoption across all businesses, at least in the short term. Because of the recession, most vehicle companies, for example, are unable to invest in IoT initiatives. As a consequence, we look at COVID-19's impact on IoT adoption in different sectors in the short, medium, and long term. Furthermore, we highlight new initiatives, issues that must be addressed, and major research topics that will allow IoT adoption in each of these businesses.

This is the first research that we are aware of that looks at the impact of COVID-19 on IoT adoption in different businesses. Since the commencement of COVID-19, a slew of publications addressing IoT and COVID-19 have been released. In the following crucial areas, however, our work varies significantly. To begin with, the great majority of current research is limited to IoT in the healthcare sector. Given that COVID-19 is a public health emergency, this is predictable. COVID-19, on the other hand, has impacted almost every aspect of our life, and we provide the first research on its influence on IoT in a number of major areas, including healthcare. Second, most of the present research focuses on how the Internet of Things (IoT) and other digital technologies may (or are) be used to combat COVID-19.

On the other hand, in the aftermath of COVID-19, we not only provide an overview of existing IoT initiatives across numerous sectors, but we also examine the impact of COVID-19 on IoT adoption in these areas. To put it another way, current research focuses on how the Internet of Things (IoT) may or should impact COVID-19, while we examine how COVID-19 affects (or is expected to effect) the IoT sectors. Finally, many of the existing COVID-19 research focus only on current and/or future IoT applications. In this paper, we also look at the impact of COVID-19 on IoT installations as well as the research topics that need to be solved in order to boost IoT adoption in different sectors.

The fast growth of the population has posed several challenges for health care, ultimately leading to a scarcity of medical resources. Given the limited resources available, it is vital to address these difficulties and provide a rapid response. IoT, mobile, and network connections are attractive solutions because to their cheap cost and simplicity of usage. IoT-based healthcare services seek to provide a rich user experience at a low cost while simultaneously enhancing quality of life. The fundamental goal of the Internet of Things is to connect older individuals with chronic diseases to readily available medical resources and to provide trustworthy, efficient, and intelligent healthcare services. Smart healthcare systems, which are often made up of smart sensors, a remote server, and a network, are introduced to the medical industry via the Internet of Things (IoT). This system is intended to provide multi-dimensional monitoring as well as basic therapeutic advice.

In turn, mobile computing provides IoT services via mobile phone services, apps, and the m-health care system. Compactness, IP connectivity, low power consumption, and security are all aspects that e health contributes to the Internet of Things. Many applications have lately been developed in the area of healthcare with the purpose of providing customers with mobile-based services. Patients may use smartphone applications to learn about their conditions after an inquiry in the ends of gynaecology and paediatrics. In healthcare, there are two kinds of IoT applications: single condition apps and clustered condition apps. Only a few of the applications discussed in this article include glucose level sensing, blood pressure monitoring, body temperature monitoring, oxygen saturation monitoring, ECG (electrocardiogram) monitoring, wheelchair management, and rehabilitation. There are several papers on IoT in healthcare that are available, however they are all on IoT in healthcare. The proposed study, on the other hand, is a comprehensive evaluation of existing research on IoT in healthcare using the concept of mobile computing. The contribution of the proposed study is to provide a systematic literature review protocol for examining how mobile computing aids IoTapplications in healthcare, contributes to current and future IoT research work in the healthcare system, provides privacy and security in health IoT devices, and impacts IoT in the healthcare system. To support the proposed research, a total of 116 key papers were included, and the recommended study shows the articles that were included based on the filtering technique and contents. After that, the publications were examined for research concerns that would be addressed in the planned study.

A list of the selected research publications is also included in this section. This part also contains a qualitative and quantitative analysis as well as a related graphic. The third section of this page organises a summary of the selected studies as well as details on the study subjects. Based on the study inquiry, the fourth portion of this article outlines numerous types of constraints. Several ideas for strengthening the IoT are provided at the end of this article. Clinical, financial, and operational data must now be managed and integrated in all health-care organisations, regardless of size. In the current regulatory and economic context, hospitals must focus their efforts on performance criteria that are significant in the short term but will also be critical for long-term success. By giving the relevant information to the appropriate person at the right time, any organisation may improve the delivery of healthcare services and make operations more effective. This is the process through which data becomes intelligence. Different smart gadgets that are currently available and will be accessible in the future must be employed to change a hospital management system into a smart hospital management system. These many devices will help the corporation maintain a seamless flow of data across various systems and corporate divisions, enabling it to function at both a high and low level. At the macroscopic and microscopic levels, patients, caregivers, and attendants may all benefit from increased treatment and satisfaction.

SMART HOSPITAL NETWORKS

Rather than only the absence of sickness, health is described as a full state of physical, mental, and social well-being. The desire for a better existence is inextricably tied to one's physical well-being. Unfortunately, the global health crisis has created a paradox for a variety of reasons, including insufficient health services, large gaps between rural and urban areas, and physician and nurse shortages at vital periods. The Internet of Things (IoT) has been labelled the next technological revolution since it has made every thing inherently connected during the previous decade. Smart health monitoring systems, smart parking, smart homes, smart cities, smart climate, industrial places, and agricultural regions are all examples of IoT applications. Healthcare management, which utilises IoT to monitor health and environmental factors, is the most major use of IoT. IoT refers to the process of using sensors and networks to link computers to the internet. Health-monitoring systems might make use of these interrelated components. M2M, which comprises machinery for computers, machines for people, portable devices, and smartphones, is then used to send the data to distant locations. It's a simple, energy-efficient, more smarter, scalable, and interoperable approach of monitoring and optimising therapy for any health condition. To assist individuals live wiser lives, modern systems now incorporate a customised interface, helpful gadgets, and mental health management.

Heart rate and body temperature are the two most significant indicators of human health. The number of heartbeats per minute, often known as the pulse rate, is the heart rate. By detecting the increase in blood flow volume, calculating the pulses may be utilised to calculate the pulse rate. A typical heart rate for healthy people is between 60 and 100 beats per minute. Adult men's resting heart rates are about 70 beats per minute, whereas adult women's resting heart rates are around 75 beats per minute. Females above the age of 12 had a higher incidence of cardiac disease than men. The quantity of heat released by the body is estimated scientifically, and the temperature of the human body is just the body's heat. A lot of factors impact a person's body temperature, including ambient temperature, gender, and eating habits. In healthy people, it is most likely to be between 97.8 °F (36.5 °C) and 99 °F (37.2 °C). The flu, low-temperature hypothermia, or any other ailment may induce a change in body temperature. Fever is a sign of almost every illness.

There are invasive and noninvasive methods for assessing heart rate and body temperature. Consumers have found noninvasive approaches to be accurate and convenient over time. It is important that a healthcare institution provide patients with pleasant room conditions. Factors such as room humidity, CO2 levels, and other gases may influence the quality of a room's atmosphere. Patients are at risk from toxic chemicals and particular humidity levels. For best comfort, the room humidity should be between 30 and 65 percent. Some studies are carried out only for the objective of creating a smart home, rather than for specialised healthcare. There are many severe diseases in the medical industry, such as heart disease, diabetes, breast cancer, liver disease, and so on, but the fundamental goal of our system is to track the basic symptoms of all patients as well as the patient's room environment. This article proposes a customised healthcare system that employs sensors to monitor patients' pulse and body temperature, as well as room humidity, CO, and CO2 gas levels, and communicates the data through Wi-Fi to medical workers. Apart from customising essential health-related criteria, the developed solution addresses the problem of maintaining a single patient database at hospitals through a web server.

In this system, the gas sensor is used to identify an unexpected occurrence by comparing performance to a threshold and generating a PPM signal if the output value exceeds the threshold. A smart city differs from traditional metropolitan areas in that it combines cutting-edge technology (such as big data, the Internet of Things, machine learning, sensor networks, 2G, 3G, and 4G connectivity, and high-performance computing equipment) with innovative ideas to improve the lives of its residents. Risks (increased temperature, air pollution, lack of transportation infrastructure, disaster conditions, traffic, and dramatic changes in the landscapes, ferocity, crime, and unemployment) are currently confronting urban areas with the current infrastructure and resources, which are barely adequate to meet the rapidly expanding urban population. Information and communication technology (ICT) as well as a combination of creative ideas may be used to tackle the difficulties. This kind of innovation assists in the interface and integration of the city's systems, as well as its services, in order to boost the citizens' personal pleasure. As a consequence, smarter cities make it simpler to make better use of existing infrastructure and resources. The Internet of Things (IoT) concept is built on the power of smart, self-configuring items that are closely connected via a global network foundation. The Internet of Things (IoT) is often defined as a physical item with limited storage capabilities, broadly dispersed and handling capacities, as well as the security and dependability of smart city frameworks. The following paper evaluates IoT-based smart city data from relevant publications based on this basis.

The Internet of Things is made up of three layers: an application layer, a network layer, and a perception layer. The perception layer is made up of a group of internet-connected devices that can gather data, recognise things, perceive information, and exchange it with other devices through the internet. Cameras, radio frequency identification devices (RFID), global positioning systems (GPS), and sensors are examples of perception layer devices. The network layer's responsibilities include delivering data from the perception layer to the application layer while staying within network, device, and application constraints. IoT systems communicate data from perception devices to a nearby gateway using a combination of short-range network communication protocols including ZigBee and Bluetooth, depending on the communication parties' capabilities. Internet technologies such as 4G, Wifi, 5G, and power line connection (PLC) transport data across huge distances depending on the implementation.

The data is received and processed at the application layer since the purpose of applications is to develop smart cities, power system monitoring, smart homes, demand-side energy management, renewable energy generator integration, and distributed power storage coordination. As a consequence, we'll be able to create more efficient power distribution and management techniques. The smart health illness monitoring system interacts with the smart health care system. The key objectives of this monitoring are smart IoT devices and smart backbone devices. This is very beneficial to cloud computing and significant server systems in hospitals. Based on a personal poll and a global response, the World Health Organization (WHO) has announced plans to establish the Disease Intelligence Unit, which will function independently. The backbone network, which is today's most urgent demand, has been attained through trends and analysis. Smart disease surveillance is a revolutionary new way to speeding up the present monitoring process and achieving the highest levels of accuracy and real-time database. Smart disease monitoring is an epidemiological technology that enables epidemics to be tracked and spread. The primary responsibility is to predict and monitor threats to people's lives. Organizations like the World Health Organization (WHO) and disease control centres, for example, may now report using more advanced and complex tools like the "smart grid" and smart devices like heart monitors, biochips, and transponders.

CONCLUSION

The smart backbone relies on smart servers to keep track of time and give information. A smart health-care system is necessary due to a lack of information, limited facilities, and undeveloped technology in the current health-care system. On-network services at the hospital aid patients and clinicians with remote service delivery. Smart phone applications connected to the health care system may provide patients with advise on which decisions to make. IoT enables the tagging of any patient and the retrieval of health-care data through an address or database associated with a particular RFID tag (Radio frequency identification). RFID tags attach to goods are automatically identified and tracked using electromagnetic waves. Diagnosis, treatment, health professionals, and policies are the most important aspects of health care, with medical issues and public health tossed in for good measure. The phrase "individual health system" refers to how individuals, institutions, and resources are organised to offer health-care services in order to meet the need for smart health-care. The smart health care system based on IOT includes ehealth and smart devices as upgrade tools, as well as future smart healthcare technologies.

REFERENCES

Ahn, B. G., Noh, Y. H., & Jeong, D. U. (2015). *Smart chair based on multi heart rate detection system.* IEEE Sensors.

Almotiri, S. H., Khan, M. A., & Alghamdi, M. A. (2016). Mobile health (m-health) system in the context of iot. *2016 IEEE 4th International Conference on Future Internet of Things and Cloud Workshops (FiCloudW)*, 39–42.

Barger, T. S., Brown, D. E., & Alwan, M. (2005). Health-status monitoring through analysis of behavioral patterns. *IEEE Transactions on Systems, Man, and Cybernetics. Part A, Systems and Humans*, *5*(1), 22–27. doi:10.1109/TSMCA.2004.838474

Chiuchisan, I., Costin, H. N., & Geman, O. (2014). Adopting the internet of things technologies in health care systems. *2014 International Conference and Exposition on Electrical and Power Engineering (EPE)*, 532–535. 10.1109/ICEPE.2014.6969965

Dwivedi, A., Bali, R. K., Belsis, M. A., Naguib, R. N. G., Every, P., & Nassar, N. S. (2003). Towards a practical healthcare information security model for healthcare institutions. *4th International IEEE EMBS Special Topic Conference on Information Technology Applications in Biomedicine*, 114–117. 10.1109/ITAB.2003.1222486

Gupta, M. S. D., Patchava, V., & Menezes, V. (2015). Healthcare based on iot using raspberry pi. *2015 International Conference on Green Computing and Internet of Things (ICGCIoT)*, 796–799. 10.1109/ICGCIoT.2015.7380571

He, C., Fan, X., & Li, Y. (2013). Toward Ubiquitous Healthcare Services With a Novel Efficient Cloud Platform. *IEEE Transactions on Biomedical Engineering*, *60*(1), 230–234. doi:10.1109/TBME.2012.2222404 PMID:23060318

Istepanaian, R. S. H., & Zhang, Y.-T. (2012). Guest editorial introduction to the special section: 4 G health—The long-term evolution of m-health. *IEEE Transactions on Information Technology in Biomedicine*, *16*(1), 1–5. doi:10.1109/TITB.2012.2183269 PMID:22271836

Kakousis, K., Paspallis, N., & Papadopoulos, G. A. (2010). A survey of software adaptation in mobile and ubiquitous computing. *Enterprise Information Systems*, *4*(4), 355–389. doi:10.1080/17517575.2010.509814

Kang, W., Kapitanova, K., & Son, S. H. (2012). RDDS: A real-time data distribution service for cyber-physical systems. *IEEE Transactions on Industrial Informatics*, *8*(2), 393–405. doi:10.1109/TII.2012.2183878

Kyusakov, R., Eliasson, J., Delsing, J., Deventer, J. V., & Gustafsson, J. (2013). Integration of wireless sensor and actuator nodes with IT infrastructure using service-oriented architecture. *IEEE Transactions on Industrial Informatics*, *9*(1), 43–51. doi:10.1109/TII.2012.2198655

Li, S., Xu, L., Wang, X., & Wang, J. (2012). Integration of hybrid wireless networks in cloud services oriented enterprise information systems. *Enterprise Information Systems*, *6*(2), 165–187. doi:10.1080/17517575.2011.654266

Pereira, N., Andersson, B., & Tovar, E. (2007). WiDom:Adominance protocol for wireless medium access. *IEEE Transactions on Industrial Informatics*, *3*(2), 120–130. doi:10.1109/TII.2007.898461

Valls, M. G., & Val, P. B. (2013). Usage of DDS data-centric middleware for remote monitoring and control laboratories. *IEEE Transactions on Industrial Informatics*, *9*(1), 567–574. doi:10.1109/TII.2012.2211028

Wang, K., Bai, X., Li, J., & Ding, C. (2010). A service-based framework for pharmacogenomics data integration. *Enterprise Information Systems*, *4*(3), 225–245. doi:10.1080/17517575.2010.498525

Chapter 8
Monitoring Supply Chain Management in Healthcare Using Wireless Sensor Networks

Amit Chugh
IMS Engineering College, Ghaziabad, India

Supriya P. Panda
https://orcid.org/0000-0001-8054-8567
Manav Rachna International Institute of Research and Studies, Faridabad, India

ABSTRACT

The healthcare system is transforming from traditional medication to smart healthcare. Smart healthcare plays a vital role in urban development. Medicines and injections are the key building blocks of the healthcare system. Environmental conditions like temperature, pressure, and humidity can adversely affect the quality of medicines and injections. So, maintaining proper temperature and humidity is a must to keep them safe. There is need of continuous monitoring of medicines and injections during their supply chain. The wireless sensor network (WSN) strives to detect surrounding parameters and relay sensed data to the base station without any human deployment. Supply chain management (SCM) in healthcare system is also one of the applications, which requires a different type of monitoring, supervision, and handling at different levels. WSN adds a contribution in the making of smart healthcare, as it uses the smart way (sensors) of monitoring the medicines and injections in the supply chain.

INTRODUCTION

Sensor networks have a wide range of applications (Muduli et al., 2018; Ramson, 2017; Rashid & Rehmani, 2016). Sensor networks are in use to make monitoring efficient whether in environment or health science or habitat or Industry. Out of many plication areas, supply chain management (SCM) is the one which is touching everyone's life. Sensors were limited with the challenge of tracking so the idea is to combine sensors with Radio Frequency Identification (RFID) have given the benefit of tracking

DOI: 10.4018/978-1-6684-2508-4.ch008

along with monitoring (Zhang & Wang, 2006). The integration of RFID and sensor nodes can be done by multiple ways one of them is RFID tags along with sensors, the other can be special hardware in the sensor or third option can be a combination of all. The combination of RFID and sensor nodes brings the next leaf in contrast to the tradition Wireless Sensor Network (WSN) or network of RFID (Clauberg, 2004). The author Clueberg has worked on funded research by combining sensors for monitoring and RFID for identification to show improved supply chain management (Clauberg, 2004). In the designed network Actuator Unit (AU) and Sensor Unit (SU) communicate observations to central servers through Gateways. This combination of the sensor along with RFID can work to make better management of the supply chain. SCM deals with opportunities and threats to integrate supply and demand to ensure successful coordination. It reduces the total cost and also improves operational efficiency. Out of many reasons of importance to monitor SCM, one is user awareness as they are always keen to have the best quality (Alfian et al., 2017; Wang et al., 2015). So, it can be said that user awareness about health is also a driving force that quality of food items during supply should also be monitored so that standards could meet the expectation. Without any doubt it can be said that monitored SCM could lead to improve quality assurance, and integrity in food products along a guarantee food safety (Alfian et al., 2017; Gomez et al., 2012; Wang et al., 2013). Authors Gong li and Jing shi have explored the application of WSN for service innovation in SCM (Li & Shi, 2010).

RELATED WORK

Authors Evers et al. have shown the role of WSN in SCM automation (Evers & Havinga, 2007). This work is a demonstration of the Sensor Scheme to show the work of sensors in the supply chain. For simulation purposes, the shipment of bananas from one stop to another location had been considered. Throughout the complete supply chain, the sensors are placed to perform various tasks. Sensors are attached to pallets in which bananas are kept. Here the first task of the sensor is to monitor whether the temperature is sufficiently cold or not. In the next step, their placement is considered. Further, their location is tracked like where the shipment is now and has it reached the proper destination or not? Complete tracking is aimed in such a manner that even a single wrong step will trigger an alarm. This alarm can let the business authorities know about unusual or unexpected scenarios during the supply chain. This paper alarm is shown by the use of a red LED and successful transmission is by a green LED.

The paper (Alfian et al., 2017) describes the food traceability system that achieves customer confidence by assisting the assurance of quality and safety of food along the supply chain. The paper (Alfian et al., 2017) discussed the use of sensor networks in pedigree food chain supply systems. The author has combined WSN, RFID, Data Mining, and multilayer perceptron to make a successful system, out of which WSN is playing the role of temperature monitoring. The benefit of this integration is multifold. for example, the cost of deployment will be reduced because now sensors will be collecting data, second benefit can be in terms of delay time, which can be surely reduced by applying appropriate routing or clustering in WSNs. Sensors are mainly focusing on temperature and humidity. In the case of perishable food products, temperature plays a vital role in affecting the quality and safety of the same. Sensor nodes that constitute the WSN monitor environmental conditions like temperature, pressure, and humidity. WSN plays an important part in the traceability system, as it monitors the conditions of perishable food items and can help to maintain the safety and quality of such food products in the supply chain. During transportation in the supply chain, there can be a possibility that the sensors may not successfully transmit the data due to network communication problems or a lesser battery lifetime. Data mining techniques can be used to predict the missing sensor data and a traceable system will ensure the complete history of temperature and humidity during that phase of the supply chain. Further, the supply chain is controlled with the use of RFID with prediction based on the multilayer perceptron model. This proposed model has benefited both managers and customers by providing a web-based interface for real-time location through RFID and temperature and humidity control with sensors.

Li introduced the concept of Hybrid Sensor Node (HSN) which is a combination of RFID tag, reduced function RFID reader (RFRR), and sensor unit (Li et al., 2008). RFRR is an exceptional sensor node that reads the tag information of neighbor HSN's and writes that into their tag. The sensor unit monitors the environmental condition and writes in its tag. So, every HSN node has its surrounding information and its neighbor HSNs as well. The advantage of using HSN is that the RFID reader's channel congestion can be reduced, as it is not required for every HSN to be in the range of the reader. It also reduces the cost of deployment as there is no requirement to use multiple readers or high-quality readers. HSN can be in active or sleep mode. In an active mode, its sensor unit will monitor the environment & write it into the tag. Tag information of its neighbor node can also be read and written in its tag during this mode. In sleep mode the node will not perform any function, however, its tag information can be read by its neighboring nodes. The time frame for active and sleep mode will depend upon the need for application, as the critical application requires frequent data updating and trivial applications can work on low-frequency data updations.

Paper (Evers, 2007) defines supply chain automation with wireless sensors by introducing a system named Sensor Scheme. The proposed work is proving greater efficiency along with security. The author used sensors as Active Transport Tracking Devices (ATTD) fixed on Returnable Transport Items (RTIs) to enhance the quality of service. ATTD will be performing various tasks throughout the supply chain of goods. For example, in the first step sensors say ATTD will be monitoring temperature for perseverance, in the next step, they will be monitoring surrounding for perseverance. Further, they along with RFID will allow tracking of the items. ATTD which is attached to RTI can ensure no leakage of material and also proper placement of containers. During the complete journey of supply, sensors can do different types of verifications which will lead to an improvement in the quality of service. Sensor Scheme is a runtime system well programmed for transport monitoring and fault detection in the supply chain.

Paper (Molka-Danielsen et al., 2018) has discussed the integration of Big Data (BD) and Industrial Internet-of-Things (IIOT) with WSN for Logistics Shipping Base. The work is done for Air Quality Monitoring with the help of Sensor nodes. The comfort and health of workers largely depend on Air quality wherever they are working. Various studies support that production quality is not independent of workers' safety. After all, this can't be ignored that ensuring production quality is the first step of a successful supply chain. The authors researched pilot monitoring of the air quality of two buildings. Sensor units are placed at height and will be measuring atmospheric parameters including gases present, the surrounding temperature, humidity in the environment, etc. This Monitoring could benefit in a way to give workers a safe working place which further results in enhanced productivity and employee effectiveness. This monitored data will be considered big data that will be worked with IIOT in decision-making for the health and safety of the workplace. The integration of WSN with BD and IIOT can make automation better for Industry 4.0 era.

Similarly, WSN with RFID help to monitor & track the supply chain of drugs and injections in the healthcare system. As the health of the patient cannot be compromised at any cost, for the same it is of utmost urgency to maintain the quality of medicines and injections during its supply chain. Temperature and humidity are the factors that could affect the quality of medicines and injections, so it is important to keep them at adequate temperature and humidity. WSN will help in monitoring the environmental conditions and will generate required alarms for unwanted conditions. These raised alarms will be the key to maintaining the quality of the lifesaving products and will provide social and economic benefits. RFID can be beneficial in tracking the location of critical medicines and injections. That will help in calculating the estimated time of arrival in case of emergency and necessary actions can be taken accordingly. So WSN with RFID will play a crucial role in attaining urban development in the healthcare sector.

MEDC with Relay Nodes in SCM For Healthcare

Researchers in Paper (Alfian et al., 2017; Chugh & Panda, 2019) have discussed the issue of data loss on the sensor side. The sensor may lose sensed information due to multiple reasons; battery level is a major of them. There can be many energy-saving solutions that can ensure prolonged battery life, in other words, WSN with a more lifetime (Chugh & Panda, 2019). One Proposed solution Mutual Exclusive Distributive Clustering (MEDC) with relay nodes in paper (Chugh & Panda, 2018) can also become a clear solution for power saving. Before the concept of the relay node, MEDC clustering was solving the issue the first hand by taking away the need for transmission via every sensor (Singh & Chugh, 2013). Only the cluster head will take the charge of transmission of sensed information to the base station. Later the energy of cluster head can be saved by delegating the role of forwarding to another node within the cluster. The selection of cluster head is done based on residual energy. After every iteration, a node with the highest residual energy in the cluster is given the responsibility of forwarding the data. The Introduction of the concept of the relay node is to reduce the burden over the cluster head. As the cluster head is burdened with both the responsibility of collecting the sensed data and forwarding the same to the base station, the relay node will take the responsibility of forwarding the data and reducing the burden on the cluster head. The relay node will be selected in the same fashion as the cluster head. A node with the highest residual energy will be the cluster head and the second-highest energy node in the cluster will be elected as a relay node. In the next iteration, the same process will repeat and the selection of cluster head and relay nodes will be done. This concept will help out in reducing the energy loss of WSN and the network could sustain for a longer period of time. Monitoring of healthcare products in SCM through MEDC and MEDC with the relay in WSN is simulated in MATLAB 9.0 environment. Various ranges of communication like 15, 20, and 25 are been taken to compare the lifetime time of sensor nodes in MEDC and MEDC with the relay. The result corresponding to range 15 is shown in Figure 1. It clearly shows that MEDC with relay nodes sustains for a longer period of time. In the same fashion comparison on range 20 is given in Figure 2 and MEDC with relay sustains up to 700 rounds however the MEDC network gets down around 600 rounds. Similarly, on range 25, MEDC with relay has more live sensor nodes at 500 rounds however there is no live node in MEDC even at 400 rounds and the same is shown in Figure 3.

In supply chain management, there can be a requirement for long-distance transportation of medical products. To monitor the same, there is a requirement for a WSN that utilizes the energy of sensor nodes effectively so that network could sustain during long transportation in SCM. MEDC with relay nodes will help out in the above scenarios by supporting the network to utilize the energy efficiently and be live for a longer period of time. With this proposed solution it has been shown that network lifetime has improved by 10-30 percent (Chugh & Panda, 2020; Chugh & Panda, 2022). The benefit of this can be taken in supply chain Management also. It was observed many times that SCM monitoring gets compromised due to dead sensor nodes with a reason of battery power. So can be concluded if clustering can be programmed then all sensor cluster members can save energy by giving their sensed information to the cluster head. The relay nodes can help further to save the energy of cluster heads.

So, sensors will keep sensing and monitoring after that cluster heads will aggregate the sensed information, and the relay node will take the task of forwarding this information. In this way, communication will be less energy-consuming and there will be fewer dead nodes. So, we can say better Monitoring of the supply chain could be done.

Figure 1. Comparison of MEDC and MEDC with Relay in SCM at RC 15

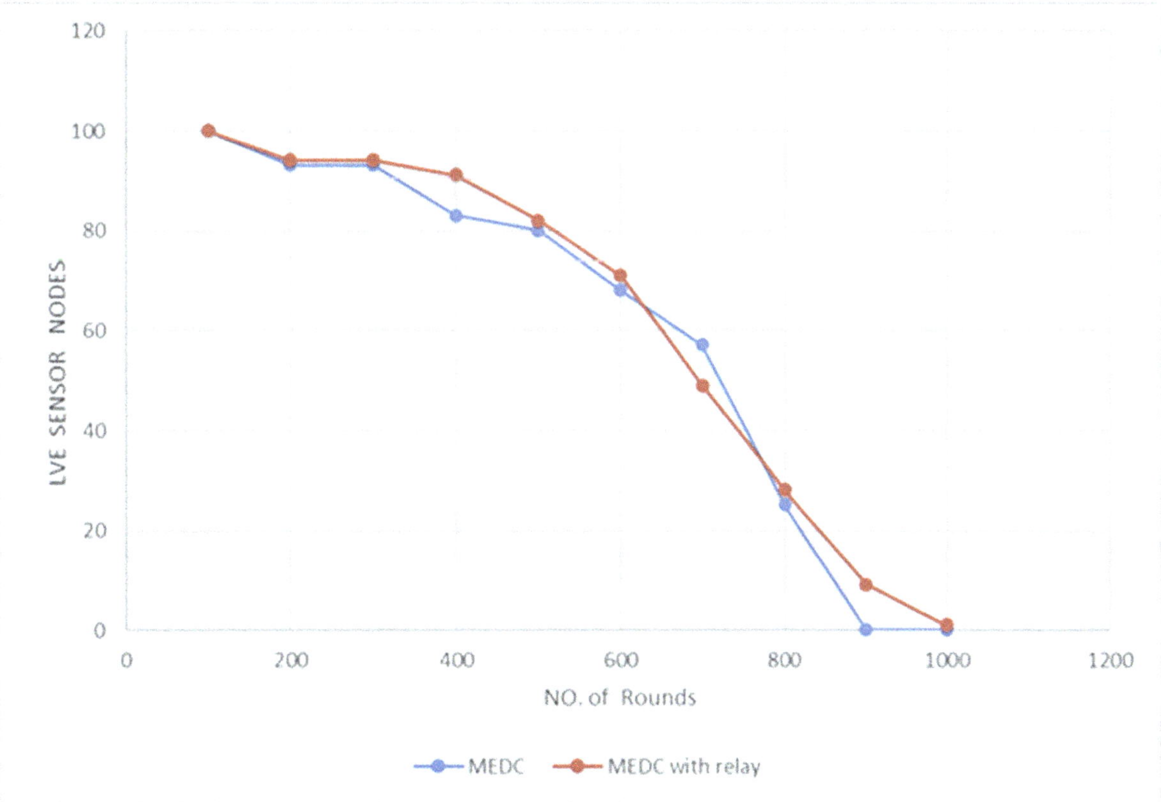

Figure 2. Comparison of MEDC and MEDC with Relay in SCM at RC 20

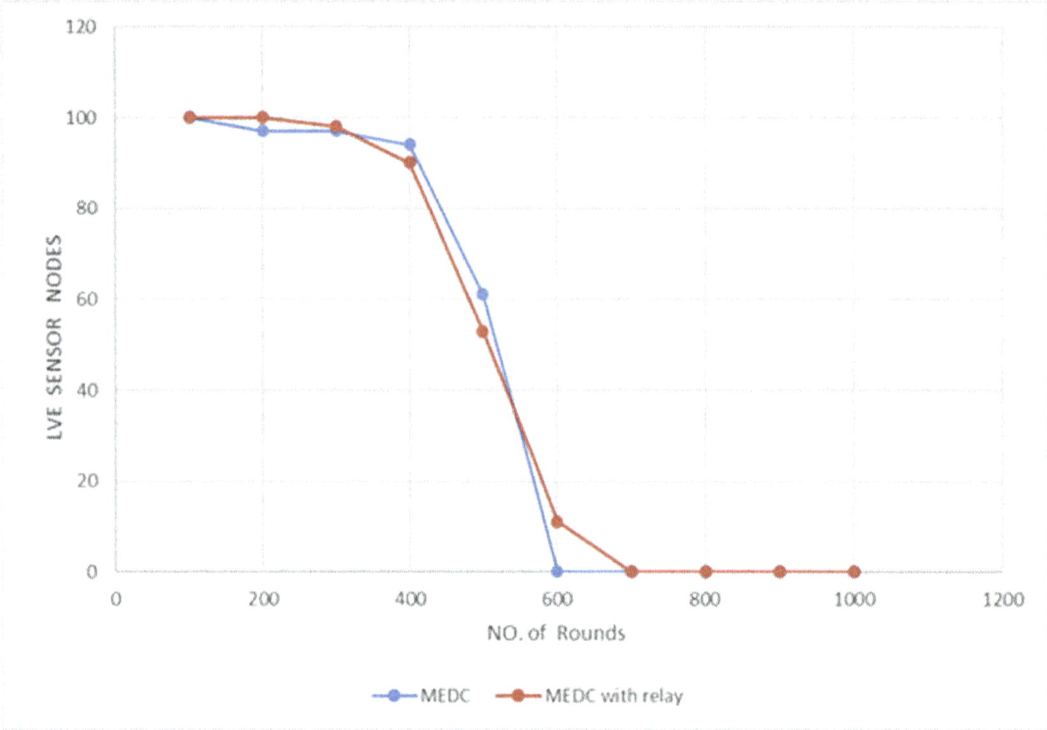

Figure 3. Comparison of MEDC and MEDC with Relay in SCM at RC 25

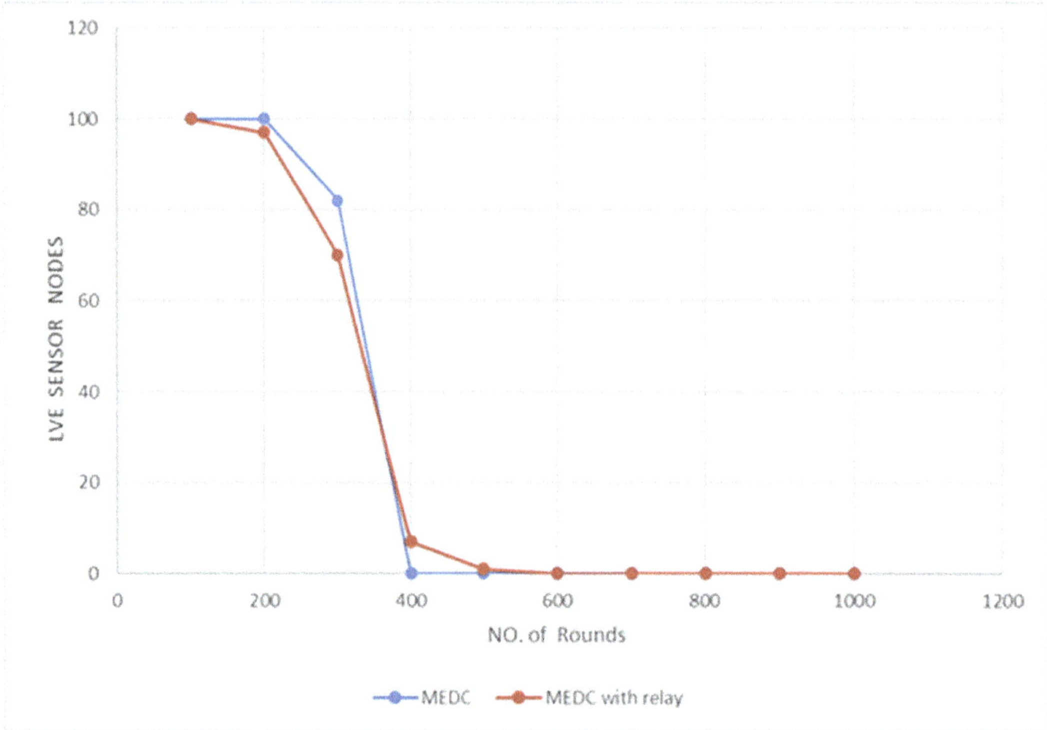

CONCLUSION

RFID combined with WSN can play a significant role in the monitoring of healthcare products in supply chain management. Monitoring the temperature and humidity of medicines and injections helps in maintaining the quality and value of healthcare products. Monitoring SCM not only leads to quality and cost-effectiveness but also enhances customer belief. One challenge in monitoring through WSN can be the battery of sensors. Low battery power can be one of the concerns in WSN when the product is to be transported for a longer distance. MEDC with relay nodes in WSN can be one of the solutions that can help to utilize energy in effective manner and make the network live for a longer period of period. By using this solution energy of cluster members will be saved by communicating to near cluster head instead of far located base station and also the energy of cluster heads will be further saved by delegating forwarding tasks to relay nodes. So, it can be concluded that the proposed solution could supports the network to work uninterrupted even for long transportation in supply chain management.

REFERENCES

Alfian, G., Rhee, J., Ahn, H., Lee, J., Farooq, U., Ijaz, M. F., & Syaekhoni, M. A. (2017). Integration of RFID, wireless sensor networks, and data mining in an e-pedigree food traceability system. *Journal of Food Engineering*, *212*, 65–75. doi:10.1016/j.jfoodeng.2017.05.008

Chugh, A., & Panda, S. (2018). Strengthening clustering through relay nodes in sensor networks. *Procedia Computer Science*, *132*, 689–695. doi:10.1016/j.procs.2018.05.072

Chugh, A., & Panda, S. (2019). Energy efficient techniques in wireless sensor networks. *Recent Patents on Engineering*, *13*(1), 13–19. doi:10.2174/1872212112666180731114046

Chugh, A., & Panda, S. (2020). Relay Node Employment for Performance Enhancement of MEDC in Wireless Sensor Network. *International Journal of Innovative Technology and Exploring Engineering*, *9*(6), 835–839. doi:10.35940/ijitee.F3943.049620

Chugh, A., & Panda, S. P. (2022). Improved MEDC Protocol through Relay Nodes in Wireless Sensor Networks. In *Futuristic Sustainable Energy & Technology: Proceedings of the International Conference on Futuristic Sustainable Energy &Technology (ICFSE, 2021)* (p. 259). CRC Press. 10.1201/9781003272328-30

Clauberg, R. (2004). RFID and sensor networks. *Proc. RFID Workshop*.

Evers, L. (2007). Sensorscheme: Supply chain management automation using wireless sensor networks. In *2007 IEEE Conference on Emerging Technologies and Factory Automation (EFTA 2007)*. IEEE. 10.1109/EFTA.2007.4416802

Evers, L., & Havinga, P. (2007). Supply chain management automation using wireless sensor networks. In *2007 IEEE International Conference on Mobile Adhoc and Sensor Systems*. IEEE. 10.1109/MOBHOC.2007.4428689

Gomez, Laurent, & El Moustaine. (2012). Risk assessment along supply chain: A RFID and wireless sensor network integration approach. *Sensors & Transducers, 14*(2), 269.

Li, G., & Shi, J. (2010). Wireless sensor network technology and its application potentials for service innovation in supply chain management. *International Journal of Applied Logistics*, *1*(4), 30–51. doi:10.4018/jal.2010100103

Li, Z., Shen, H., & Alsaify, B. (2008). Integrating RFID with wireless sensor networks for inhabitant, environment and health monitoring. In *2008 14th IEEE International Conference on Parallel and Distributed Systems*. IEEE. 10.1109/ICPADS.2008.66

Molka-Danielsen, J., Engelseth, P., & Wang, H. (2018). Large scale integration of wireless sensor network technologies for air quality monitoring at a logistics shipping base. *Journal of Industrial Information Integration*, *10*, 20–28. doi:10.1016/j.jii.2018.02.001

Muduli, L., Mishra, D. P., & Jana, P. K. (2018). Application of wireless sensor network for environmental monitoring in underground coal mines: A systematic review. *Journal of Network and Computer Applications*, *106*, 48–67. doi:10.1016/j.jnca.2017.12.022

Ramson, S. R. (2017). *Applications of wireless sensor networks—A survey. In 2017 international conference on innovations in electrical, electronics, instrumentation and media technology (ICEEIMT)*. IEEE.

Rashid, B., & Rehmani, M. H. (2016). Applications of wireless sensor networks for urban areas: A survey. *Journal of Network and Computer Applications*, *60*, 192–219. doi:10.1016/j.jnca.2015.09.008

Singh, Y., & Chugh, U. (2013). Mutual Exclusive Distributive Clustering (MEDC) Protocol for Wireless Sensor Networks. *International Journal of Sensors, Wireless Communications and Control*, *3*(2), 101–107. doi:10.2174/22103279030214050510025 3

Wang, J., Wang, H., He, J., Li, L., Shen, M., Tan, X., Min, H., & Zheng, L. (2015). Wireless sensor network for real-time perishable food supply chain management. *Computers and Electronics in Agriculture*, *110*, 196–207. doi:10.1016/j.compag.2014.11.009

Wang, L., Da Xu, L., Bi, Z., & Xu, Y. (2013). Data cleaning for RFID and WSN integration. *IEEE Transactions on Industrial Informatics*, *10*(1), 408–418. doi:10.1109/TII.2013.2250510

Zhang, L., & Wang, Z. (2006). Integration of RFID into wireless sensor networks: architectures, opportunities and challenging problems. In *2006 Fifth international conference on grid and cooperative computing workshops* (pp. 463-469). IEEE. 10.1109/GCCW.2006.58

Chapter 9
Design and Implementation of Smart and Safety Device for Women and Children

Vijayakumari B.
https://orcid.org/0000-0003-0564-1301
Mepco Schlenk Engineering College, India

Benitha V. S.
Mepco Schlenk Engineering College, India

Shabna R. M.
Mepco Schlenk Engineering College, India

Siva Sundari T.
Mepco Schlenk Engineering College, India

Manonmani T.
Mepco Schlenk Engineering College, India

ABSTRACT

In modern India, with the government surveys, it is clearly agreed upon that still women are the major victims of violent crimes and harassment. Since most of the women employees are there in all the fields, women have to travel a long distance lonely and during late hours also. Thus, women's safety is a much desired need of this hour. This chapter focuses to provide safety for women and to reduce the number of crimes to some extent and provides security exclusively for women employees. The ultimate aim of the device is to transmit the emergency situation of the victim along with their current location to parents and the police for help. The location is traced using GPS and a message is sent via GSM to the pre-defined numbers. When women sense that they are in danger they can manually press the button so that their current location along with an alert message is sent to the predefined numbers. The device can involuntarily detect the emergency situation by fall detection sensor and heart rate sensor. This module can also send an alert using medical emergency.

DOI: 10.4018/978-1-6684-2508-4.ch009

1 INTRODUCTION

In the modern civilization there is a saying that 'Men and women should be treated equally'. Today they are no more homemakers. Women can help the society in all aspects from space to sports. But the truth is that women are not safe. For every single minute a baby girl to woman are getting harassed. The proposed device is a safety device which can be used in case of emergency. It is a personal safety device which makes you and your friends safer for 24/7. The ultimate aim of the device is to intimate the parents and police that the girl is in danger. The device can be operated in two ways either by manually or automatically. The ultimate aim of the device is to clannish the emergency situation of the victim along with their current location to parents and the police for sudden help. The system that we have proposed is manual cum automatic device that may help victim in case of emergency and also provides medical alert in case of emergency. The objective is to provide wearable security device that needs to be compact and henceforth the module is controlled using Arduino Nano.

2 RELATED WORK

Yi Shu et al. (2015) designed a device which is used to measure the heart rate using polymer based pressure sensor. (Bandana and Ajit Kumar, 2016 a) designed a device for the monitoring of heart rate continuously and supervise the woman for any abnormalities, if any change in the range, an immediate alert message is sent to the rescue team. Higher level of heart rate is notified by the increased level of epinephrine hormone. This device can be miniaturized in future and can be implanted in jewelries, mobile phones, etc. Monisha et al. (2016 b) proposed a mobile based device if the volume button is pressed once, then message will be sent and if it is pressed twice, message and audio will be sent and if the button is pressed long time, then it makes a call to police. The main characteristics is that all the wearable devices are in the form of armband, the reason is that, it is much easier to detect the fall. Holovatyy et al. (2017 a) developed a model for the low cost and rapid device Modification for the principle of Analysis of Vibration Acceleration Spectrum(MANVAS). Aihua Mao et al. (2017 b) designed a device which can measure a fall which in turn uses tri-axis accelerometer to detect whether the women is fall or not, which indirectly implies that the victim is not in the position to turn on the switch. Javier Medina Quero et al. (2017 c) designed a wrist based device which in turn used to improve the quality of heart rate sensors and applications and also uses a fuzzy model for real time monitoring. R.A. Mahajan et al. (2017 d) designed a device which sends the message either in online or offline based on the victim's network connectivity. If the victim is in online, it records audio which is converted to text and the message will be sent and in case if offline, the SMS will sent to the numbers which contains alert messages along with location.

Darshik et al.(2017 e) proposed a device for the communication of the alarming situation to the police and parents is successfully achieved by GPS & GSM/GPRS. (Roshini and Mohan, 2018 a) innovated a device that has the access to the GPS and messaging services which is preprogrammed in such a way that whenever it receives an emergency alert, it can immediately intimate nearby radius police station for the quick recovery. Arunachalam et al. (2018 b) designed a device to sense the vigorous falling which indirectly indicates that the victim is badly attacked and also not in a position to manually press the switch and it is further improvised by Diana et al. (2018 c) for the monitoring of elderly people. At present several solutions has been proposed for the fall detection, and they are categorized into three types based on the sensor technology: Non-wearable based systems (NWS), Wearable based system (WS) and Fusion or Hybrid based systems (FS). Samad et al.(2018 d) proposed the accelerometer-based fall detection for the evidential in the detection of a Valid fall occurrence. Self-defense mechanism is also included in the armband for the short term prevention. Rosaria et al. (2018 e) designed a device which detects both static falls (standing) and dynamic falls (walking) which can be achieved by accelerometer sensor that detects potential falls.

This paper proposes the module which provides safety in case of any emergency situations for women. This paper is organized into six chapters include introduction, Relater work, Proposed system, hardware requirements, Results and implementation and finally concluded.

3 PROPOSED SYSTEM

3.1 System Architecture

This module composed of GPS, GSM/GPRS, Accelerometer sensor, Heart rate sensor, siren, flash light and Shock circuit.

The proposed system uses three modules:

(I) Switch
(II) Accelerometer sensor
(III) Heart rate sensor

The overall performance is controlled by Arduino Nano. The system is based on non-Android which makes easier for the children to operate. The overall system is shown in Fig.1.

Figure 1. Block diagram of armband

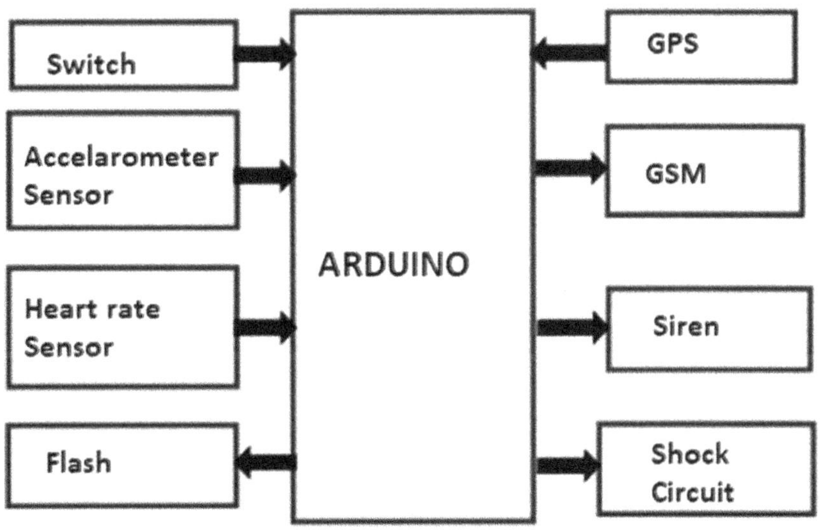

3.2 System Design

The proposed system for the safety armband has facility of activations of both manual and automatic methods. This has been constructed in the point of view that women may be pushed into any kind of situations that she can be attacked expectedly or by unexpectedly. The working of module doesn't end only with the simple notification. Though women are brave and mentally strong, they need some physical support for safeguarding themselves until the arrival of police. This has additional improved feature like self-defense mechanism which can help the victim to safeguard themselves until the arrival of police for their rescue.

The proposed system works on the flow such that when the victim feels that she is in danger she can hand operate the module by pressing the button so that the current location of the victim gets tracked and it is get transmitted in the form of a text message to the parents and cops. If the victim is attacked unexpectedly and is not in a stable condition to voluntarily press the switch, the module can be operated on the basis of sensor values. The sensors used in the modules are accelerometer sensor and heart rate sensor. The sudden and heavy fall can be traced by accelerometer sensor and the danger situation is intimated via SMS. The heart rate sensor traces the heart beat in which it may rise vigorously due to some frustrations or any heart disease.

This is also intimated through SMS. The text message consists of the current site of the victim so that the police can reach the spot immediately. Until the arrival of the police the victim needs to be safeguarding herself. For that, this module have siren and Flash which can cover the nearby people's attention for help. The proposed flow is shown in Figure 2.

4 HARDWARE DESCRIPTION

Controller Unit

Arduino nano is a small, flexible and compact microcontroller board developed by arduino.cc, based on AT mega 328p.Arduino nano board is similar to arduino Uno board but quite in small size. The operating voltage is 5V.However the input voltage varies between 7V to 12V.Arduino nano pinout contains 8 analog pins, 14 digital pins, 2 reset pins & 6 power pins. It consists of a crystal oscillator of frequency 16MHZ.Tiny size and breadboard friendly nature of arduino nano make this device as an ideal choice for most of the applications.

Location Tracking Unit

The current location of women is tracked by GPS NEO6M module. The GPS NEO6M is compatible with all microcontroller boards. The module has four pins: VCC, TX, RX & GND. The module can communicate with arduino through TX and RX pins. It is highly sensible for indoor application.

Figure 2. Flow diagram of the prototype working

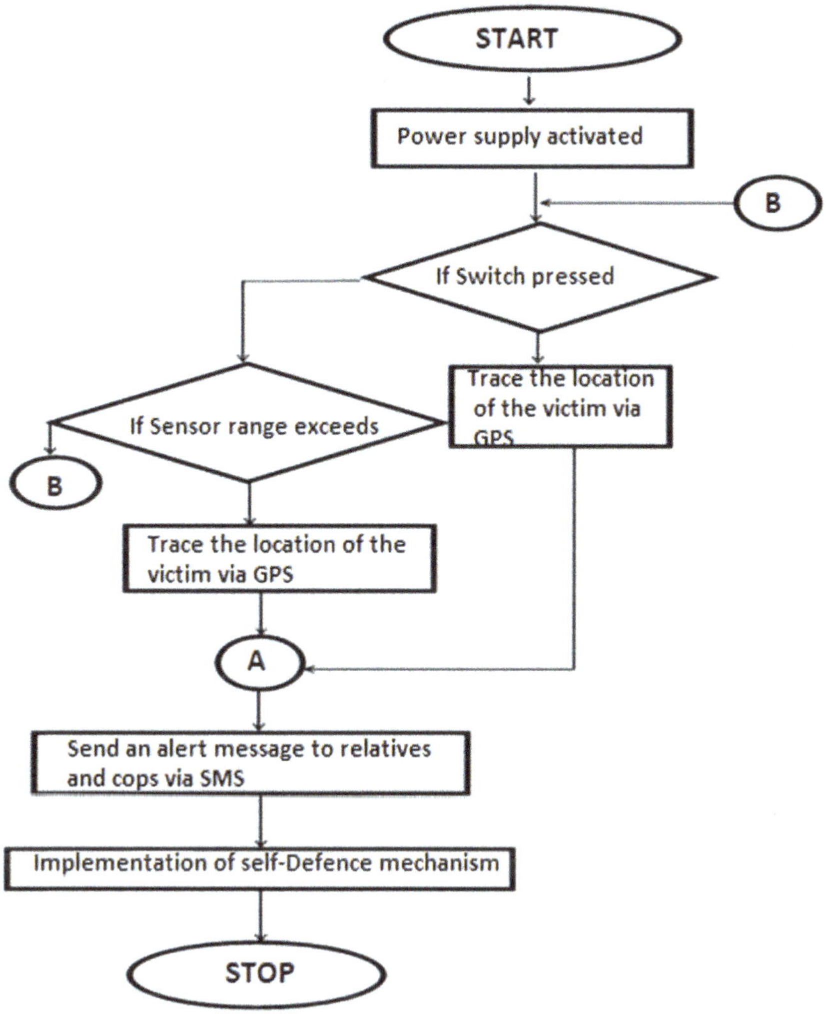

Cellular Messaging Unit

The cellular messaging unit used in this device is GSM SIM800C. SIM 800C is a complete Quad-band GSM/GPRS solution in SMT type. With the tiny size of it, this can be readily fit into compact design of customer's application. It is suitable for the transmission of SMS, Voice and DATA transfer applications in M2M interface.

Sensing Unit

Accelerometer sensor: Accelerometer sensor is an electromechanical device which is used to measure acceleration. ADXL 345 is a small, thin, ultralow power, 3-axis accelerometer with high resolution of 13 bit measurement. It is well suited for mobile application. Because of its compact structure, it is well suited in the implantation of armband.

Heart rate sensor: Heart rate sensor or pulse sensor is a plug and play sensor for arduino. The principle behind the heart rate sensor is photo phlethysmography. The measured pulse rate decides the rate of flow of blood volume, since blood absorbs the light and the signal pulses are equivalent to heart rate pulses.

Usage of heart rate sensor is straight forward, the proper positioning of the sensor matters. The flat side of the sensor should be placed on the veins and it needs the little press for the correct data.

5 IMPLEMENTATION AND RESULTS

The prototype have been implemented with the help of arduino Nano and results have been verified for manual operation if victim is in a position to turn ON the system in case of emergency otherwise a simple fall which is detected by fall detection sensor that may also initiate the system automatically. In need of medical alert, if heart beat is very high above prescribed range, then the system will be turned ON. After the system turned ON, location will be tracked by GPS module and panic message along with location will be sent to cops and numbers that is predefined. For self defense, we make use of Flash circuit that may blur the attackers for few minutes. The designed prototype is shown in Figure 3 and Figure 4.

Figure 3. Interfacing of GPS Module with Arduino nano

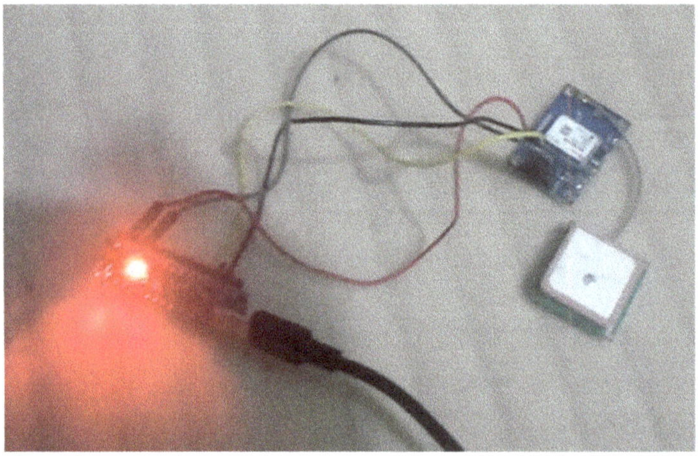

The prototype developed in the Embedded lab of Mepco Schlenk Engineering College is sown in Figure 6. The results have been tested for different positions and corresponding implementation have been checked in accelerometer sensor and the position include normal position, walking, running and pressing. The corresponding graph have been plotted using matlab and with the help of the graph, threshold values have been set. For pulse rate sensor, maximum pulse is detected using formula:

Maximum pulse rate=220-Age→ (1)

Figure 4. Located values of GPS

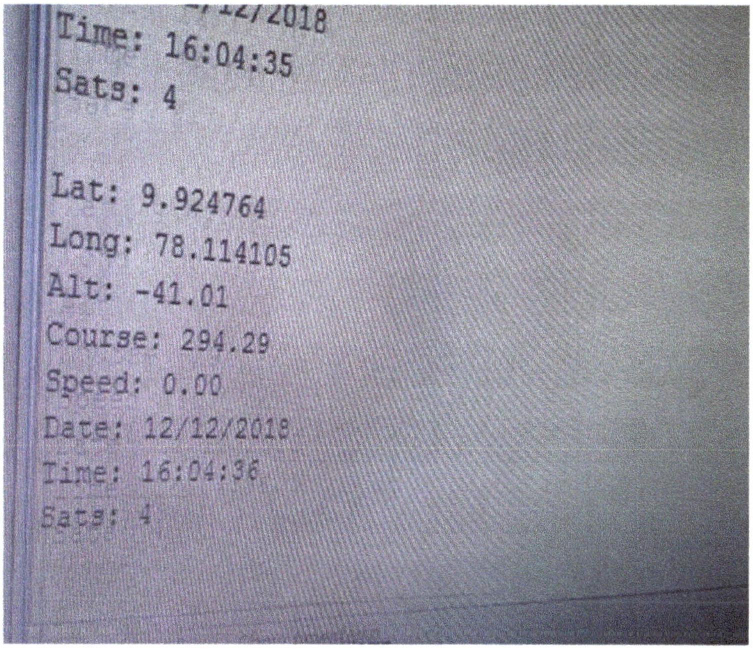

Figure 5. Display of SMS when switch is pressed

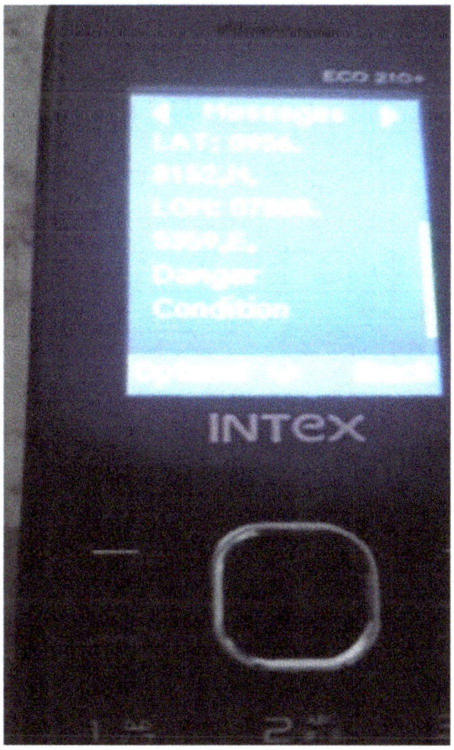

Figure 6. Display of SMS when vigorous falling

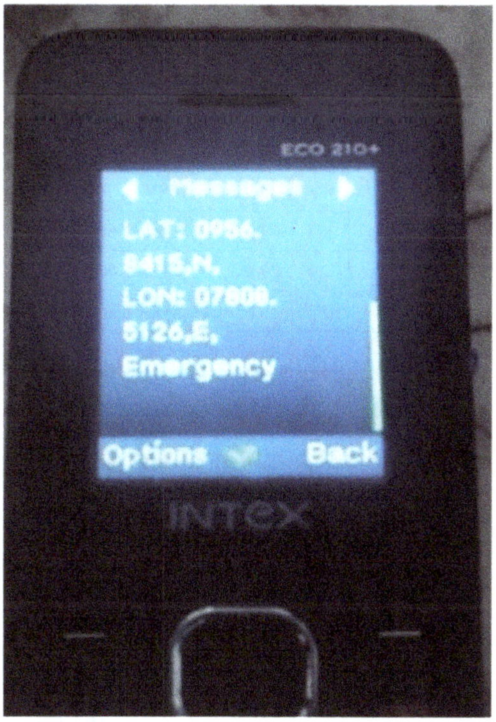

Figure 7. Prototype of the armband

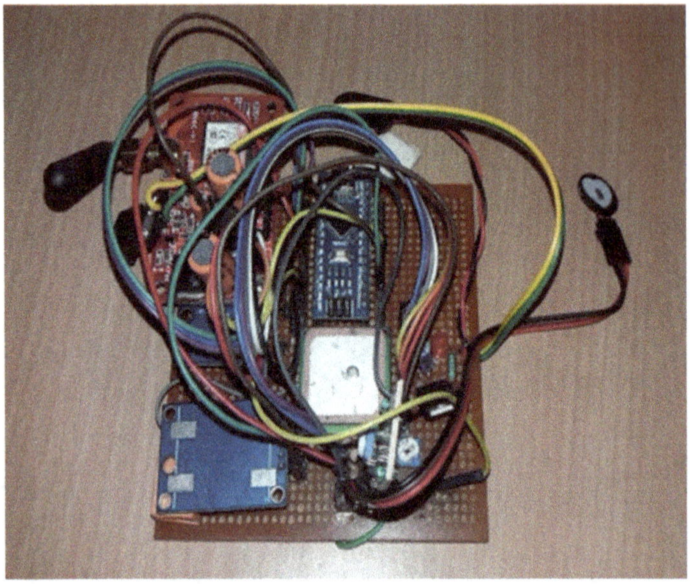

The digital output of heart beat sensor value is obtained and whenever pulse value is above maximum pulse rate, message will be sent with location. The smart system is designed that can be turned on both manually and automatically.

Table 1. Tabulation of vibration values of ADXL 345 with force and time

ACTIONS	5S		10S		15S		20S		25S		30S	
	SV	FV(mG)	SV	FV(mG)	SV	FV(mG)	SV	FV(mG)	SV	FV(mG)	SV	FV(mG)
Normal	283	69.05	281	68.56	289	70.52	291	71	287	70.03	287	70.02
Walking	319	77.8	329	80.27	312	76.13	308	75.15	320	78.08	325	79.3
Running	355	88.62	353	86.13	355	86.62	366	89.3	378	92.23	371	90.52
Pressing	396	96.62	404	98.57	392	95.65	436	106.38	418	102	397	96.87

Where, **SV**→Sensor value, **FV**→Force value

$$FV = SV * (0.244) \quad (2)$$

The monitoring of accelerometer sensor for the falling is further declared with the inclusion of the paramater force. The relation of time and sensor values are recorded and plotted as in Figure 9. Figure 9 describes the three dimensional view of force, time and corresponding sensor value. Because for each action force varies. In normal works the amount of force is comparitively less tan that of hard working work. This statement is clearly viewed with the help of 3D surface plots for various actions as shown in Figures 8, 10, 11, 12.

Figure 8. 3D plot for various actions

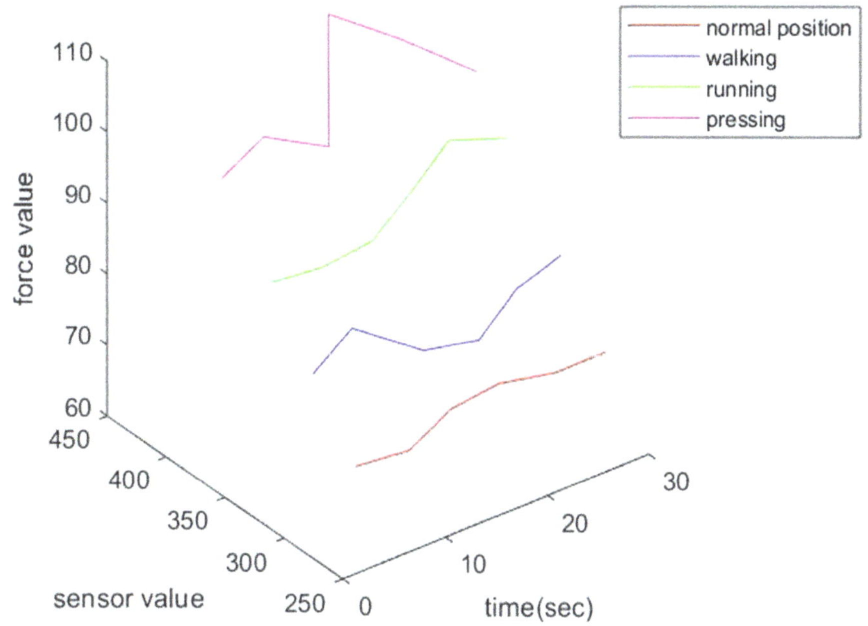

Figure 9. 3D Surface plot for normal position

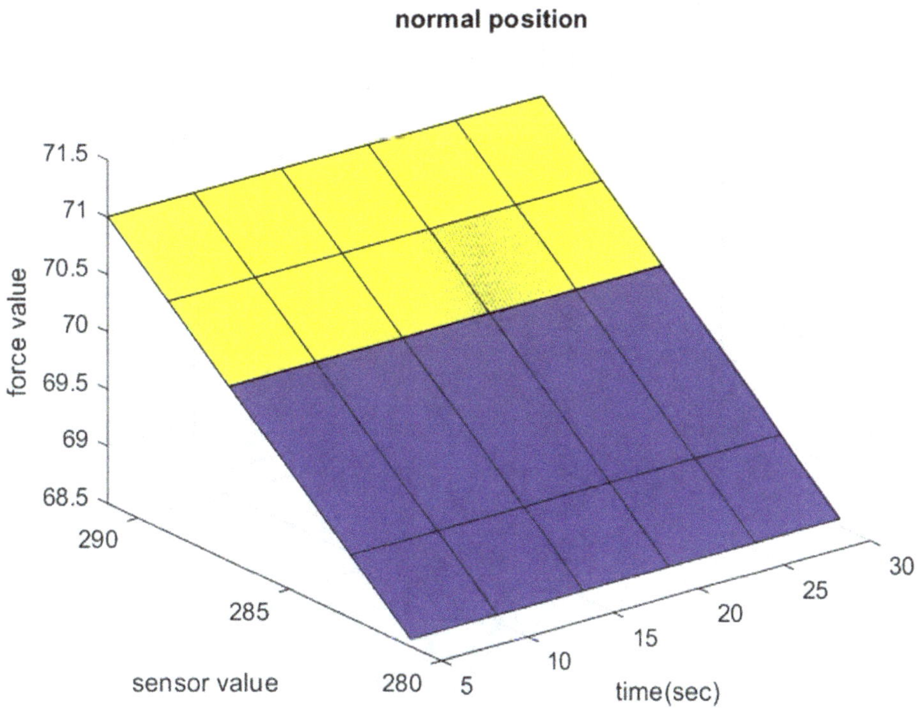

Figure 10. 2D plot for various actions

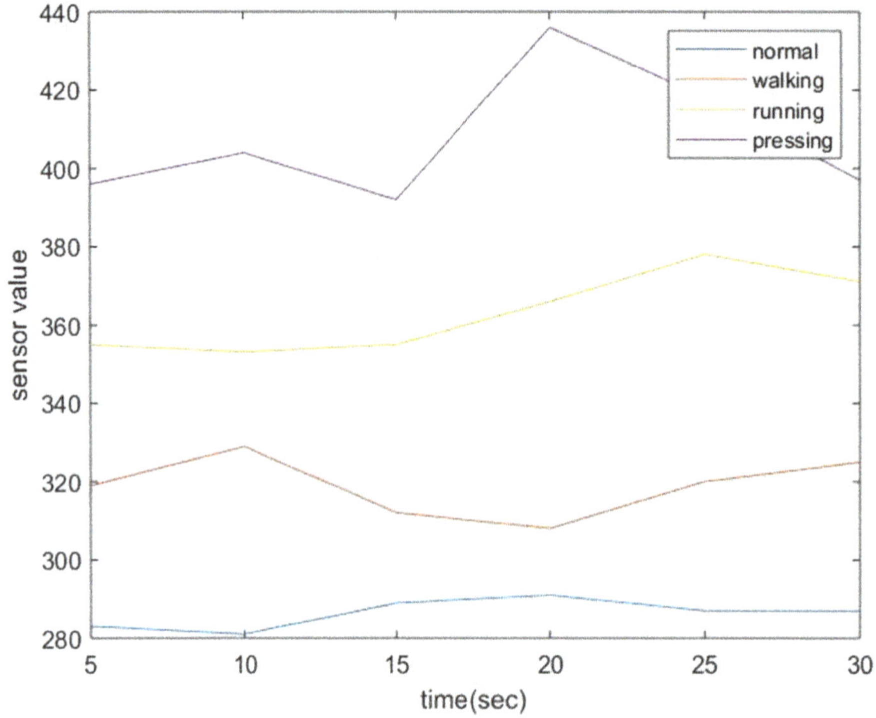

Figure 11. 3D Surface plot for walking

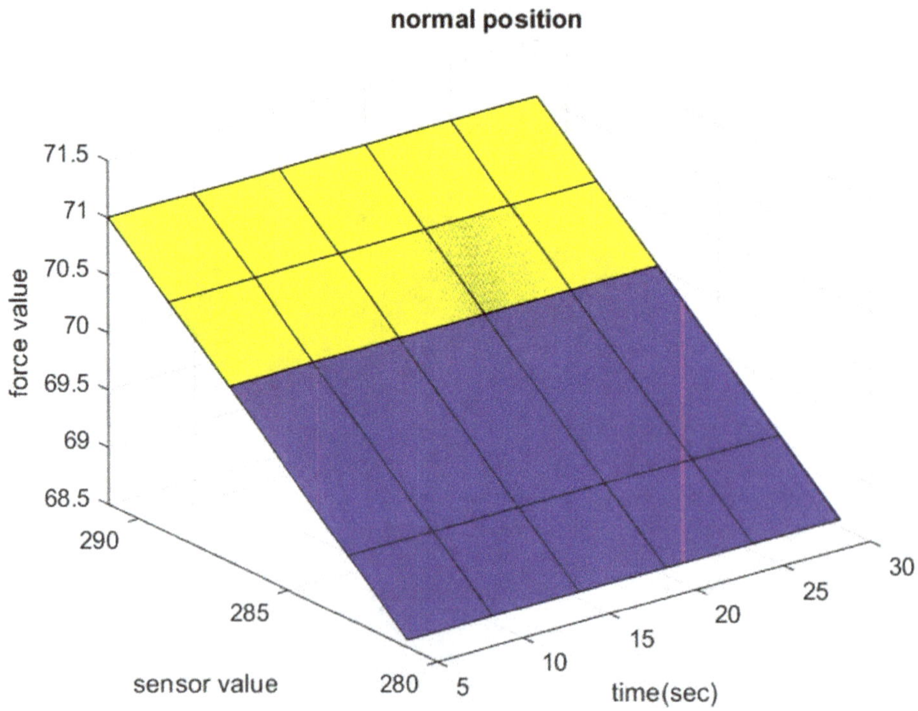

Figure 12. 3D Surface plot for running

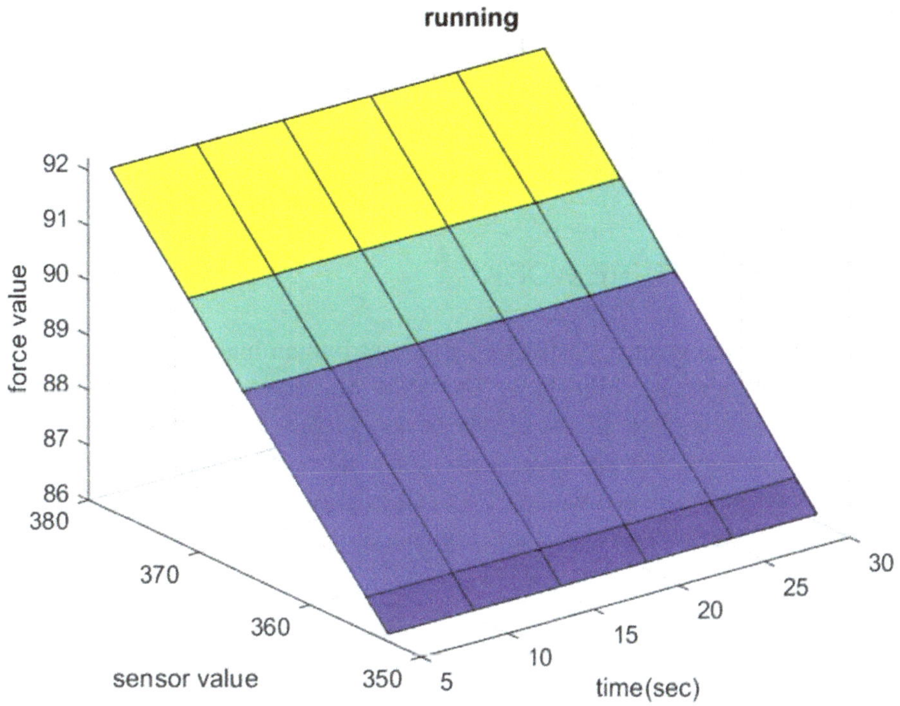

Figure 13. 3D Surface plot for pressing

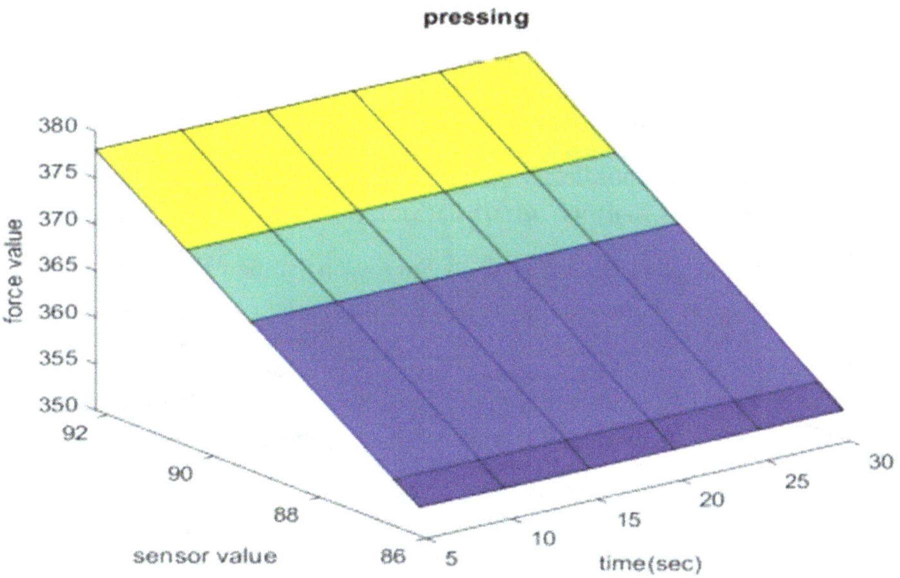

The prototype of the proposed model is done with the interfacing of arduino Nano. The speciality of the set up is that it can be activated on both manual and automatic basis. As explained earlier a switch is responsible for the manual operation. The model uses the accelerometer sensor for the automatic analysis of falling. The range for the vigourous falling is declared after undergoing several experimental check up. Thus this set up does intimate the false falling. Heart rate sensor takes the responsible for the checking of frustration.

6. CONCLUSION AND FUTURE WORK

The security measures for the women's safety is turned out into an intelligent innovative idea in controlling the women harassment and child abuse. The GSM modem with a SIM card helps to locate the exact position of women to cops for their rescue. The developed prototype can be further more improved in future in an advanced way with the camera interfacing which can provide evidences to trace out the culprit. In addition it can be developed wit MEMS devices to get compact set up. The application can be further more extend for the safety of military soldiers.

REFERENCES

Arunachalam, A. R., & Michael, G. (2018). An efficient system for posture recognition based fall detection system and health monitoring. *International Journal of Pure and Applied Mathematics*, *118*(18), 1019–1027.

Holovatyy, A., Teslyuk, A. V., Iwaniec, M., & Mashevska, M. (2017). Development of the system for monitoring vibration accelerations based on the RaspberryPi microcontroller and the ADXL345 Accelerometer. *Eastern-European Journal of Enterprise Technologies*, *6*(9), 52–61. doi:10.15587/1729-4061.2017.116082

Khojasteh, S., Villar, J., Chira, C., González, V., & de la Cal, E. (2018). Improving fall detection using an On-wrist Wearable Accelerometer. *Sensors (Basel)*, *18*(5), 1350. doi:10.339018051350 PMID:29701721

Mahajan, Lavhate, Waghmare, & Pingale. (2017). A Survey on Women's Security System Using GPS and GSM. *International Journal of Innovative Research in Computer and Communication Engineering*, *5*(2), 1560–1563.

Mallick, B., & Patro, A. K. (2016). Heart rate monitoring system using finger tip through arduino and processing software. *International Journal of Science Engineering and Technology Research*, *5*(1), 84–89.

Mao, Ma, He, & Luo. (2017). Highly Portable, Sensor-Based System for Human Fall Monitoring. *Sensors, 17*(9). . doi:10.3390/s17092096

Monisha, D. G., Monisha, M., Pavithra, G., & Subhashini, R. (2016). Women Safety Device and Application-FEMME. *Indian Journal of Science and Technology*, *9*(10), 1–6. doi:10.17485/ijst/2016/v9i10/88898

Paradkar, A., & Sharma, D. (2015). All in one Intelligent Safety System for Women Security. *International Journal of Computers and Applications*, *130*(11), 33–40. doi:10.5120/ijca2015907144

Quero, Olmo, Aguilera, & Estévez. (2017). Real-Time Monitoring in Home-Based Cardiac Rehabilitation Using Wrist-Worn Heart Rate Devices. *Sensors, 17*(12).

Rajput, Mohd, Shinde, Parathe, & Sahu. (2017). Design and implementaion of safety armband for women and children using ARM7. *International Journal of Engineering Technology Science and Research, 4*(4), 161-165.

Roshni, Sune, & Nerkar. (2018). Internet of Things Based Women Tracking And Security with Auto-defender System. *International Journal of Innovative Research in Computerand Communication Engineering*, *6*(6), 63–68.

Rucco, Sorriso, Liparoti, Ferraioli, Sorrentino, Ambrosanio, & Baselice. (2018). Type and Location of Wearable Sensors for Monitoring Falls during Static and Dynamic Tasks in Healthy Elderly: A Review. *Sensors, 18*(5), 1-20.

Shu, Li, Wang, Mi, Li, & Ren. (2015). A Pressure Sensing System for Monitoring with Polymer-Based Pressure Sensors and an Anti-Interference Post Processing Heart Rate Circuit. *Sensors, 15*(2), 3224-35.

Yacchirema, D., Suarez de Puga, J., Palau, C., & Esteve, M. (2018). Fall detection system for elderly people using Iot and Big Data. *Procedia Computer Science*, *130*, 603–610. doi:10.1016/j.procs.2018.04.110

Chapter 10
Smart Interactive System for the Hearing and Speech Impaired

Rohan Saini
J.C. Bose University of Science and Technology, YMCA, India

Sonali Gupta
https://orcid.org/0000-0001-5885-0612
J.C. Bose University of Science and Technology, YMCA, India

ABSTRACT

The deaf face far more difficulties than normal people in day-to-day life, and sign language acts as the most important communication tool for them. Though a lot of books are available as a learning resource for this language, it's not common amongst a major section of the Indian population. An important area of concern is when they need to seek healthcare facilities. The doctors and other hospital staff struggle to understand their issues, and they themselves also put in much effort and time to communicate it to the doctors. Irrespective of joint efforts put in by both the communities, they are unable to get proper health benefits and the services of world-class doctors. In order to solve this problem, SISD, which is a smart interactive system for differently abled persons, based on Indian Sign Language has been proposed. It works similarly to the interactive voice response (IVR) system. SISD provides the user with choices (animations/videos of signs) and recognizes the user's choice via a sign language recognition system.

I. INTRODUCTION

Deaf and dumb people communicate using sign language. Sign language is the most natural language for a deaf and dumb person because even when a child is born he learns gesture until he is been able to speak. Sign language consists of gestures like facial expressions, body postures, and primarily hand gestures, combination of these make a particular sign. There are more than 300 sign languages present all across the globe. According to WHO (World Health Organization), over 5% of the world's population suffers from hearing or speech loss (3playmedia, n.d.). India is the second-largest country to have more than 63 million people who are suffering from full deafness or partial deafness including 50lakh

DOI: 10.4018/978-1-6684-2508-4.ch010

children (Hindustan Times, n.d.). Details of hearing and speech impaired people is given in table 1. Their inability to communicate with hearing people holds them back and creates a large gap between deaf society and the rest of the world. Not every person around them understands sign language due to which these people struggle to get proper health, education, and jobs.

Table 1. Hearing And Speech Impaired Population According To Census 2011, India.

Disability	*Persons*	*Males*	*Females*
Hearing	50,72,914	26,78,584	23,94,330
Speech	19,98,692	11,22,987	8,75,705
Multiple Disability	21,16,698	11,62,712	9,53,986
Total	91,88,304	49,64,283	42,24,021

Health care is the basic necessity that everyone should have. But due to the communication gap between deaf society and hearing people they struggle to get proper healthcare. It is also not feasible for a deaf or dumb person to have a human translator with them all the time. So, there is a need for an automatic sign language translator system that can translate sign language to a form that can be easily understood by fully-abled or normal people. An automatic sign language recognition system helps deaf and dumb people to interact with computer devices and express their feelings and thoughts which can be further converted to a human-readable form or speech as well.

Some of the common challenges faced by deaf and dumb people are:

1. Public Announcement: They miss out important information on public announcements.
2. Slow talkers: When normal people see sign language users they slow down their speaking, which makes it difficult for deaf and dumb person for lip reading.
3. Gesture misunderstanding: This is a very common issues among deaf society. This happens very often when both sign language users uses different sign languages.
4. Interviews: Interviews are already a tense environment, for a deaf and dumb person it could be more difficult when it comes to job interviews. In most of the cases they need to bring a sign language translator.
5. Being in the dark: A deaf and dumb person may find it difficult to analyse gestures in dark.

There are majorly two approaches for SLR (Sign Language Recognition) first one is vision-based and another is physical sensor based.

Vision based SLR: This approach is called vision based because primary source of input data is a camera unit. There are several types of cameras has been used in SLR like digital cameras, stereo cameras, web cameras etc. Kinect and Leap Motion Controller (LMC) are some of the most advanced camera devises used in SLR domain. Images/frames captured from camera unit are then modified to reduce the size and noise from the image which makes it easier for further processing.

After processing these images relevant information is extracted and fed to a classification algorithm like SVM (Support Vector Machine), KNN (K-Nearest Neighbor)or CNN (Convolutional neural network) to classify/recognize user's sign (Bantupalli & Xie, 2018; Liu & Xiao, 2015; Revanth & Raja, 2019).

Figure 1. Camera devices used in SLR kinect(left), webcam(middle),LMC(right)

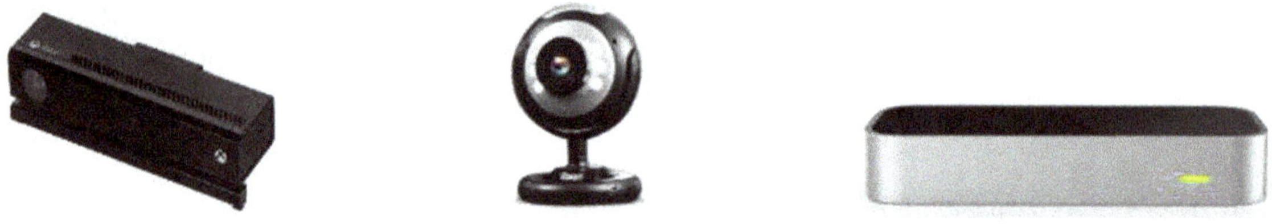

Main advantage of using a vision based approach is user doesn't have to wear sensors or data glove for sign language recognition. Also Cameras are cheaper and highly available to general public now days. Most of daily used gadgets like laptop and smartphone have high end cameras available. Although it has some disadvantages also, like picture quality and orientation can really affects the classification task for example light source, camera angle, background, etc.

Physical Sensor Based SLR: The primary source of data accumulation is a set of sensors like IMU (Inertial Measurement Units), EMG (Electromyography), strain sensor, etc. These sensors are attached to the user's hand or wrist to capture their gestures then this data. Mostly these sensors are attached to a glove which is famously known as data glove. Data glove makes it easier for the user to wear these sensors. Then all the data captured from this data glove is transferred to a computing device for data pre-processing. After pre-processing data it will be fed to a classification algorithm like SVM (Support Vector Machine), KNN (K-Nearest Neighbor), Linear Discriminant Analysis (LDA),

Hidden Markov Models (HMMs), Artificial Neural Networks (ANN), etc. to recognize sign (Abdullah et al., 2020; Barioul et al., 2020; Wu et al., 2016).

Figure 2. Sensor based approach for SLR: IMU based data glove (left), EMG based armband (right)

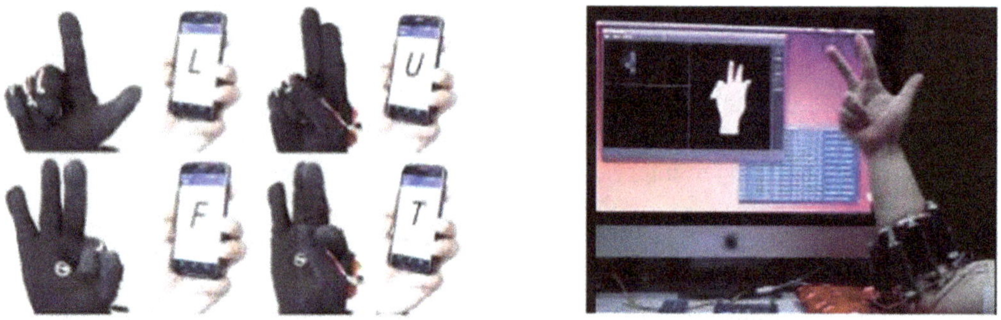

The major advantage of physical sensor based approach over vision based is that it directly provides the relevant information in terms of signals, thus eliminating the need to process raw data into meaningful data and removes huge computing overhead.

II. LITERATURE SURVEY

As we have discussed above that there are two major approaches in sign language recognition task one is physical sensor based and another is vision based, from these two we chose vision based because of the fact that user would not have to wear any sensors for making gestures.

Also looking at the recent pandemic, vision base approach is more appropriate. For the past few years many researchers have come up with different methods for vision base SLR.

Some of the papers are worth mentioning in the field of SLR that is very helpful in the context of health care and automated communication systems for deaf and dumb. Kanchon Kanti Podder et al (Podder et al., 2021) introduced a sign language transformer (SLT) that converts sign language to text and speech and converts back from speech to sign language they have used 3D-CNN+LSTM model for sign language recognition and for conversion of sign language to text and speech they have used NLP. This will help in communication between a doctor and a deaf and dumb patient. Another paper by Veronica Lopez et al (López-Ludeña et al., 2013) in which converts speech into sign language here they first extract sign language-related keywords from speech then pass them to an animation module which then recognizes these keywords and animates them using a 3D avatar. Also, it is very important to recognize the gesture accurately. SISD is the first of its kind smart system proposed by us in the field of sign language recognition. By considering the fact that most of the deaf and dumb people remain illiterate due to communication gap between them and the hearing society. We have proposed a system similar to IVR, which can be easily used by deaf and dumb person.

III. SISD ARCHITECTURE

SISD is divided into 3 main modules namely Query module, SLR module, and NLP module.

Figure 3.

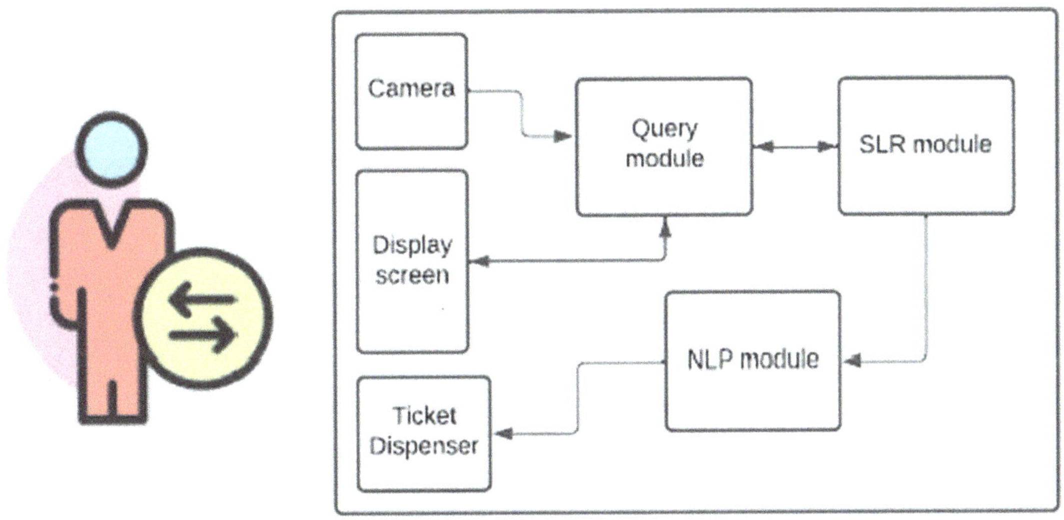

SISD has 3 physical units and 3 logical units.

Physical units: The physical components attached to SISD are

1. Display Screen: This unit is responsible for displaying sign language videos/animation (query videos) and other information to the user.
2. Camera: This unit is responsible for capturing user's response. The captured response then will be forwarded to the logical unit for further processing.
3. Ticket Dispenser: This unit is responsible for dispensing a physical transcript of the whole session so that doctors or other hospital staff can easily understand patient's problem.

Logical units: These are responsible for performing logical operations such as data processing, sign language recognition, sign language to text conversion etc.

1. Query module: This module is responsible for query management. This module has a list of queries with options stored in the form of videos jus like telephone IVR system that uses predefined options associated with a number ranges from 0 to 9 . Some of the stored queries like "Type of issue you have" or "what is your age" etc. Every query includes options like in query "Type of issue you have" has following options "1 for skin-related issue, 2 for dental and so on". These queries are in the form of sign language video i.e. pre-recorded videos of these queries in sign language. It works similar like decision tree where every next query is based on previous query's answer. Then the system will wait for the user's response, the user has to respond to the form of numbers (1, 2, 3…) through sign language. Query module then checks the user response with the help of the SLR module and accordingly it keeps going on depending on the user's input. At last, it will show a combination of videos/animations to guide the user to the concerned department and room number. The user can then collects a manual transcript produced from SISD and hand it over to the doctor so that doctor can diagnose further. The main function of this module is to probe the user. At last user will receive an option for detailed response where user can explain whole issue in detail. All the details captured will be converted into plain text and will be printed on the transcript produced by SISD.

Figure 4.

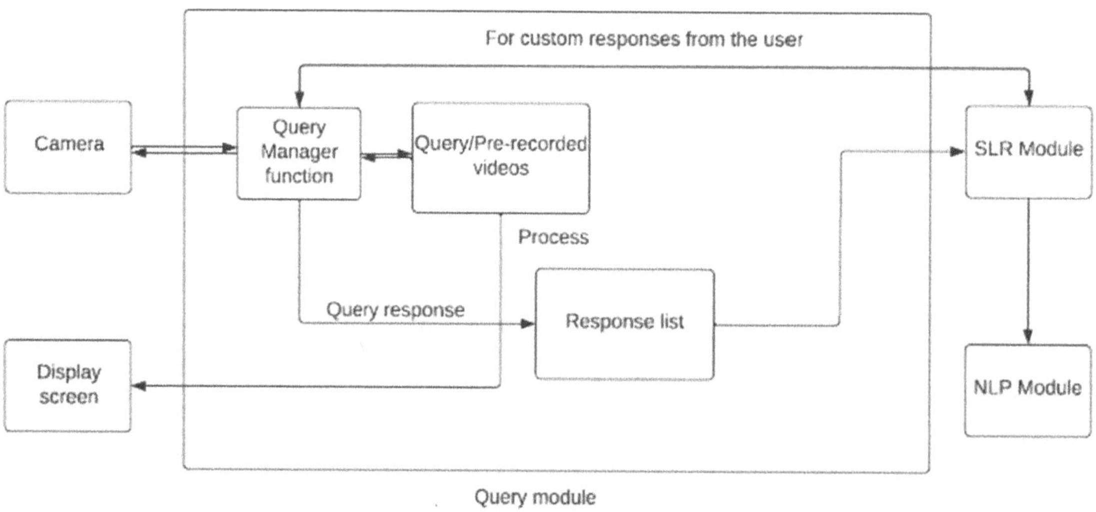

2. SLR module: This module is responsible for recognizing the user's sign and providing the user's response to the query module. It includes a real-time sign language recognition system that captures users' signs, pre-processes them, and feeds these frames to a neural network-based image classifier like CNN and recognizes the signs. As we have used deep learning model so image segmentation and feature extraction is automatically done with the help of CNN model. We have discussed all the SLR models we have used in the following section.

Figure 5. Typical SLR process

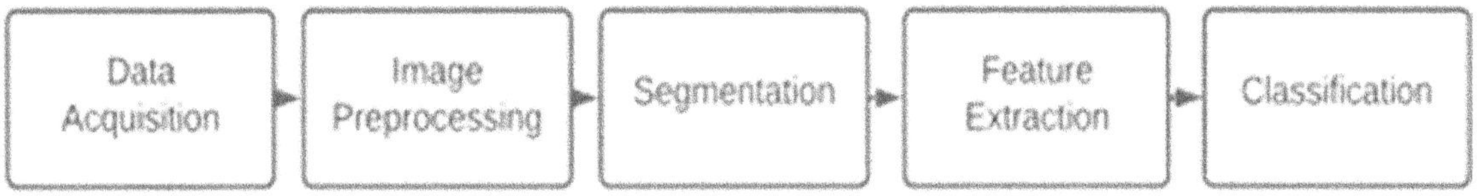

Table. 2. Hearing and speech impaired population according to census 2011, India.

Sr No.	Sign	Instances
1	Allergy	25
2	Appointment	25
3	Bandage	35
4	Blood	42
5	Dcaf	36
6	Dumb	35
7	Doctor	35
8	Help	23
9	Obese	41
10	Operation	40
11	Pain	40
12	Skin	42
13	Heart	37
14	Dental	35
15	1 (One)	40
16	2 (Two)	40
17	3 (Three)	40
18	4 (Four)	40
19	5 (Five)	40
20	6 (Six)	40
21	7 (Seven)	40
22	8 (Eight)	40
23	9 (Nine)	40
24	10 (Ten)	40

Data Acquisition

Since unavailability of dataset for Indian sign language words related to healthcare, we created the dataset for 25 signs by ourselves. This self-created dataset includes 14 words related to healthcare and 10 numerals from Indian sign language.

These words are referenced from (Indian Sign Language, n.d.). Some of the videos are taken from internet but mostly are created by us using a smartphone. Duration of these videos is kept between 2 - 8 sec.

Image Pre-Processing

In this step images/frames are processed and modified in a form that can be easily and efficiently handled by the classifier. Image preprocessing requires several operations to be performed on the original image to enhance the quality of image by removing non relevant information from the image, such as noise removal, colour conversion, etc. Some of the image preprocessing techniques are:

1. Colour conversion: Images captured by the camera unit is generally in coloured (RGB) format which is quite tough to process. Conversion of image to formats like grayscale not just reduce the size of image but makes it easier to process them.
2. Image restoration and Enhancement: To restore the image different kinds of filters are applied to the image such as Median filter or Gaussian filter to reduce the noise in images. To enhance the image i.e. increasing or decreasing brightness, contrast, sharpness etc. some of the enhancement techniques are Histogram Equalization (HE), Contrast Limited Adaptive Histogram Equalization (CLAHE), Adaptive

Histogram Equalization (AHE), and logarithmic transformation.

Figure 6. Image restoration: Median filter (left), Gaussian filter (right)

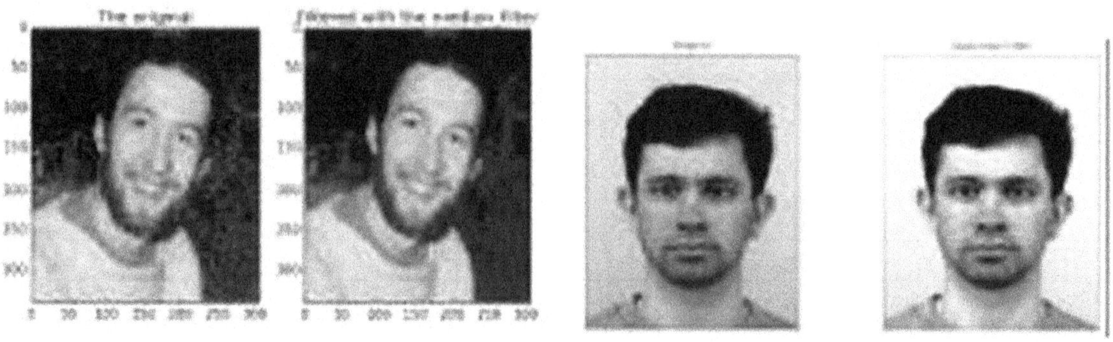

Figure 7. Image enhancement: Histogram equalization (left), Contrast limited adaptive histogram equalization (right)

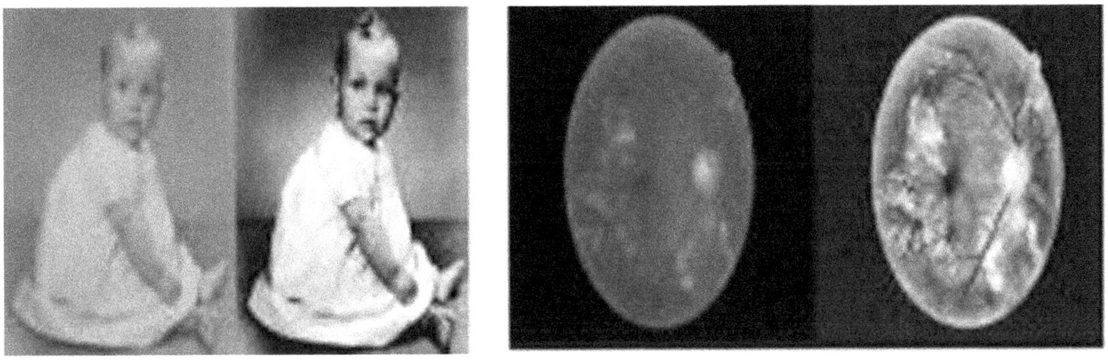

Proposed Models

A. CNN+LSTM

This approach uses combination of CNN and LSTM for predicting gestures/signs from the captured images. CNN will be used for handling spatial features and LSTM is used for handling temporal features. We have used VGG-16 pre-trained model for better recognition. The technique of transfer learning has reduced computation overhead to quiet some extent and also removes the need of building image recognition model from scratch. Data was acquired through a smartphone camera and all the details are mentioned in previous section. First we have applied data augmentation to our dataset to increase dataset.

After data augmentation, our dataset has been tripled in size. Then dataset was split into training and test part followed by frame extraction and pre-processing. Next we have removed last layer from the pretrained model (VGG-16) to get features extracted from dataset. Then these extracted features have been passed to the LSTM model for temporal data sequencing and prediction.

B. Mediapipe+LSTM

Mediapipe is an open-source multi modal pose detection and estimation framework. It uses hand, face and body landmarks to mask the region of interest. It can generate more than 540 landmarks including face, pose and both hands. Mediapipe finds some predefined landmarks on human body in order to create a pose graph in terms of numpy array, after that these array works as input to the image classifier for prediction. We calculated landmarks for all the frames passed to mediapipe, and then we extracted these key points and store them in the form of numpy arrays followed by pre-processing of the data extracted.

C. LSTM

Long Short-Term Memory (LSTM) is used to find the temporal sequences in the input data. For each class LSTM will find temporal information with the help of frames extracted from the previous process. Our LSTM model has 9 layers from which initial 6 layers include lstm layers followed by dropout layers. Then 2 dense layers were added and finally a softmax layer was added with 20 units.

Figure 8. Some frames extracted from Allergy sign video

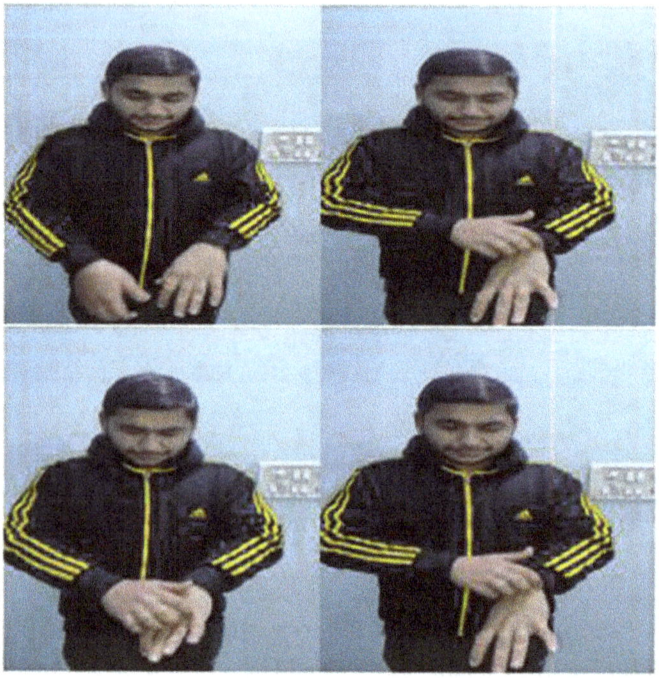

Figure 9. Keypoints generated by mediapipe

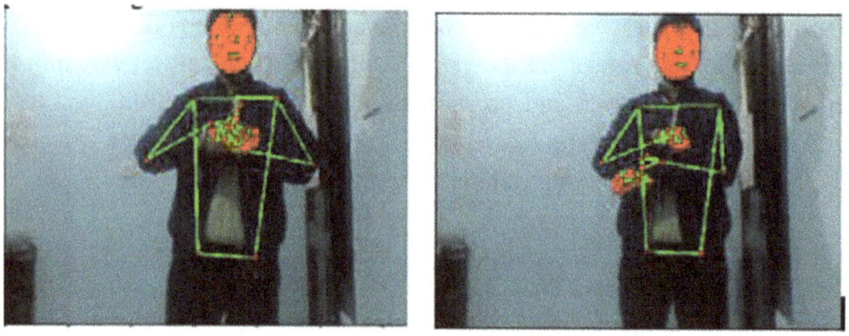

D. NLP Module

This module is responsible for converting sign language to text. There is a grammatical difference between sign language and spoken language. so, to deal with this problem, this module first takes the keyword generated from corresponding gestures by SLR module and sequence of these keywords are recorded and, then with the help of Natural Language Processing, these keywords will be converted to a human-readable form (keywords to sentences). Everything converted from sign to text will be printed to the transcript to help the doctor better understand the patient's problem.

Figure 10. LSTM model architecture

Layer (type)	Output Shape	Param #
lstm (LSTM)	(None, 12, 256)	468992
dropout (Dropout)	(None, 12, 256)	0
lstm_1 (LSTM)	(None, 12, 128)	197120
dropout_1 (Dropout)	(None, 12, 128)	0
lstm_2 (LSTM)	(None, 64)	49408
dropout_2 (Dropout)	(None, 64)	0
dense (Dense)	(None, 64)	4160
dense_1 (Dense)	(None, 64)	4160
dense_2 (Dense)	(None, 20)	1300

Figure 11. Final transcript example

```
What is your issue: Dental
Any previous checkup: Yes
custom note: Dental pain 2 days bleeding
```

IV. RESULTS AND OUTPUT

Query module is a set of functions written in python language that keeps on showing query videos using loops and function calls. SLR module is the main module in SISD for which we have proposed 2 models, CNN+LSTM and Mediapipe+LSTM.This module is responsible for recognizing signs received from user as an input. The recognized response will trigger another option from query module in front of user and then user can go forward accordingly.

Model performance related information is shown in table no.3.Although mediapipe + LSTM model has done a better job in recognizing gestures. Performance of our SLR model could have been better but there are some issues, like self-created dataset which contains low resolution images and also variable background could be a reason for poor performance.

At last the NLP module which concatenates and generates new string using keywords from the custom input of user. Although query responses are already fed into the system and can be easily fetched and printed on the final transcript. But when user puts custom remarks our module lags sometime creating meaningful sentences. This is something we are looking to work upon in the near future

Table.3. Result analysis of SLR methods

Sr No	Method	Model Name	Accuracy
1.	CNN+LSTM	VGG-16	60 ± 7%
2.	Mediapipe+LSTM	-	83 ± 2%

V. CONCLUSION

In this paper, we have designed an automatic sign language recognition system SISD that can help deaf patients to express their issues to the doctor. SISD is a machine consisting of a camera for capturing sign language data and a touch screen that can assist the user by showing sign videos and other information. It also generates the transcript at the end of the conversation. The main aim of SISD is to provide deaf and dumb patients with an automatic recognition system that can understand their problem and save their time and efforts in emergency situations. This is the first novel approach for creating a healthcare interaction system using a concept of IVR. Our main goal is to reduce interaction time and efforts by the user and hospital staff. Using concept of IVR also helps when user is illiterate because even illiterate deaf would know basics like numerals in sign language. Our future aim will be to add a graphical user interface (GUI) to SISD for better representation and make it more easy and interactive for user.

REFERENCES

3playmedia. (n.d.). https://www.3playmedia.com/blog/growing-population-hearing-loss/

Abdullah, A., Abdul-Kadir, N. A., & Che, H. F. K. (2020). An Optimization of IMU Sensors-Based Approach for Malaysian Sign Language Recognition. In *2020 6th International Conference on Computing Engineering and Design (ICCED). 2020 6th International Conference on Computing Engineering and Design (ICCED).* IEEE. 10.1109/ICCED51276.2020.9415838

Bantupalli, K., & Xie, Y. (2018). American Sign Language Recognition using Deep Learning and Computer Vision. In *2018 IEEE International Conference on Big Data (Big Data). 2018 IEEE International Conference on Big Data (Big Data).* IEEE. 10.1109/BigData.2018.8622141

Barioul, R., Ghribi, S. F., Ben Jmaa Derbel, H., & Kanoun, O. (2020). Four Sensors Bracelet for American Sign Language Recognition based on Wrist Force Myography. In *2020 IEEE International Conference on Computational Intelligence and Virtual Environments for Measurement Systems and Applications (CIVEMSA).* IEEE. 10.1109/CIVEMSA48639.2020.9132742

Hindustan Times. (n.d.). https://www.hindustantimes.com/analysis/breach-the-wall-of-silence-give-state-recognition-to-indian-sign-language/story-hg7lj7LTWzfKgYB19prOhP.html

Indian Sign Language. (n.d.). https://indiansignlanguage.org/

Liu, S., & Xiao, Q. (2015). A Signer-Independent Sign Language Recognition System Based on the Weighted KNN/HMM. In *2015 7th International Conference on Intelligent Human-Machine Systems and Cybernetics. 2015 7th International Conference on Intelligent Human-Machine Systems and Cybernetics (IHMSC).* IEEE. 10.1109/IHMSC.2015.71

López-Ludeña, V., San-Segundo, R., González Morcillo, C., López, J. C., & Pardo Muñoz, J. M. (2013). Increasing adaptability of a speech into sign language translation system. In Expert Systems with Applications (Vol. 40, Issue 4, pp. 1312–1322). Elsevier BV. doi:10.1016/j.eswa.2012.08.059

Podder, K. K., Tabassum, S., Khan, L. E., Salam, K. M. A., Maruf, R. I., & Ahmed, A. (2021). *Design of a Sign Language Transformer to Enable the Participation of Persons with Disabilities in Remote Healthcare Systems for Ensuring Universal Healthcare Coverage. In 2021 IEEE Technology & Engineering Management Conference - Europe (TEMSCON-EUR).* IEEE. doi:10.1109/TEMSCON-EUR52034.2021.9488605

Revanth, K. K., & Raja, N. S. M. (2019). Comprehensive SVM based Indian Sign Language Recognition. In *2019 IEEE International Conference on System, Computation, Automation and Networking (ICSCAN).* IEEE. 10.1109/ICSCAN.2019.8878787

Wu, J., Sun, L., & Jafari, R. (2016). A Wearable System for Recognizing American Sign Language in Real-Time Using IMU and Surface EMG Sensors. IEEE Journal of Biomedical and Health Informatics, 20(5), 1281–1290. doi:10.1109/JBHI.2016.2598302

Chapter 11
Reformation of the Healthcare Sector With Innovation and Entrepreneurial Approaches

Sunishtha S. Yadav
Amity Institute of Biotechnology, Amity University, Noida, India

Swapnaneel S. Mazumder
Amity Institute of Biotechnology, Amity University, Noida, India

Nishi Arora
Amity Institute of Biotechnology, Amity University, Noida, India

Seneha Santoshi
https://orcid.org/0000-0001-8893-2221
Amity Institute of Biotechnology, Amity University, Noida, India

Vandana Chauhan
https://orcid.org/0000-0001-9447-0422
Amity Institute of Biotechnology, Amity University, Noida, India

ABSTRACT

The COVID-19 pandemic has been an eye-opener towards human lifestyle and the healthcare sector. During this phase, a new factor witnessed by humankind is the economic and social impact of the healthcare sector. Due to this rising concern in the healthcare sector, new market segments, niches, and micro-niches are created, which have given some abundant opportunities for entrepreneurs to execute new business models, ideas, and technological implementations. This definitely will add uniqueness and will revolutionize the healthcare sector. Adding up, the new normal at this moment is artificial intelligence, machine learning, and virtual reality, which together have changed the perspective of the healthcare sector. So, keeping all these factors in mind, this chapter focuses on transformations in the healthcare sector during the pandemic followed by discussing various innovations and entrepreneurial ideas in the same with all the overcoming challenges. Furthermore, the significant innovations which have improvised the understanding of novel biological threats will also be discussed.

DOI: 10.4018/978-1-6684-2508-4.ch011

INTRODUCTION

With the rising concern over recent times, technology and life sciences have broadened their parameters of advancement. Not just healthcare has got a boon during the pandemic but also other opportunities associated along, like entrepreneurship and innovative ideas to open up wide horizons for economic collectively by impacting the business, market, strategies, planning, etc. (Melder et al., 2018; Suryavanshi et al., 2020). The developing skillset and wider imaginations have been a positive point in setting up new ventures and startups. Entrepreneurship is a revolutionary involvement not just for ideologies but even for the working class with plenty of options and job opportunities. To make it more logical it has been witnessed that during the pandemic although there was a heavy backlash in business, the segments of healthcare got explored and are still receiving various exploration options that are further being a new concept or a new business model leading to increment in both national and international economy. Hence, entrepreneurs in the field of life sciences and healthcare have received the scope of innovations and advancements to help humankind (Wiig et al., 2020; Chen et al., 2020).

With the advancement & integration of technology in the life sciences and the healthcare sector, a new paradigm took over the conventional methods. People are getting versed with The picture that has transformed over the years, not only technologically but also in healthcare. People do not trust to doctors for getting blood pressure checked or even their sugar checked, the portable solutions exist, which are easy and pocket-friendly at the same time. Furthermore, the production of industrial insulin by Eli Lilly and the Company is another factor. Diabetic patients have a defensive move now leading to innovations like in dialysis, where the survival rate has now gotten better (Wiig et al., 2020; Chen et al., 2020).

Gene therapy is another one on the list that has advanced a lot over the decades. Starting right from gene splicing using siRNA, that is a potential cure to severe disease like 4th Stage cancer. The emergence of machine learning and artificial intelligence has changed the whole story of the health sector. The rising influence of genomics is a way to develop personalized medicines now. The scope of innovations is also vast with options like virtual reality in anatomical visuals, 3D- printing, etc. are some available options for entrepreneurs. With all these advancements as of now, as per the recent reports of April 2021, India single-handedly has witnessed a hype of 59% in pharmaceutical while it was 16% back in March 2020 (Schwartz et al., 2010; Coorevits et al., 2013; Liu et al., 2020).

Is COVID-19 an Eye-Opener for Healthcare and Life Sciences?

The novel coronavirus has not only affected the healthcare sector but every domain of life, starting right from schooling to jobs; from children to adults; some physical health to mental health; from National crisis to an international emergency. Introducing sanitizers and facemask as the "new normal" along with social distancing, the entire perspective of human life has been hampered. COVID-19 is one of the most devastating healthcare emergencies the world has experienced up till now. While the whole world struggle gets has adapted to the crisis and has started to face it off with more strength. This strength factor includes innovations, improvising, collaborative approach, and entrepreneurship boost (Wiig et al., 2020; Chen et al., 2020; Liu et al., 2020).

Being the epicenter for the pandemic, both healthcare and life sciences have started to evolve to get better right from testing ability to beds requirement and other resources availability. The pandemic has changed the story but a new one is being written now and the availability of vaccines is the proof. Furthermore, the pandemic has made the authorities understand the importance and need of innovations in life sciences for better healthcare crisis management along with entrepreneurship ideas to build in an impact. While making concerns incline towards healthcare and life sciences, the pandemic has also defined the risks, intensity, and regulations associated along. Hence, versatile advancements and entrepreneurial approaches are required from time to time. With the rise in scientific complexities and barriers, this sector of huge market entrants across the globe dominates the large incumbent ventures from the west (Wiig et al., 2020; Chen et al., 2020; Liu et al., 2020).

The Rising Pharmaceutical Sector

Usually, North America and Europe have been the hub for advanced medical facilities and a source to other countries as well because of their ancient embark of innovations, gripped markets, and talent exposure. Whereas other countries like India have recently discovered the niche of pharmaceuticals. Few of the remarkable inventions as that of X-Ray and penicillin have been a boost for the industry followed by second-generation drugs and super genetics (Davenport & Kalakota, 2019).

While we particularly highlight the Indian pharmaceutical industry, it has been a world leader by introducing generic drugs at a much pocket-friendly value. Followed by this is the introduction of biosimilars for global Healthcare industries. Based on these advancements, the future seems much brighter above biosimilars and generics. The influence of the entrepreneurial approach in 2 life sciences and Healthcare would be a progression in the existing ecosystem of India. These progressions are like, the translational method used therapies, improved genome Sequencing, the influence of Precision medicines, etc. (Wiig et al., 2020; Chen et al., 2020; Liu et al., 2020).

Precision Medicine and Artificial Intelligence in the Healthcare and Pharma Industry

Precision medicine, as the definition goes, approaches healthcare through treatment and prevention by taking into consideration the lifestyle data of an individual, genomic information, and environmental factors. Looking at the current scenario brought up by the pandemic, the pharma industry and healthcare sector need to make drug discovery fast, efficient, and cost-effective. From an industry point of view, the process of drug discovery and development has always been a complex, sensitive and costly process which time and again keeps challenging the healthcare sector and pharmaceutical industry in terms of efficiency and R&D costs (Workman, Antolin, and Al-Lazikani, 2019; Filipp, 2019). The ongoing pandemic has only added to the challenges and has led to an urgent demand to keep in pace and apply the latest technologies for the same. Especially if a disease is approached for treatment and prevention using precision, the drug discovery process in the healthcare sector needs advancement in terms of the latest technologies. This new era has made it more important to use biomedical data via Precision medicine for drug discovery as it provides us with an insight into the mechanism and potential treatment options of a patient's disease. We will understand in this portion how the Drug discovery process has been enabled by AI for effective and timely precision medicine delivery (Chen et al., 2018; Anastasopoulos et al., 2020).

Involvement of Artificial intelligence is possible from the bench to the bedside as it can assist in decision making during various iterative phases of drug discovery, it can help to determine the effective and appropriate therapy for a patient, and most importantly assist in managing the clinical data generated and use it for future drug development (Duch et al., 2007; Vyas et al., 2018). In totality, the drug discovery opportunities are completely different from the earlier times. Based on individual genetic variations, clinical, environmental, and lifestyle data new therapeutic targets need to be located along with accelerated development of novel drugs or repurposed candidates and co-development of diagnostic tools for efficacious treatment of patient groups (Baronzio, Parmar and Baronzio, 2015; Blasiak, Khong and Kee, 2020).

In the current times Artificial intelligence has led us to understand human biology better and faster, which is indeed the need of the hour. The incorporation of AI is not only helping the healthcare industry in better and faster analysis of biomedical data but in coming times is going to help speed up the development of precision medicine. Various statistical and deep learning methods are currently being used not only for analysis of Covid related data but also data related to multiple diseases. The pandemic has given rise to a lot of data which needs to be analyzed and interpretation will pave a way for the diagnosis and classification of diseases and disease subtypes among patients. The use of machine learning, clustering, and feature finding methods has increased the possibility of identification of drug targets for covid 19 and other disease targets in an accurate and fast manner (Sellwood et al., 2018; Mak and Pichika, 2019). The use of technologies and processes like neural networks, big data, and data mining algorithms along with enhanced statistical analysis on experimental data leads to the enhancement of de novo drug design which is the need of the hour in the fast-changing pharma industry. Use of genetic markers and accessible and improved patient information systems, repurposing and combination therapies of drugs holds the promise to will improve the area of precision medicine as well, in fact, the COVID 19 and its allied problems can be better dealt with Precision medicine and holds great opportunity for a better healthcare system. The health care and Pharma industry are gearing up for AI-driven faster, efficient, and reliable research processes to meet the challenges of the market.

With the promise of providing better healthcare to the patients and as a way forward towards precision medicine, a new sync has started developing between pharmaceutical companies and AI companies. Pharmaceutical companies, hospitals, and other healthcare agencies have started to work long with AI companies in the hopes of developing better healthcare tools. The joint ventures to improve the diagnosis through biomarkers, target identification, and novel drug design have already begun through tool development, data analysis, and data exchange with the aim of (Mak and Pichika, 2019).

AI has shown great promise in the rapidly evolving drug design process through accurate and fast predictions of the existing as well as newly designed compounds and better exploration of drug targets. These advancements will serve as the most important contributing factors for the betterment of healthcare services, improvement in terms of efficiency in clinical trials, enhancement in stratified medicine, and more. Presently, drug discovery costs billions and takes around 12 to 15 years to complete. This trend is unsustainable in this fast-changing world, positive change is extremely essential (Paul et al., 2020). These collaborations will help to not only improve upon the existing design space but to discover and explore rare molecules which have properties of extreme importance, which were impossible to identify by solely relying on conventional methods. In the present scenario, it is a challenge to develop a drug, especially while including the genetic/genomic information, environmental factors, and lifestyle of individuals for precision medicine development. It takes thousands of studies to analyze known side effects and unknown interactions. However, once available, such an AI algorithm approach, would prove invaluable in further hastening drug development efforts. AI will revolutionize how drugs are discovered and will reinvent the pharmaceutical industry along with precision medicine.

Electronic Health Record

Execution of EHR in a medical service isn't just about as simple as it sounds. There are various likely difficulties in executing an electronic wellbeing records framework (Mak and Pichika, 2019). Some of the major problems faced while implementing EHR could be:

1. Implementation of Cost: It should come as no surprise that EHR implementation is costly. The determination, execution, and advancement of EHR will remove a lot of the arranged capital spending venture. Even sometimes just finding the financial resources could be a major problem (Yadav et al., 2020).
2. Staff Resistance: Not everyone on the medical team is on board with the concept of implementing technology in the hospital. Furthermore, some health professionals are skeptical of the effectiveness of electronic health records. They might be hesitant to abandon the documentation process (Yadav et al., 2020).
3. Lack of Usability: Physicians find it difficult to adapt to an EHR scheme that does not fit with their current workflow. The one-size-fits-all rule does not apply to EHR systems since a dentist's workflow varies from that of a cardiologist, and vice versa. The software's ease of use is hampered by design defects or insufficient preparation.
4. Lack of Communication: To develop an EHR framework that delivers the desired results, effective communication between the healthcare provider and the IT vendor is required. It is a continuous operation, not a one-time task, to ensure that all parties needs are met (Yadav et al., 2020).

Electronic Health Records in India: India is giving quality medical services of worldwide principles at a generally minimal effort and has pulled in patients from across the globe. Rules depended on the suggestions made by the EMR guidelines advisory group, which was comprised of a request for the Ministry of Health and Family Welfare. It was composed by the Federation of Indian Chambers of Commerce and Industry for its sake. The rules prescribe a set of guidelines to be trailed by various medical services specialist organizations in India and thus that clinical information gets compact and effectively transferable. India having a populace of 1.27 billion individuals with just 160 million web clients' upkeep of EHR is an overwhelming undertaking, however with the interest and backing of the Government of India in its usage, it will a triumph soon (Yadav et al., 2020).

The Backlash Amidst COVID-19 in Healthcare and Life Sciences

The COVID-19 pandemic has been a roller coaster for the health sector and life sciences worldwide. Encountering the immense crisis in management and delivering resources, it had a threat to collapse but fortunately with the conversion of challenges into opportunities by providing a cure, pumping facilities, the failure was rescued. COVID-19 hasn't just been a threat to health care but majorly to humankind, because life is what matters. The Global crisis witnessed the lack of oxygen, medicine, beds, food, shelter, and every basic entity that is required for survival (Gillman-Wells et al., 2021).

After the outbreak of the novel coronavirus, a drug named Viraffin by Zydus Cadila and 2D- glucose from DRDO, which were a treatment for the virus took longer for production to get available in the market for the people. Even the vaccination had a higher demand and the supply was insufficient for the population of 140 crores in India. Organizations like Bharat Biotech and Serum Institute of India were gathered up to pump the production at a great speed with a huge margin to overcome the scarcity. The COVID-19 pandemic exposes the reality of the degrading Healthcare sector of India in almost no time. The failures highlighted were patients being sent back, lack of supportive supplies, exhausting doctors and health care in personal protective equipment (PPE) kits after hours of work, lack of oxygen supply, and the list continues further. With the Indian population of 140 crores, the pre-preparedness had a question mark towards availability of beds, Intensive Care units (ICUs), ventilators, workers, experts, etc. The disease dynamics challenged the Healthcare system in totality (Consolidated FDI Policy, 2021).

Adding on to this challenge, a way to overcome was entrepreneurship by sanctioning projects for innovations and delivery, financial aids being provided, etc. to switch to collaborative and transitional outcome approaches in healthcare and life sciences.

Innovation and Entrepreneurial Approach: A Ladder of Improvement during COVID- 19

There has been a massive difference line between pre-covid and in current covid scenarios concerning the healthcare sector and life sciences. Also, a mindset change has been observed towards entrepreneurs in healthcare and life sciences for innovations. Some of these options emerging is mentioned in figure 1.

Figure 1. Emerging trends in healthcare industry

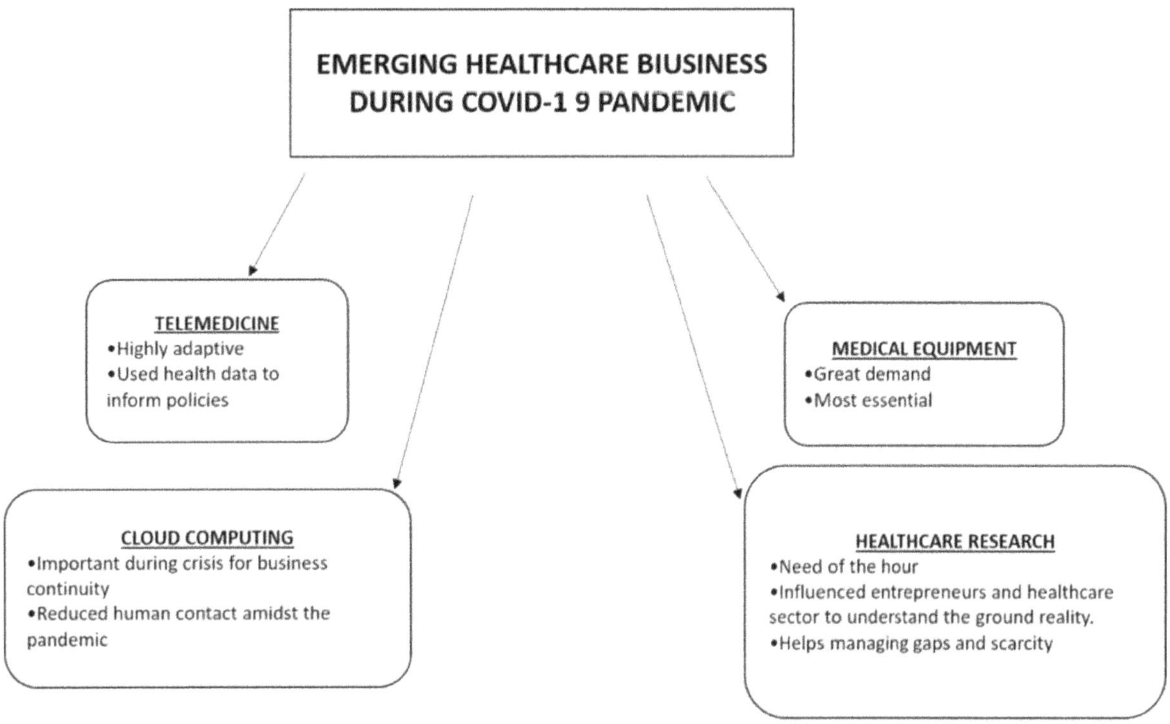

Undoubtedly, innovations have broad in the aspects of entrepreneurial implementation and Exploration of new business ideas in the field of healthcare and life sciences. Financial guides, government initiative, and execution have been a boost up for these benches uplifting the Healthcare sector and field of life sciences which wasn't taken more seriously before the pandemic (Portnoy et al., 2020; Niang et al., 2021).

DISCUSSION

Covid-19 has made healthcare and life sciences received their due credit by providing a reality check, especially the one witnessed in India. Due to this very reason, revolutionary changes are required by letting leaders and minds of innovators come up, that are entrepreneurs, to get a goal gaining long-term shot in the sector. It is high time to understand the ability of such a mind for the growth of the nation on the front. And hence, this stands as a sole reason for the introduction of various pharmaceutical companies that have balanced the economy from the different dips the previous year. Yet, after many twists and turns, India was able to provide all the necessary supplies during the pandemic at a much affordable price (Das, 2020; Rawat et al., 2021; Royal et al., 2021).

The influence of government is one of the primary concerns to accelerate any domain. Henceforth, it is a must for the authorities to level up innovations and entrepreneurial approaches. Biotechnology is a better tomorrow and hence required concern for advancements. Followed with the influence of the IT sector, which has experienced almost no harm during the pandemic can lift the technological aspects of adaptation that include Machine Learning, Artificial Intelligence, and Virtual Reality. It is the need of the hour not just for humans but for various domains of life as well. It will also uplift the entrepreneurial influence and approaches in the upcoming years towards innovations and startups (Das, 2020; Rawat et al., 2021; Royal et al., 2021). If the development goes exponentially inclined, then it won't be a dream to see India as one of the most dominant entities in the healthcare and life sciences sector.

The inherent complexities of machine learning science, technical difficulties in implementation, and consideration of adoption obstacles as well as required sociocultural or pathway changes are all key challenges for the translation of AI systems in healthcare. The gold standard for evidence production should be a robust peer-reviewed clinical assessment as part of randomized controlled trials, although this is not always acceptable or practical in practice. The aim of performance measurements should be to capture real clinical applicability while still being understandable to the intended audience. To ensure that patients are not subjected to harmful treatments or denied access to beneficial technologies, a regulation that balances the speed of innovation with the potential for harm, as well as thoughtful post-market surveillance, is needed. Mechanisms for direct comparisons of AI systems, such as the use of autonomous, local, and representative test sets, must be created. Dataset change, unintentional fitting of confounders, unintended discriminatory prejudice, the challenges of generalization to new populations, and the unintended negative effects of new algorithms on health outcomes are all possible hazards that AI algorithm developers must be aware of (Chen et al., 2018; Workman, Antolin and Al-Lazikani, 2019; Filipp, 2019; Anastasopoulos et al., 2020)).

CONCLUSION AND FUTURE PERSPECTIVE

While we conclude concerning the current scenario, specifically the ongoing covid-19 pandemic, humankind has learned the value of healthcare and life sciences. Also, how innovations are crucial key to providing the best to them while fighting the novel biological threats. Adding on with life sciences and health care is entrepreneurship that is accelerating the bedding ideas into notions. Even the government is financing and finding such projects to deliver products and services that could be a helping hand in a medical emergency. Although there are various challenges to overcome like resource management, production unit setup, and distribution of the products and services, yet a brighter future is readily visible in the domain of life sciences, healthcare, and entrepreneurship going hand in hand.

REFERENCES

Anastasopoulos, C., Weikert, T., Yang, S., Abdulkadir, A., Schmülling, L., Bühler, C., Paciolla, F., Sexauer, R., Cyriac, J., Nesic, I., Twerenbold, R., Bremerich, J., Stieltjes, B., Sauter, A. W., & Sommer, G. (2020). Development and clinical implementation of tailored image analysis tools for COVID-19 amid the pandemic: The synergetic effect of an open, clinically embedded software development platform and machine learning. *European Journal of Radiology*, *131*, 109233. doi:10.1016/j.ejrad.2020.109233 PMID:32927416

Baronzio, G., Parmar, G., & Baronzio, M. (2015). Overview of methods for overcoming hindrance to drug delivery to tumors, with special attention to tumor interstitial fluid. *Frontiers in Oncology*, *5*. Advance online publication. doi:10.3389/fonc.2015.00165 PMID:26258072

Chen, H., Engkvist, O., Wang, Y., Olivecrona, M., & Blaschke, T. (2018). The rise of deep learning in drug discovery. *Drug Discovery Today*, *23*(6), 1241–1250. Advance online publication. doi:10.1016/j.drudis.2018.01.039 PMID:29366762

Chen, S., Zhang, Z., Yang, J., Wang, J., Zhai, X., Bärnighausen, T., & Wang, C. (2020). Fangcang shelter hospitals: A novel concept for responding to public health emergencies. *Lancet*, *395*(10232), 1305–1314. doi:10.1016/S0140-6736(20)30744-3 PMID:32247320

Consolidated F. D. I. Policy, Press Information Bureau (PIB), Media Reports, Pharmaceuticals Export Promotion Council, AIOCD-AWACS, IQVIA. (n.d.). https://www.ibef.org/industry/pharmaceutical-india.aspx

Coorevits, P., Sundgren, M., Klein, G. O., Bahr, A., Claerhout, B., Daniel, C., Dugas, M., Dupont, D., Schmidt, A., Singleton, P., De Moor, G., & Kalra, D. (2013). Electronic health records: New opportunities for clinical research. *Journal of Internal Medicine*, *274*(6), 547–560. doi:10.1111/joim.12119 PMID:23952476

Das, A. (2020). Challenges faced by healthcare-related sectors in India during COVID-19 pandemic: A review. *International Journal of Advanced Research*, *8*(8), 639–641. doi:10.21474/IJAR01/11536

Davenport, T., & Kalakota, R. (2019). The potential for artificial intelligence in healthcare. *Future Healthcare Journal*, *6*(2), 94–98. doi:10.7861/futurehosp.6-2-94 PMID:31363513

Duch, W., Swaminathan, K., & Meller, J. (2007). Artificial Intelligence Approaches for Rational Drug Design and Discovery. *Current Pharmaceutical Design*, *13*(14), 1497–1508. Advance online publication. doi:10.2174/138161207780765954 PMID:17504169

Filipp, F. V. (2019). Opportunities for Artificial Intelligence in Advancing Precision Medicine. *Current Genetic Medicine Reports*, *7*(4), 208–213. doi:10.100740142-019-00177-4 PMID:31871830

Finset, A. (2021). Challenges for healthcare communication during the COVID-19 pandemic. *Patient Education and Counseling*, *104*(2), 215–216. doi:10.1016/j.pec.2021.01.006 PMID:33518199

Gillman-Wells, C. C., Sankar, T. K., & Vadodaria, S. (2021). COVID-19 Reducing the Risks: Telemedicine is the New Norm for Surgical Consultations and Communications. *Aesthetic Plastic Surgery*, *45*(1), 343–348. doi:10.100700266-020-01907-8 PMID:32885319

Liu, Y., Lee, J. M., & Lee, C. (2020). The challenges and opportunities of a global health crisis: The management and business implications of COVID-19 from an Asian perspective. *Asian Business & Management*, *19*(3), 277–297. doi:10.105741291-020-00119-x

Mak, K. K., & Pichika, M. R. (2019). Artificial intelligence in drug development: Present status and future prospects. *Drug Discovery Today*, *24*(3), 773–780. Advance online publication. doi:10.1016/j.drudis.2018.11.014 PMID:30472429

Melder, A., Burns, P., Mcloughlin, I., & Teede, H. (2018). Examining 'institutional entrepreneurship' in healthcare redesign and improvement through comparative case study research: A study protocol. *BMJ Open*, *8*(8), e020807. doi:10.1136/bmjopen-2017-020807 PMID:30082347

Niang, M., Dupéré, S., Alami, H., & Gagnon, M. P. (2021). Why is repositioning public health innovation towards a social paradigm necessary? A reflection on the field of public health through the examples of Ebola and Covid-19. *Globalization and Health*, *17*(1), 46. doi:10.118612992-021-00695-3 PMID:33853631

Paul, D. (2020). *'Artificial intelligence in drug discovery and development', Drug Discovery Today*. Elsevier Ltd. doi:10.1016/j.drudis.2020.10.010

Portnoy, J., Waller, M., & Elliott, T. (2020). Telemedicine in the Era of COVID-19. *The Journal of Allergy and Clinical Immunology. In Practice*, *8*(5), 1489–1491. doi:10.1016/j.jaip.2020.03.008 PMID:32220575

Rawat, K., Kumari, P., & Saha, L. (2021). COVID-19 vaccine: A recent update in pipeline vaccines, their design, and development strategies. *European Journal of Pharmacology*, *892*, 173751. doi:10.1016/j.ejphar.2020.173751 PMID:33245898

Royal, A., Mali, M. A., Kumar, V., Wagh, I. A., Bhushan, S., Mokal, A. N., Mehta, K., & Bhattacharya, S. (2021). Harnessing the potential of the primary healthcare facilities in India to respond COVID-19 pandemic: A scoping evidence-based research synthesis. *Journal of Family Medicine and Primary Care*, *10*(1), 116–121. doi:10.4103/jfmpc.jfmpc_1609_20 PMID:34017712

Schwartz, K., & Huff, B. (2010). *The story of Eli Lilly's open innovation journey—How one company developed a mature model*. PDMA Visions.

Sellwood, M. A., Ahmed, M., Segler, M. H. S., & Brown, N. (2018). Artificial intelligence in drug discovery. *Future Medicinal Chemistry*, *10*(17), 2025–2028. Advance online publication. doi:10.4155/fmc-2018-0212 PMID:30101607

Suryavanshi, T., Lambert, S., Lal, S., Chin, A., & Chan, T. M. (2020). Entrepreneurship and Innovation in Health Sciences Education: A Scoping Review. *Medical Science Educator*, *30*(4), 1797–1809. doi:10.100740670-020-01050-8 PMID:34457846

Vyas, M. (2018). Artificial intelligence: The beginning of a new era in pharmacy profession. *Asian Journal of Pharmaceutics*.

Wiig, S., Aase, K., Billett, S., Canfield, C., Røise, O., Njå, O., Guise, V., Haraldseid-Driftland, C., Ree, E., Anderson, J. E., & Macrae, C. (2020). Defining the boundaries and operational concepts of resilience in the resilience in the healthcare research program. *BMC Health Services Research*, *20*(1), 330. doi:10.118612913-020-05224-3 PMID:32306981

Workman, P., Antolin, A. A., & Al-Lazikani, B. (2019). Transforming cancer drug discovery with Big Data and AI. *Expert Opinion on Drug Discovery*, *14*(11), 1089–1095. Advance online publication. doi:10.1080/17460441.2019.1637414 PMID:31284790

Yadav, S., Soni, J., Porwal, S., Chauhan, V., Rashid, S., & Jain, A. (2020). Tally Education in Covid-19 Era: Impact on Health, Cancer Care and Education Sectors. *Asian Pacific Journal of Cancer Care*, *5*(S1), 95–99. doi:10.31557/apjcc.2020.5.S1.95-99

Chapter 12
Spark-Based Deep Learning for Recognition of Epileptic Seizures With Multimodal Brain Waves

Ashish Bhagchandani
https://orcid.org/0000-0001-7638-1661
Gandhinagar Institute of Technology, India

ABSTRACT

In this chapter, electrical activity in the brain is measured with the help of brain sensors. Further, electrical activity is stored and analyzed for two different datasets: first, for the epileptic seizure, and second, for brain activity. Next, both epileptic seizure and brain activity datasets are used for deep learning models interfacing with Apache Spark. The deep learning model has a feed-forward neural network, which helps determine features from the epileptic seizure dataset that are important and fit in the hidden patterns among them. Further, FFNN is interfaced with Apache Spark to analyze how it can be beneficial with processing of the deep learning model. The results of the accuracy of deep learning model and processing time caused by Apache Spark help determine how effective the FFNN is for predicting the seizure activity in the brain and how Apache Spark can be applied with a deep learning model to increase its effectiveness for different types of datasets.

INTRODUCTION

The brain is the body's control center and part of the nervous system, including an extensive network of neurons and the spinal cord. Brain disorders can affect our body functionalities, including a person's memory, personality, and sensation. The conditions that cause such disorders can be 1) Illness, 2) Genetics, or 3) Traumatic injury. An Epileptic seizure is one such brain disorder caused by the above conditions. Around 1% of the world's population gets affected by epileptic seizures. Of this 1%, two-thirds get cured of antiepileptic drugs. Another 7-8% get cured by epileptic surgery, but at the same time, it is

DOI: 10.4018/978-1-6684-2508-4.ch012

challenging to diagnose seizures in patients. Therefore, around 25% of patients with epilepsy seizures are severe to discover and thus are uncontrollable (Litt & Echauz, 2002). Due to seizure activity, anxiety becomes part of a patient's life and affects them in their routine activities. Seizure activity is so harmful that it causes irreversible changes in the brain, which sometimes remain unprovoked. Consequently, this has been a significant concern among clinical researchers and a substantial area of interest in epileptic disorder (Sun et al., 2018).

Recording a patient's EEG could help the clinician to detect seizure activity. Before, EEG could only be performed in a hospitalized environment, but portable EEG systems were introduced due to the technological advancement of pervasive sensors (Waterhouse, 2003). Nevertheless, it becomes difficult to study the EEG recording of an epileptic patient due to its size and complexity, which requires highly trained professionals at the clinical level. It also becomes an arduous and time-consuming task to detect seizure activity from the EEG dataset (Mormann et al., 2006). The complexity of the EEG recording dataset has inspired researchers to find a procedure that can detect epileptic seizures automatically, which can match the precision of any clinical professional. These machine learning algorithms find patterns between the attributes of the EEG dataset and perform iterations in a closed loop to make the model more accurate toward precision.

Literature survey- This section outlines various previous approaches for seizure activity prediction in an epilepsy patient. All of these technologies have impacted clinical research in multiple ways. After critically analyzing recent research on seizure activity prediction that has used machine learning algorithms, it can be said that modern technologies have been introduced to the world of neuroscience to improve the clinical sector. Brinkmann et al. (2015) showed that the preictal state of epilepsy was diagnosed from continuous ECoG in dogs with the help of Support Vector Machines (SVM). Zhang et al. (2016) showed the extension of this technique by introducing the pre-processing of ECoG data and then having it classified from the Kalman filter, which improved the input data for the SVM linear classifier. Wang et al. (2015) proposed the processing time by decreasing the redundancy in the dataset. Doing further refining by using the global features of datasets were easily classified. A specialized seizure detection with EEG scalp was introduced by Vidyaratne et al. (2016), which was automated with the help of a novel Deep Recurrent Neural Network (DRNN) and was patient-specific. For seizure detection, Turner et al. (2014) worked with high resolution and multichannel EEG data using the Deep Belief Network (DBN). Yuan et al. (2017) identify abnormalities for seizure detection using multichannel epileptic EEG signals.

Golmohammadi et al. (2017) used multiple machine learning algorithms to categorize the EEG attributes with various arrangements. Chaovalitwongse et al. (2014) introduced the time-series classification to identify epileptogenicity from the EEG dataset. A Bayesian network was built by He et al. (2016), which differentiates EEG waves from a BCI system. The New Feature extraction method was used by D Rafik & B Larbi (2019), which used EDA and a Multi-Layer Perceptron Neural Network. Hadi Ratham Al Ghayab et al. (2018) used the Information Gain technique to frequency domain of EEG data and, with the help of Fast Fourier Transform (FFT) and LS-SVM, classified the features of epileptic seizure data for the seizure prediction. S Raghu et al. (2020) used cross-database evaluation for EEG data pre-processing and used different classification techniques while using AM-FBC for the classifier output to detect the seizure activity. R Hussein et al. (2019) used Fully Connected Layer to classify the important EEG data features for Epileptic Seizure and then applied LSTM for selected features. M Fan & C Chou (2018) characterize Temporal Synchronization Patterns in the EEG dataset of epileptic seizures. Based on that, they recorded changes in patterns that helped them detect seizure activity. Solveig Vieluf et al. (2020) proposed using Autonomic Nervous System (ANS) changes instead of the EEG dataset to detect seizure activity by applying the statistical analysis on ANS. Gaetano Zazzaro et al. (2019) build their tool using data mining techniques, including SVM to detect seizure activity in the brain. Yun S Park et al. (2020) used an invasive approach for an early finding of seizures with the help of intracortical Microelectrode Array (MEA) signals, LFP, MUA, and SVM. Walter Bomela et al. (2020) introduced a novel approach to classify EEG patterns with a multivariate time-varying method and applied graph theory for seizure detection. Clémence Alla Takam et al. (2020) used spark based framework with a deep learning model to produce low-dose image processing for CT scans. The spark framework helped them decrease the processing time with the help of map-reduce. Kuldeep Singh et al. (2022) described an approach in the fog-cloud integrated environment using a Convolution Neural Network. This helped them achieve real-time processing but was only limited to a fog-cloud integrated environment. Sai Manohar Beeraka et al. (2021) applied both convolution neural network and Bi-LSTM, getting the time-frequency analysis of EEG segments from STFT and further feeding it to the Bi-LSTM and CNN model. Omaima Ouichka et al. (2022) used five different deep learning approaches based on CNN from the five 3-CNN, and 4-CNN gave the best results, but processing the model was a significant concern in the approach. Syed Muhammad Usman et al. (2021) proposed ensemble learning and bandpass filtering technique for noise removal. They also used Generative Adversarial Networks to solve the class imbalance problem, the feature set of the dataset was further used on an ensemble classifier, which had SVM, CNN, and LSTM using agnostic meta-learning. Mehmet Akif Ozdemir et al. (2021) designed a novel approach of Fourier-based Synchrosqueezing Transform (SST) and the output of it is feed into a CNN model which further detects the epileptic seizure by analysing the TF plane from the SST.

Challenges- Machine learning for seizure recognition has created a new research area for clinical use. The approaches provided by machine learning algorithm make it possible to study patterns between the hidden pre-ictal characteristics. The initial steps of Machine learning involve classification, feature extraction, and pre-processing, which help to analyze the structure of epilepsy patient's EEG datasets (Shin, 2015). These steps help us understand which features in data play a substantial role in seizure detection and can be applied for dimensionality reduction; this can ease the classification process. Lately, deep learning has created an impact in the field of neuroscience and has proved to be better among various machine learning algorithms (Min et al., 2016). A multi-layer neural network can be created with machine learning approaches that can easily extract the hidden features and pre-process data; this could increase the computational power and decrease the training time of deep learning models (Hinton & Salakhutdinov, 2006; Bengio et al., 2013). Despite various advancements in the neuroscience field due to deep learning, there are still complex challenges that create difficulties implementing any deep learning model on the EEG dataset of an epileptic seizure. First, feature selection from the epilepsy dataset becomes difficult as the problems faced by one patient can be different from another patient, and therefore, feature selection becomes more patient-specific. Second, how each feature is related to each other, and the hidden patterns between them is difficult to identify as the epileptic seizure dataset can contain more than 150 features. Third, handling such a tremendous amount of data becomes very difficult as it increases the processing time and decreases the deep learning model efficiency. It will take days, and even after that, it is uncertain that the DL model will still provide the utmost accuracy.

An epileptic seizure is a chronic disorder that can be recognized with the study of seizure activity from multimodal brain waves of a particular person. The following research solves the above three challenges using deep learning with Apache Spark. First, two types of multimodal brain wave recordings have been stored as a dataset, which includes an epileptic seizure dataset and the brain activity dataset. These data sets vary exceedingly in size, as the dataset on epileptic seizures has 178 input parameters, whereas the dataset on average person brain activity has only three input parameters. Second, the Deep learning model is designed for both datasets to predict seizure and brain activity. The following deep learning model consists of FFNN, whose activation function and parameters are tuned to produce the utmost accuracy. This deep learning model will automatically choose important features from the EEG dataset which will most impact the result. The FFNN in this deep learning model is extensive enough to accommodate all the hidden patterns among the features. Third, this deep learning model has been used with and without Apache Spark to evaluate the result of how Apache Spark can be beneficiary with processing time and handling such a massive dataset. This approach will also help us understand how FFNN will produce compelling predictions when used with Apache Spark.

DEEP LEARNING WITH APACHE SPARK: SYSTEMML

1. Machine Learning Algorithm and SystemML

The growing amount of data has put up new challenges for data scientists. It becomes challenging to train machine learning algorithms on such massive datasets from the healthcare, manufacturing, mobile, and automotive industries. Due to this, the need for distributed and parallel data systems like Map Reduce (MP), Spark, and Flink can satisfy performance and scalability on cost-effective commodity clusters (Boehm et al., 2016).

Apache SystemML uses declarative ML to solve the above challenges. High-level specifications of ML algorithms are targeted by the declarative ML, which separates the algorithm semantics from runtime execution plans, and data representations (Boehm et al., 2016) and therefore increases the development and deployment of ML algorithms over such massive data.

2. Apache Spark and SystemML

Implementing ML algorithms directly on the Spark environment requires tremendous effort, and even the functionality of declarative ML reduces substantially, this can be understood from the Fig.1 cycle. SystemML omits the above two possibilities as it can be integrated with the Apache Spark ecosystem by (1) seamless integration of Spark APIs, and (2) compilation of ML algorithms for efficient execution plans on top of Spark automatically. Without performing any changes, the ML algorithm transition can be performed from MR to YARN and Spark with the help of declarative ML (Boehm et al., 2016).

The cycle represented in Fig.1 needs to follow when SystemML is absent. Due to the increase in the amount of data, industries prefer to store their data on big data platforms. Data scientists need to modify the ML algorithm written in python/R to work with significant distributed systems using Scala-like language. The above process is a very time-consuming and tedious job, as for every change made in the ML algorithm, the cycle repeats.

SystemML tries to solve this issue faced in Fig.1 by eliminating the need for system programmers and Scala-like language. In Fig.2, SystemML uses Declarative Machine learning scripts and compiles them into distributed jobs and mixed drivers. There is no need for modification of ML algorithms. They can directly run on the drivers or Apache Spark cluster as SystemML can run on Apache Spark.

Figure 1. Developing algorithm for distributed platform

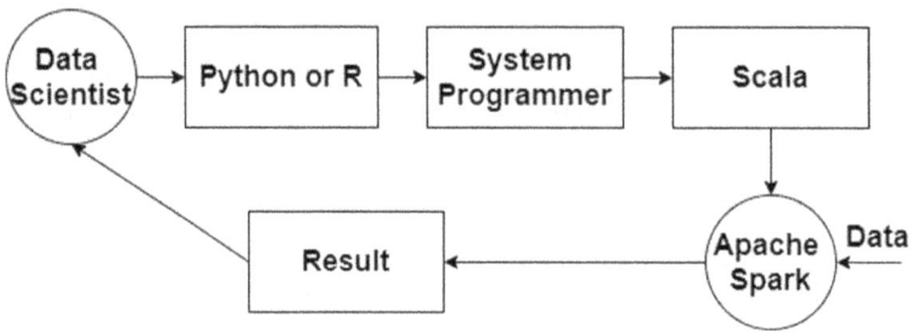

Figure 2. Developing algorithm for distributed platform using SystemML

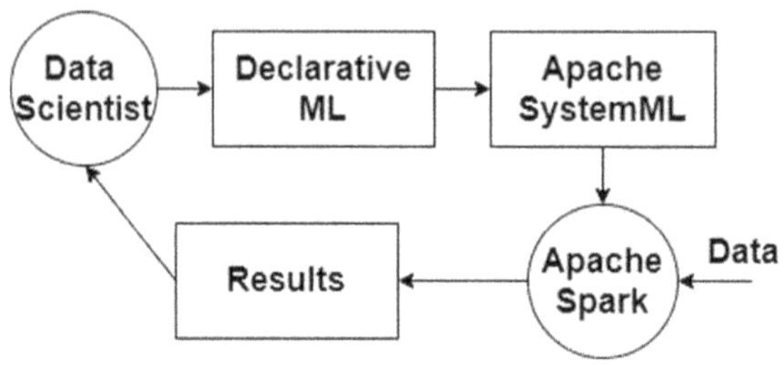

3. Use of SystemML in this Chapter

By analyzing Fig.3, it can be understood that the application of SystemML in this chapter follows various stages, i.e., Language, Compiler, and Runtime. These stages will connect the declarative ML scripts with Apache Spark.

Language: The deep learning models built for epileptic seizures and brain activity datasets are written in python, with DML-like syntax. The language block in SystemML architecture parses the DML script of FFNN to check semantic validations, syntactic analysis, and live variable analysis by building a hierarchical model of statement blocks and control structures (Apache, 2016).

Compiler: Compiler of SystemML will work on FFNNs generated by HOPs and DAGs. In the activation function in the FFNN, all the parameters and performance metrics will be compiled with the help of HOPs and DAGs (Boehm et al., 2014). Memory computations are estimated with the use of generated HOPs to set the requirement of in-memory single-node operations or the Apache Spark instances. Individual HOPs and DAGs are compiled and are set to Low-Level Operators (LOPs) (Boehm et al., 2014). Instructions are set with each LOPs with their runtime implementations. By this, the compiler will generate an executable runtime program for the deep learning model, which could run on top of Apache Spark.

Runtime: After generating runtime programs, they are executed locally in the Control Program (CP). The CP drive handles if the recompilation occurs, it also contains a memory buffer pool and Spark jobs

Figure 3. SystemML- Spark Architecture

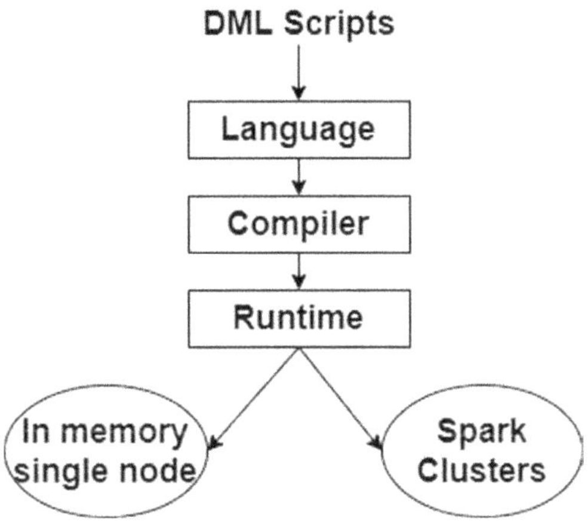

due to distributed computation, informing of Spark jobs. The memory will hold matrices with the help of a buffer pool and evict them if necessary for further operation by this, backend data exchange happens between local and Spark platforms. The adaptive matrix block library is the core of 'SystemML's runtime instruction. It performs continuous operations with CP and distributed processes with matrix blocks. Therefore, the SystemML will perform runtime execution of the deep learning model on Apache Spark instances, initiating plan adaptation addressing initial unknowns, dynamic recompilation for runtime, and parallel for-loops for task-parallel computations.

PROPOSED WORK

1. Material

I. Brain Activity Dataset

The brain activity dataset is the result of the continuous thoughts emerging in the brain. This dataset is generated with the help of two electrode brain sensors. The nerve impulse is generated when there is a change in the voltage between the membranes. This nerve impulse is also known as the action potential. These pulses are further captured and displayed as a waveform known as brain wave or brain rhythm. Due to this, the brain sensor records the changes and shows them as attention and meditation values with timestamps. Attention values are responsible for the beta waves, which are caused by problem-solving or decision-making. In contrast, meditation values are responsible for alpha waves, which cause calm and learning processes.

Fig. 4 & Fig.5 are the frequency-time graphs of the EEG brain waves. These graphs help differentiate meditation and attention values easily by mapping their frequency values to time. From the low frequency to time, Fig.4 gives the idea of meditation waves, and from high frequency to time, Fig.5 shows an idea of attention waves.

Figure 4 Alpha waves (Meditation)

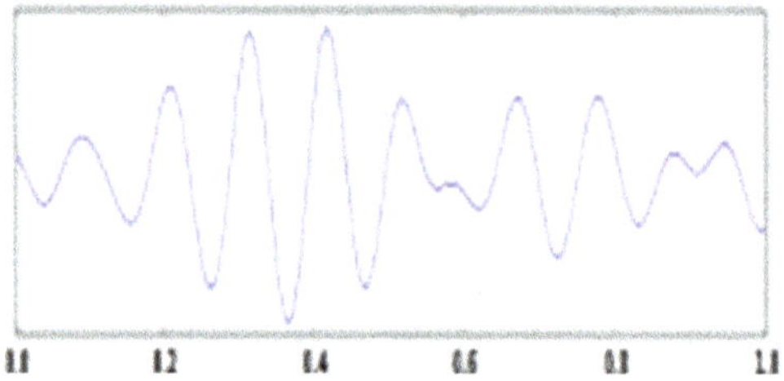

Figure 5. Beta waves (Attention)

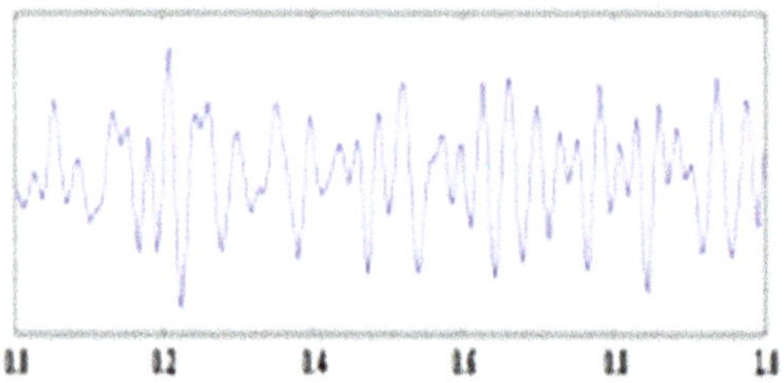

a. Dataset Evaluation

The EEG recordings of brain activity datasets can be used to analyze how Apache Spark can be useful in developing deep learning models for small and large datasets. EEG dataset of brain activity is a small dataset that has only three features, which are input to the deep learning model, i.e., Attention values, Meditation values, and Time Since Last Packet (TSLP), the dataset has 6758 instances. The dataset's output or label feature is the resulting brain activity representing the particular set of attention and meditation values. The output label feature is classified into ten different cases of brain activity.

b. Data Acquisition

Data acquisition is possible with the help of EEG sensors (brain sense). The sensor has two electrodes attached to the band, one electrode is placed on the forehead, and another is used as a clip to the earlobe. The sensor operates at 3.3V and uses Bluetooth v2.0+ to transfer sampled data to the connected device.

c. Data Storing

The brainwaves data are transferred to neuroview with the help of a Bluetooth connection. Further, neuroview helps to record the EEG waves and store them in the form of numerical data with each timestamp in CSV format. The CSV files generated by neuroview are raw_data, filtered_data, powerspectrum_data, meditation_data and attention_data.

d. Data Pre-Processing

The data is further pre-processed for efficient training of deep learning models. The input features are sampled and scaled between 0 to 1 values. The scaling of data will produce efficient results as noise will be reduced in features and even fewer outliers. After sampling and scaling input features, the Output label is divided into different class labels with the help of One Hot Encoding (OHE). After performing OHE, the ten different cases present in the label feature are divided into ten different features of the labeled class with values of 0 and 1 representing false or true, respectively for a particular case to happen. After completing the pre-processing of data, the pre-processed data is shuffled randomly and then divided into training and test data for deep learning models. The random shuffling of data omits the case of bias results from a deep learning model.

II. Epileptic Seizure Dataset

This is the primary dataset used in this research. The dataset is mentioned as the Epileptic seizure recognition dataset. It is a vast dataset with 179 total features. The epileptic seizure dataset helps test Apache Spark's specification over such an EEG dataset and see how effective it can be with a deep learning model to produce efficient results.

a. Dataset Evaluation

The EEG dataset of epileptic seizures comprises five different folders with 100 files each. To which each file represents a person/patient. Each file consists of an EEG recording for 23.6 seconds. Within that time, a total of 4097 data instances were recorded. After combining the data of 500 people/patients for every 23.6 seconds and 4097 cases, we get a total of 2,048,500 data instances.

The data has 178 features of multimodal brain waves captured from different parts of the brain and an output label feature which defines 5 cases based on the result from 178 features of multimodal brainwaves. The cases involved with the output of the epileptic seizure dataset are,

Table 1. Output cases (Epileptic Seizure dataset)

Case	Description
1	Recording of seizure activity
2	Previously had a brain tumor
3	Region identified in the brain for previously located tumor, and now the brain is healthy
4	EEG recording when person/patient eyes are closed
5	EEG recording when person/patient eyes are open

From the above table, the patient/person having cases 2, 3, 4, and 5 do not have any seizure activity, and only the patient/person having case 1 has an epileptic seizure.

b. Data Pre-Processing

The epileptic seizure data collected is further pre-processed so that the deep learning model can train itself efficiently. The data set is a collection of 178 input features and one output feature. Patient ID is dropped from the dataset; as such, it is irrelevant to the prediction method. Further, one hot encoding (OHE) is performed over the output of epileptic features. Performing OHE will divide the output feature into five different output features, representing five other test cases individually. The values of these features will be zero and one, which will mean false or true, respectively, for a particular case. Again, to omit the deep learning model's bias prediction, the pre-processed data is shuffled randomly and then divided into train and test data into 70% and 30% of aggregate data.

2. Methods

I. Feature Importance

Feature Importance is one of the crucial aspects of feature selection. It tells which features play an essential role in predicting the final label. The research in this chapter considers feature importance in the deep learning model itself, as for individual patients, the importance of features could change depending upon their brain health. Therefore, weights decided for the Feed Forward Neural Network (FFNN) depend upon the importance of a feature; this will increase the accuracy and solve the problem of feature importance in different patients.

The weights for the most important features will be high, so their impact can be more significant on the decision process. Gradually, weights will decrease for the decrease in the importance of the features so that the less essential features do not have a predominant role in the decision process.

For feature selection in this chapter, five methods are used. They are,

a. Pearson Correlation

Pearson correlation is a filter-based method. It is defined as,

$$r = \frac{\Sigma(x-\bar{x})(y-\bar{y})}{\sqrt{\Sigma(x-\bar{x})^2(y-\bar{y})^2}} \tag{1}$$

r is the Pearson correlation, which is calculated between the target label and the features. The larger the value of r, the more is the importance of that particular feature.

b. Chi-Squared

Chi-squared is another filter-based method. It is defined as,

$$x^2 = \sum_{i=1}^{n} \frac{(O_i - E_i)}{E_i} \tag{2}$$

x^2 is the chi-squared, which measures the relationship between the target label and input features. The larger the value of x^2, the more important is the feature.

c. Recursive Feature Elimination

Recursive feature elimination is a wrapper based method. This type of method considers a group of features for testing.

The selection of smaller and smaller features by recursion is the primary goal of Recursive Feature Elimination (RFE). Coef_ and feature__importance_ are the two types of the attribute that will provide a set of features trained by estimators. After training, the least important features are removed. The above procedure is performed recursively to get the desired number of features with the maximum importance.

The estimator used in the following deep learning model for RFE is LogisticRegression and coef_ as the observer attribute.

d. Lasso Regularization

Lasso is an embedded method which uses the L1 norm of regularization.

$$\alpha \sum_{i=1}^{k} |w_i| \tag{3}$$

Lasso's norm regularization drives parameters to zero. A higher alpha value has fewer features having non-zero values in relation to target labels. Lasso, by default, forces weights used in neural networks of less important features to be zero.

e. Tree-Based Selection

The Tree-based selection technique uses an embedded method approach, as they have built-in feature selection methods. RandomForest and LightGBM are used as tree-based selection techniques in the following deep learning model.

The Tree-based selection technique uses node impurities in each decision tree. The final output is the average of all the decision trees. The difference between RandomForest and LightGBM is that RandomForest uses a horizontal approach to calculate node impurities and average, whereas LightGBM uses a vertical approach.

f. Application of all the Feature Selection Techniques on the Epileptic-Seizure Dataset

Further, all the feature selections were applied to the epileptic seizure dataset. The dataset has a total of 178 input features, and it is possible that for a particular patient, not all input features are as important as others. Therefore, the above techniques will help measure the importance of input features and arrange them in descending order of importance.

The table-2 describes the top 20 features from 178 input features based on the approval from the tested feature selection techniques, i.e., Chi-Squared (CS), LightGBM (LGBM), Logistic Regression (LR), Pearson Correlation (PCR), Recursion Feature Elimination (RFE), Random Forest (RF). IN table-2, IF is the Input Feature, and Total describes the number of the feature selection test, which approves a particular input feature for selection based on its importance with the target label.

II. Prediction Method

The following research has two Feed Forward Neural Networks (FFNN), which are built on top of SystemML to recognize both brain activity and epileptic seizure activity.

Table 2. Feature importance

Sr. No	IF	CS	LGBM	LR	PCR	RFE	RF	Total
1	X 44	T	T	T	T	T	F	5
2	X 27	T	F	T	T	T	F	4
3	X 26	T	F	T	T	T	F	4
4	X 173	T	F	T	T	T	F	4
5	X 158	T	F	F	T	T	T	4
6	X 12	T	T	T	T	F	F	4
7	X 11	T	F	T	T	T	F	4
8	X 96	T	T	F	T	F	F	3
9	X 43	T	F	T	T	F	F	3
10	X 178	F	T	T	F	T	F	3
11	X 160	T	F	F	T	F	T	3
12	X 159	T	F	F	T	F	T	3
13	X 157	T	F	F	T	F	T	3
14	X 125	F	T	T	F	T	F	3
15	X 121	F	T	T	F	T	F	3
16	X 1	F	T	T	F	T	F	3
17	X 95	T	F	F	T	F	F	2
18	X 94	T	F	F	F	T	F	2
19	X 9	T	F	F	T	F	F	2
20	X 8	T	F	F	T	F	F	2

The FFNN built for the brain activity and epileptic-seizure datasets are almost similar. The only differences are the number of input features, hidden layers, and output features, which are 3, 5, and 10, respectively. The brain activity dataset is small compared to the epileptic seizure dataset and thus is only considered to measure spark performance when dealing with the smaller dataset. The main focus of the research is on epileptic seizures.

a. FFNN Architecture

There are various parameters and hyper-parameters used in this FFNN to reach up to its utmost accuracy.

Fig. 6 represents the actual neural network used in this chapter to detect epileptic seizures. The architecture in the figure is divided into three parts, i.e., Input Features (IF), Hidden Layers (H), and Output Features (O). There are a total of 178 input features (IF) that connect the first hidden layer with 2000 hidden units. The first hidden layer links with the second hidden layer with 1800 hidden units, and this continues up to the 10th hidden layer with 200 hidden units. All the hidden layers have ReLU as their activation function. The last hidden layer links with the output layer, which uses Softmax as its activation function; this helps predict the output label's probability. The resulted output label gets predicted to have the highest probability.

The number of nodes choose for the first hidden layer is kept high generally to not miss any relation between all the attributes of the dataset. After that 200 units are decreased in each layer till it becomes 200 in the 10th hidden layer. Each hidden layer has ReLU as its activation function as it will help to normalize the values of hidden layer and give the value itself if it is positive else zero if the value is negative. This will also help to eliminate any negative values from the hidden layer. The last layer will have softmax as its activation function as it will help to detect which case the attributes of the dataset belongs to by giving the value of each case between 0 and 1, this can be regarded as the probability of each case. By this we can get the predicted case for the given 178 attributes. By this the parameters and hyper-parameters were chosen in this FFNN.

Figure 6. FFNN architecture

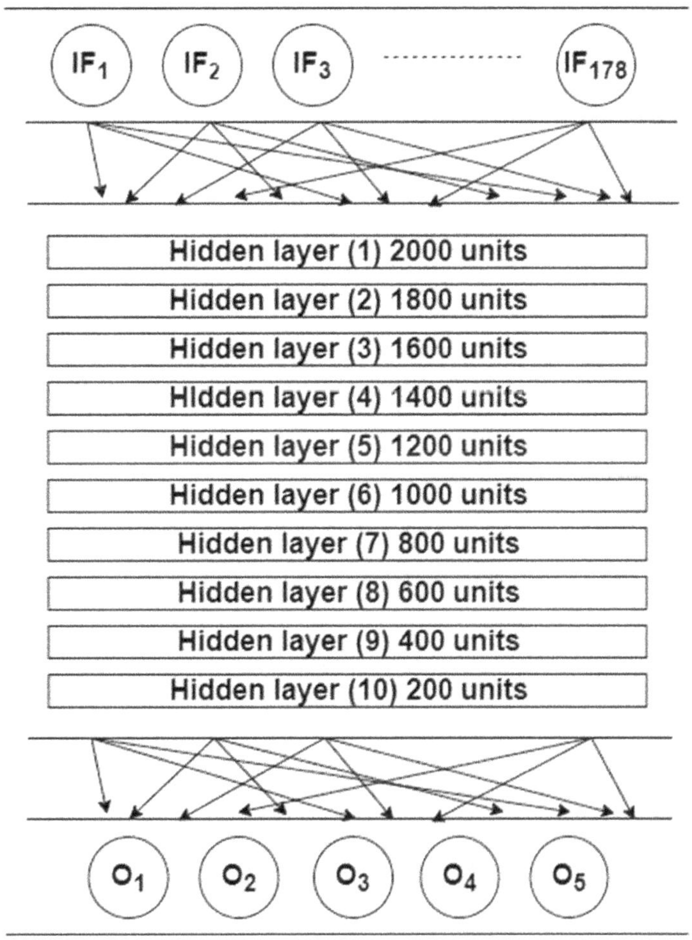

b. Activation Function

Activation function (*f*(*x*)) in Fig.7 is used to normalize the value received from the previous layer of the neural network. Activation functions used in FFNN are the Rectified Linear Unit (ReLU) for hidden layers and Softmax function for the output layer.

Figure 7. Activation function

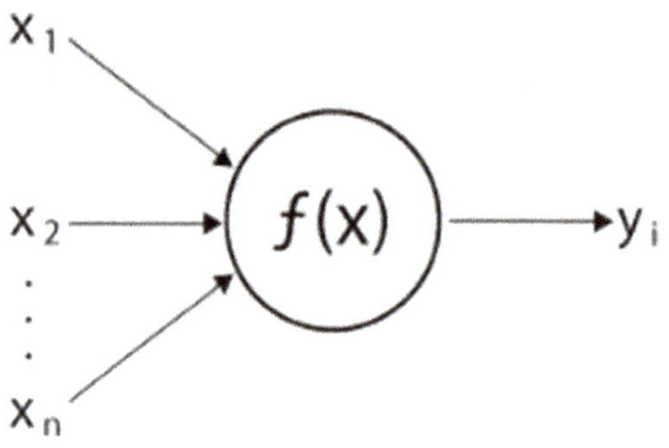

$$x = \sum_{n=1}^{10} \left(IF_n . W_n \right) \tag{4}$$

- **Rectified Linear Unit (ReLU)**

V. Nair et al. (2010) ReLU is applied to all the hidden layers in the built FFNN. It takes the value from the previously hidden layer from the eq. 5 and converts the value x to the value itself if it is positive or zero if the value is negative. This helps to normalize the hidden layer values.

$$f_{relu}(x) = \max(x,0) \tag{5}$$

Based on the eq. 5 the graph for the ReLU activation function used in FFNN is shown in Fig.8.

Figure 8. ReLU graph

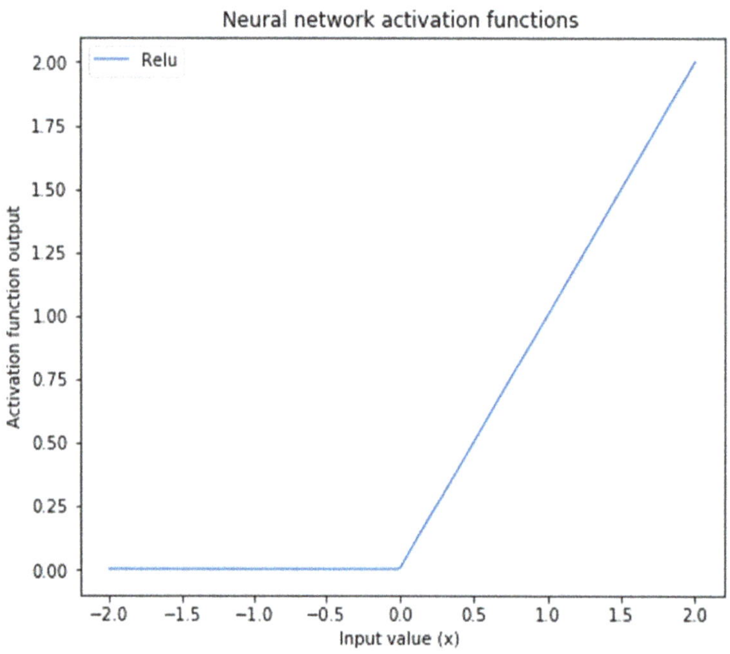

- **Softmax Function**

The softmax activation function is used only at the output layer of the FFNN. The function takes the input from the last hidden layer and converts it to 1 for the positive value and 0 for the negative value. It also formulates the probability distribution among the 5 cases of the epileptic seizure activity and chooses the case whose probability is high among all the 5 cases. Therefore because of this, it is applied to the output layer only.

$$f_{softmax} = \frac{e^{zj}}{\sum_{k=1}^{K} e^{zk}} \text{ for } j=1\ldots K \quad (6)$$

Where,

Z = vector of input to the output layer
j = number of output nodes

Based on the eq. 6, the graph for the Softmax activation function used in FFNN is shown in Fig.9.

Figure 9. Softmax graph

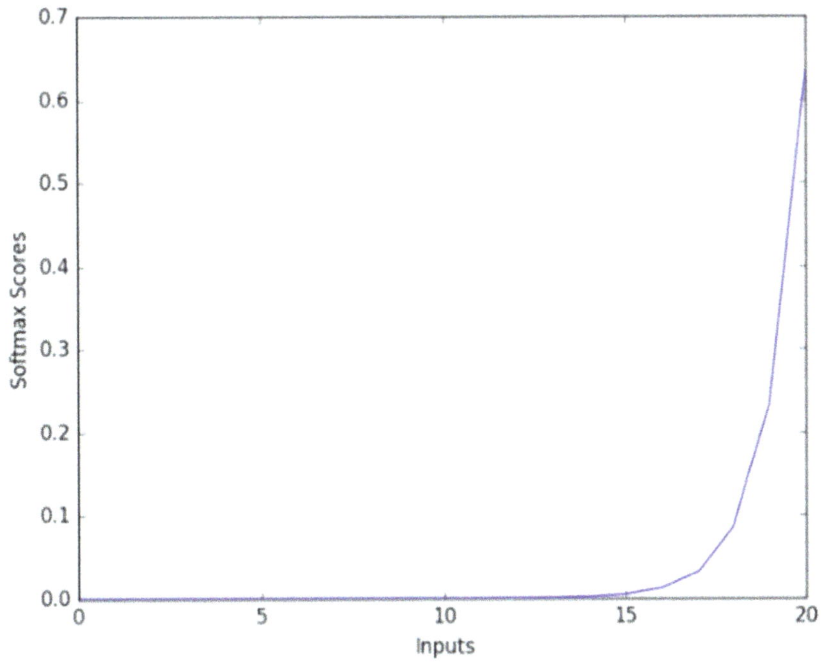

c. Performance Evaluation

The deep learning model has trained over 9200 samples and tested 2300 samples from epileptic seizure activity dataset with 100 epochs.

Figure 10. Loss graph

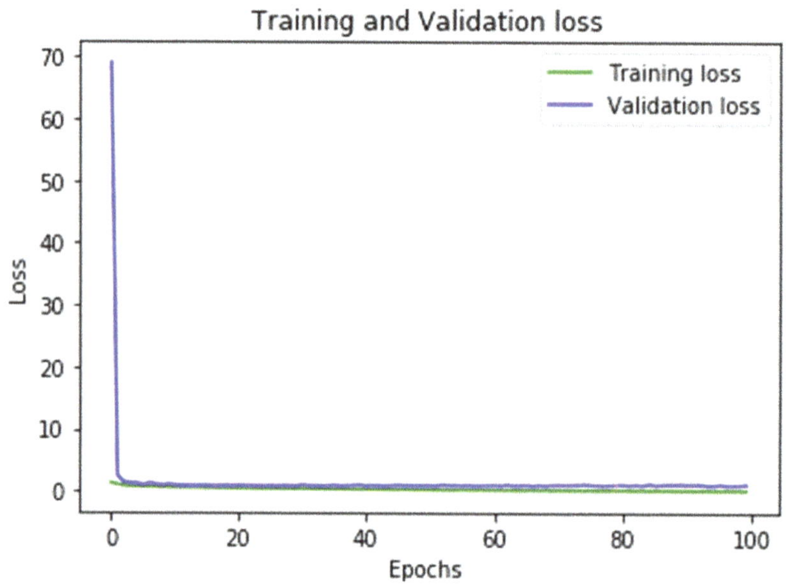

Fig. 10, shows that both training loss and validation loss decreased swiftly in the first ten epochs and then deliberated the rate of loss with an increase in the number of epochs.

Figure 11. Accuracy graph

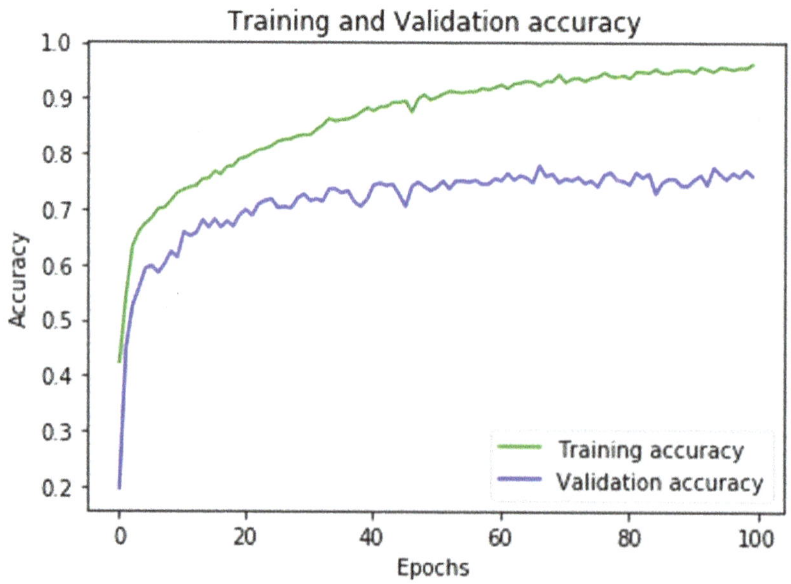

Fig. 11 shows that training accuracy steadily increased over the number of epochs, giving the final training accuracy of 96%. Validation accuracy had a steady increase till 50 epochs, and then it was stable till the 100th epoch, giving the final validation accuracy 77%.

From the above loss and accuracy graph (Fig.10 & Fig.11), it can be inferred that the FFNN model is unfettered from overfitting and underfitting, as the plot of validation accuracy and validation loss never crosses with training accuracy and training loss respectively.

d. Performance Metric

Accuracy is not only a way to measure a deep learning model's performance. Another performance metric that can be analyzed to measure the deep learning model's performance is a confusion matrix developed for the deep learning model of the epileptic seizure dataset.

Fig.12 represents the confusion matrix; this helps inspect true labels in a row and predicted labels in a column.

A confusion matrix gives a tabular representation of different types of predictions compared to its true values of different classes present in the dataset.

1. The confusion matrix is made up of x and y axis.
2. Along the y axis are the true labels of the 5 cases mentioned in the dataset.
3. Along the x axis are the predicted labels by the deep learning model of the 5 cases mentioned in the dataset.
4. The intersection of each case from the true label (y axis) and predicted label (x axis) shows the number of cases which were predicted correctly by the deep learning model.
5. For example, for case 0 which is "recording of the seizure activity" the intersection of true label and predicted label gives a total 441 cases which were predicted correctly by the deep learning model.
6. The other cases from the predicted label which is intersected by the case 0 of the true label show the number of cases which were false negative of case 0.
7. The other cases from the true label which is intersected by the case 0 of the predicted label shows the number of cases which are false positive of case 0.

The same above analysis can be applied to the other cases of the dataset.

The above confusion matrix helps us to analyze various performance metrics like Precision, Recall, and F1 measure.

1) **Precision**: The value of precision belongs between 0 and 1. It shows that percent of data predicted by the deep learning model is truly positive.

$$precision = \frac{TP}{TP + FP} \tag{7}$$

2) **Recall**: It can be regarded as True Positive Rate, which gives us the insight that what percent can be regarded as predicted positive from total positive.

Figure 12. Confusion matrix

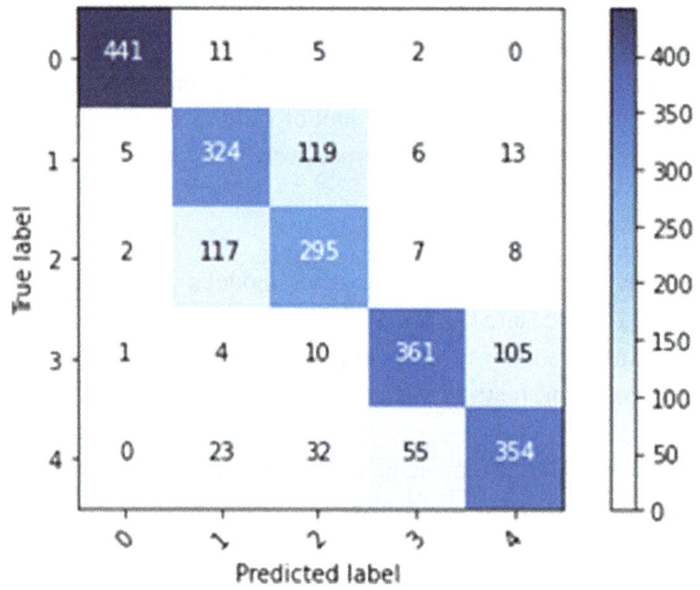

$$recall = \frac{TP}{TP + FN} \tag{8}$$

3) **F1-score**: The harmonic mean of precision and recall is know as f1-score. It is consider where the dataset is imbalance as it contains both false positive and false negative into account.

$$f1 - score = \frac{2}{\frac{1}{precision} + \frac{1}{recall}} = \frac{2 * (precision * recall)}{(precision + recall)} \tag{9}$$

Figure 13 Classification Report

	precision	recall	f1-score	support
0	0.98	0.96	0.97	459
1	0.68	0.69	0.68	467
2	0.64	0.69	0.66	429
3	0.84	0.75	0.79	481
4	0.74	0.76	0.75	464
accuracy			0.77	2300
macro avg	0.77	0.77	0.77	2300
weighted avg	0.78	0.77	0.77	2300

In the above classification report (Fig.13), 0,1,2,3, and 4 are the 5 cases of the epileptic seizure in which 0 tells regarding the seizure activity in the brain. The classification report concludes that all the performance metrics for 0 are close to 98%, which is a successful outcome of the deep learning model.

III. Apache Spark Interface with Deep Learning Model

After the successful compilation of python libraries, SystemML and PySpark are used to interface Apache Spark with the deep learning model. Further, the pipeline is built using PySpark, Keras, and SystemML that can run Apache Spark. Spark is the most salient feature in the following research, as Spark can process massive amounts of data with tremendous speed. The epileptic seizure dataset has total data instances close to 2 million, which is comparatively small as the data recorded is for only 24.6 seconds, and 500 patients/persons. Imagine that the data is recorded for two minutes, the number can quickly shift close to 10 million. To process such big data with a traditional approach can take around 5 to 10 hours and even a whole day, as EEG recording can generate thousands of data in a few seconds.

First, PySpark uses SparkSession to initiate a spark environment. Second, when using the SystemML, the code used for building the FFNN is the same as the traditional approach. Third, the deep learning model imports the SystemML library. From the SystemML library, Keras2DML class is used as a wrapper class to serialize FFNN to the Caffe model. The Caffe model again is converted to Declarative Machine Learning (DML) script, one which the Spark environment can understand. Keras2DML further uses the Spark session, input shape of the training dataset, the training samples, batch size, and FFNN to process with the number of epochs defined.

Figure 14. Keras2DML snippet

```
from systemml.mllearn import Keras2DML
import math
epochs = 100
batch_size = 220
samples =  9200
max_iter = int(epochs*math.ceil(samples/batch_size))
sysml_model = Keras2DML(spark_session, model, input_shape=(9200, 178, 1),
                        weights='weights_dir', batch_size=batch_size,
                        max_iter=max_iter, test_interval=0, display=10)
```

Fig. 14 is the code snippet from the deep learning model, which describes how FFNN uses Keras-2DML as a wrapper class.

After applying a fit method to train the Keras2DML model, the trained model shows the same performance metrics values with the validation accuracy of 77%.

RESULTS

I. Deep Learning Model on Epileptic Seizure Dataset

Various results could be concluded after applying all the appropriate data pre-processing techniques, parameters, hyper-parameters, and activation function and performance metrics.

From the fig.12 Confusion matrix,

1. Case 0, being the recording of seizure activity, has the highest correct predicted values with an accuracy of 98%.
2. Case 1 and 2 are closely related to each other due to similarities in the multimodal brainwaves.

II. Apache Spark and Deep Learning

1) Comparison of accuracy for cases,

Figure 15. Accuracy comparison

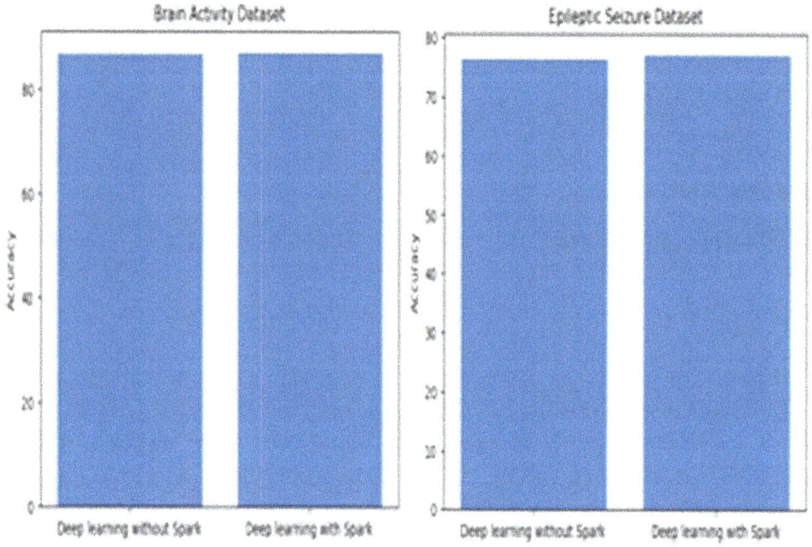

In Fig. 15 the accuracy comparison is showed when the deep learning model is trained with the help of apache spark and without apache spark. By seeing both graph of both the datasets we can see that there is minor increase in the accuracy when the deep learning model is trained on apache spark. The table 3 and 4 can further show the slight increase in the accuracy.

2) Comparison of time taken for cases

Table 3. Brain Activity dataset (Accuracy)

	"Deep learning without Apache Spark"	"Deep learning with Apache Spark"
Accuracy	86.56	86.76

Table 4. Epileptic seizure dataset (Accuracy)

	"Deep learning without Apache Spark"	"Deep learning with Apache Spark"
Accuracy	76.2	76.9

Figure 16. Processing time comparison

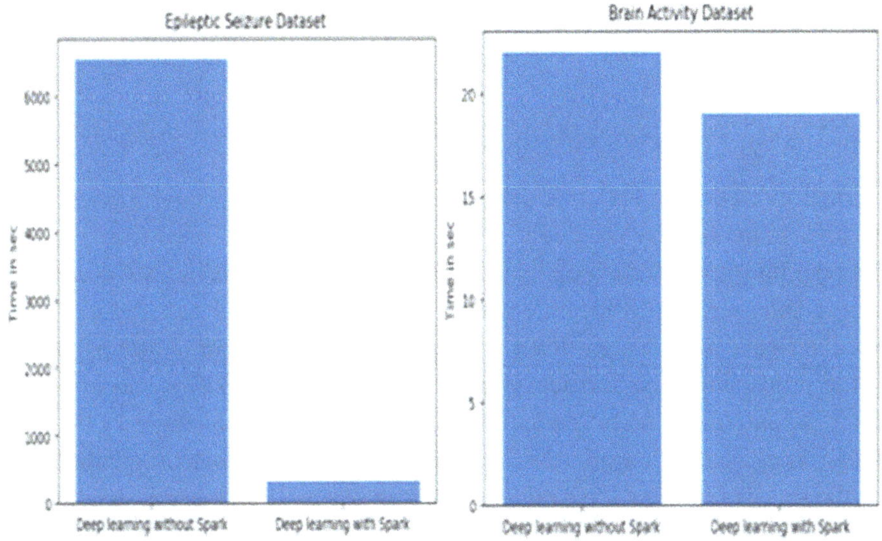

In Fig. 16 the time comparison is showed when the deep learning model is trained with the help of the apache spark and without apache spark. By seeing both the datasets we can see that there is drastic change is the time taken to train the deep learning model on apache spark for epileptic seizure dataset whereas there is slight decrease in the time taken when deep learning model is trained on apache spark for the brain activity dataset.

Table 5. Brain activity dataset (Time taken)

	"Deep learning without Apache Spark"	"Deep learning with Apache Spark"
Time taken (sec)	22	19

Table 6. Epileptic seizure dataset (Time taken)

	"Deep learning without Apache Spark"	"Deep learning with Apache Spark"
Time taken (sec)	6530	320

Various outcomes can be drawn from fig. 15 and fig.16 and table 3, table 4, table 5 and table 6,

1. There is negligible change in the accuracy concerning the involvement of Spark technology, and the dataset is chosen.
2. A drastic change in processing time to train the deep learning model can be seen in fig. 12 for epileptic seizures as processing time drops from 6530 seconds to directly 320 seconds when a deep learning model is involved with spark technology.
3. There is a slight decrease in processing time to train the deep learning model can be seen in fig. 12 for brain activity dataset as processing time drops from 22 seconds to 19 seconds.

CONCLUSION

This chapter aimed to recognize epileptic seizures using the deep learning model and observe how Apache Spark can lead to effective prediction. To which it can be concluded from this chapter that the deep learning model built for detecting epileptic seizure activity diagnoses 98% correct predictions for the seizure activity and overall 77% accurate prediction (including other cases).

Further, Apache Spark plays a significant role in processing such an enormous amount of dataset by decreasing the processing time drastically from 6530 seconds to 320 seconds. As when the deep learning model is not interfaced with Spark, the Keras model runs on a single JVM. But when a deep learning model is interfaced with spark, the Keras model adapts training on parallel Spark instances, thus increasing the speed of training the model on Spark instances. Spark is not so helpful when training small datasets such as brain activity datasets. To train a deep learning model on such a dataset, Spark uses only one of its instances, which is similar to using a single JVM. Therefore no drastic change could be noticed for a small dataset.

The main reason to use two datasets of different sizes but of same domain was to check that how effective spark play role in the training of deep learning model. Therefore, the primary dataset was epileptic seizure dataset and the secondary dataset was brain activity dataset. The deep learning model which was used for both the dataset was also same, the only difference was the size of both the datasets. Predicting epileptic seizure is a vast area of research and there are other deep learning models which can provide a decent accuracy while predicting the epileptic seizure but the processing time required is that particular models are very high. The deep learning model provided in this chapter works great with spark giving a precision of 98% and very less processing time of 320 seconds.

The final results testify that the FFNN built with the Spark technology for the epileptic seizure detection outperforms the other machine learning algorithms in both accuracy and processing time.

REFERENCES

Al Ghayab, H. R., Li, Y., Siuly, S., & Abdulla, S. (2019). Epileptic seizures detection in EEGs blending frequency domain with information gain technique. *Soft Computing*, *23*(1), 227–239. doi:10.100700500-018-3487-0

Apache. (2016). *SystemML (incubating)*. http://systemml.apache.org

Ashari, A. (2015). On Optimizing Machine Learning Workloads via Kernel Fusion. PPoPP. doi:10.1145/2688500.2688521

Beeraka, S. M., Kumar, A., Sameer, M., Ghosh, S., & Gupta, B. (2022). Accuracy Enhancement of Epileptic Seizure Detection: A Deep Learning Approach with Hardware Realization of STFT. *Circuits, Systems, and Signal Processing*, *41*(1), 461–484. doi:10.100700034-021-01789-4

Bengio, Y., Courville, A., & Vincent, P. (2013, August). Representation learning: A review and new perspectives. *IEEE Transactions on Pattern Analysis and Machine Intelligence*, *35*(8), 17981828. doi:10.1109/TPAMI.2013.50 PMID:23787338

Boehm, Dusenberry, Eriksson, Evfimievski, Manshadi, Pansare, Reinwald, Reiss, Sen, Surve, & Tatikonda. (n.d.). *SystemML: Declarative Machine Learning on Spark*. IBM Research.

Boehm. (2016). *Declarative Machine Learning - A Classification of Basic Properties and Types*. CoRR, abs/1605.05826.

Boehm. (2014). Hybrid Parallelization Strategies for Large-Scale Machine Learning in SystemML. *PVLDB, 7*(7).

Boehm. (2014). SystemML's Optimizer: Plan Generation for Large-Scale Machine Learning Programs. *IEEE Data Eng. Bull., 37*(3).

Brinkmann, B. H., Patterson, E. E., Vite, C., Vasoli, V. M., Crepeau, D., Stead, M., Howbert, J. J., Cherkassky, V., Wagenaar, J. B., Litt, B., & Worrell, G. A. (2015). Forecasting seizures using intracranial eeg measures and svm in naturally occurring canine epilepsy. *PLoS One*, *10*(8), e0133900. doi:10.1371/journal.pone.0133900 PMID:26241907

Chaovalitwongse, W. A., Fan, Y.-J., & Sachdeo, R. C. (2007). On the time series k-nearest neighbor classification of abnormal brain activity. *IEEE Transactions on Systems, Man, and Cybernetics. Part A, Systems and Humans*, *37*(6), 1005–1016. doi:10.1109/TSMCA.2007.897589

Elger, C. E. (2001). Future trends in epileptology. *Current Opinion in Neurology*, *14*(2), 185186. doi:10.1097/00019052-200104000-00008 PMID:11262733

Fan, M., & Chou, C. (2019, March). Detecting Abnormal Pattern of Epileptic Seizures via Temporal Synchronization of EEG Signals. *IEEE Transactions on Biomedical Engineering*, *66*(3), 601–608. doi:10.1109/TBME.2018.2850959 PMID:29993518

Golmohammadi, M., Ziyabari, S., Shah, V., de Diego, S. L., Obeid, I., & Picone, J. (2017). Deep architectures for automated seizure detection in scalp EEGs. https://arxiv.org/abs/1712.09776

He, L., Hu, D., Wan, M., Wen, Y., von Deneen, K. M., & Zhou, M. (2016). Common bayesian network for classification of eeg-based multiclass motor imagery bci. *IEEE Transactions on Systems, Man, and Cybernetics. Systems*, *46*(6), 843–854. doi:10.1109/TSMC.2015.2450680

Hinton, G. E., & Salakhutdinov, R. R. (2006). Reducing the dimensionality of data with neural networks. *Science*, *313*(5786), 504507. doi:10.1126cience.1127647 PMID:16873662

Hussein, R., Palangi, H., & Ward, R. K. Z. (2019). Optimized deep neural network architecture for robust detection of epileptic seizures using EEG signals. *Clinical Neurophysiology, 130*(1), 25-37. doi:10.1016/j.clinph.2018.10.010

Lin, L.-C., Chen, S. C.-J., Chiang, C.-T., Wu, H.-C., Yang, R.-C., & Ouyang, C.-S. (2016). Classification preictal and interictal stages via integrating interchannel and time-domain analysis of eeg features. *Clinical EEG and Neuroscience*. PMID:27177554

Litt, B., & Echauz, J. (2002). Prediction of epileptic seizures. *The Lancet Neurology, 1*(1), 22-30. doi:10.1016/S1474-4422(02)00003-0

Min, S., Lee, B., & Yoon, S. (2016). Deep learning in bioinformatics. *Briefings in Bioinformatics*, *18*(5), 851869. PMID:27473064

Mormann, F., Andrzejak, R. G., Elger, C. E., & Lehnertz, K. (2006). Seizure prediction: The long and winding road. *Brain*, *130*(2), 314333. PMID:17008335

Nair, V., & Hinton, G. E. (2010). *Rectified linear units improve restricted boltzmann machines*. Available https://dl.acm.org/citation.cfm

Ouichka, O., Echtioui, A., & Hamam, H. (2022). Deep Learning Models for Predicting Epileptic Seizures Using iEEG Signals. *Electronics (Basel)*, *11*(4), 605. doi:10.3390/electronics11040605

Ozdemir, M. A., Cura, O. K., & Akan, A. (2021). Epileptic EEG classification by using time-frequency images for deep learning. *International Journal of Neural Systems*, *31*(8), 2150026. doi:10.1142/S012906572150026X PMID:34039254

Park, Y. S., Cosgrove, G. R., Madsen, J. R., Eskandar, E. N., Hochberg, L. R., Cash, S. S., & Truccolo, W. (2020, March). Early Detection of Human Epileptic Seizures Based on Intracortical Microelectrode Array Signals. *IEEE Transactions on Biomedical Engineering*, *67*(3), 817–831. doi:10.1109/TBME.2019.2921448 PMID:31180831

Rafik, D., & Larbi, B. (2019). Autoregressive modeling based empirical mode decomposition (EMD) for epileptic seizures detection using EEG signals. *Traitement du Signal*, *36*(3), 273–279. doi:10.18280/ts.360311

Raghu, Sriraam, Gommer, Hilkman, Temel, Rao, Hegde, & Kubben. (2020). Cross-database evaluation of EEG based epileptic seizures detection driven by adaptive median feature baseline correction. *Clinical Neurophysiology, 131*(7), 1567-1578. doi:10.1016/j.clinph.2020.03.033

Shin, Y., Lee, S., Ahn, M., Cho, H., Jun, S. C., & Lee, H.-N. (2015, August). Noise robustness analysis of sparse representation based classification method for non-stationary EEG signal classification. *Biomedical Signal Processing and Control, 21*, 818. doi:10.1016/j.bspc.2015.05.007

Singh, K., & Malhotra, J. (2022). *Smart neurocare approach for detection of epileptic seizures using deep learning based temporal analysis of EEG patterns. Multimed Tools Appl.* doi:10.100711042-022-12512-z

Sun, M., Wang, F., Min, T., Zang, T., & Wang, Y. (2018). Prediction for High Risk Clinical Symptoms of Epilepsy Based on Deep Learning Algorithm. *IEEE Access: Practical Innovations, Open Solutions, 6*, 77596–77605. doi:10.1109/ACCESS.2018.2883562

Takam, C. A., Samba, O., Kouanou, A. T., & Tchiotsop, D. (2020). Spark Architecture for deep learning-based dose optimization in medical imaging. *Informatics in Medicine Unlocked, 19*. doi:10.1016/j.imu.2020.100335

Turner, J. T., Page, A., Mohsenin, T., & Oates, T. (2014). *Deep belief networks used on high resolution multichannel electroencephalography data for seizure detection*. Presented at the AAAI Spring Symp.

Usman, S. M., Khalid, S., & Bashir, S. (2021). A deep learning based ensemble learning method for epileptic seizure prediction. *Computers in Biology and Medicine, 136*. doi:10.1016/j.compbiomed.2021.104710

Vidyaratne, L., Glandon, A., Alam, M., & Iftekharuddin, K. M. (2016). Deep recurrent neural network for seizure detection. *Proc. Int. Joint Conf. Neural Netw. (IJCNN)*, 12021207. 10.1109/IJCNN.2016.7727334

Vieluf, S., Reinsberger, C., El Atrache, R., Jackson, M., Schubach, S., Ufongene, C., Loddenkemper, T., & Meisel, C. (2020). Autonomic nervous system changes detected with peripheral sensors in the setting of epileptic seizures. *Scientific Reports, 10*(1), 11560. doi:10.103841598-020-68434-z PMID:32665704

Walter, B., Wang, S., Chun-An, C., & Jr-Shin, L. (2020). Scientific Reports. Nature, 10(1). doi:10.103841598-020-65401-6

Wang, N., & Lyu, M. R. (2015). Extracting and selecting distinctive eeg features for efficient epileptic seizure prediction. *IEEE Journal of Biomedical and Health Informatics, 19*(5), 1648–1659. doi:10.1109/JBHI.2014.2358640 PMID:25248205

Waterhouse. (2003). New horizons in ambulatory electroencephalography. *IEEE Engineering in Medicine and Biology Magazine, 22*(3), 7480.

Yuan, Y., Xun, G., Jia, K., & Zhang, A. (2017). *A multi-view deep learning method for epileptic seizure detection using short-time Fourier transform*. Presented at the 8thACMInt. Conf. Bioinf., Comput. Biol., Health Inform., Boston, MA. 10.1145/3107411.3107419

Zazzaro, Cuomo, Martone, Montaquila, Toraldo, & Pavone. (2019). EEG signal analysis for epileptic seizures detection by applying Data Mining techniques. *Internet of Things*. doi:10.1016/j.iot.2019.03.002

Zhang, Z., & Parhi, K. K. (2016). Low-complexity seizure prediction from ieeg/seeg using spectral power and ratios of spectral power. *IEEE Transactions on Biomedical Circuits and Systems*, *10*(3), 693–706. doi:10.1109/TBCAS.2015.2477264 PMID:26529783

Chapter 13
Methods for the Recognition of Human Emotions Based on Physiological Response:
Facial Expressions

Nalini Tyagi
Delhi College of Technology and Management, Palwal, India

Mritunjay Rai
Shri Ramswaroop Memorial University, India

Probeer Sahw
https://orcid.org/0000-0003-4541-9203
Galgotias College of Engineering and Technology, India

Padmesh Tripathi
https://orcid.org/0000-0001-9455-1652
IIMT College of Engineering, India

Nitendra Kumar
https://orcid.org/0000-0001-7834-7926
IIMT College of Engineering, India

ABSTRACT

Human emotions like neutral, sad, happy, and others reveal the state of the mind of a person. This information is useful and thus finds its technical, interpersonal, and societal applications in various areas like surveillance, suicide prevention, marketing and strategy, entertainment, etc. The espousal of data science peaked the scientific interest in the detection of human emotions in the late 2000s and early 2010s. The recognition of human emotions is exigent, and it requires accurate inspection of physiological responses and/or facial expressions. Advances in the areas of bio-physiology and neuroscience have

DOI: 10.4018/978-1-6684-2508-4.ch013

introduced numerous new tools for the detection of human emotions. However, many of these tools have certain shortcomings that make their usage limited. Therefore, researchers are continuously working towards new techniques and technologies to find better solutions than the existing ones for the detection of human emotions. This chapter deals with various tools and techniques that are being used for the recognition of human emotions.

1. INTRODUCTION

Human emotions provide a glimpse into the inner thoughts of a person. Humans are capricious and their emotions fluctuate and depend upon the situation and the circumstances. It is to be noted that even the intensity of a particular emotion varies from situation to situation. An accurate assessment of emotions provides a fair idea of one's interest or disinterest in a particular product or activity and behavior in general. This knowledge may be utilized by business organizations to streamline their strategies or institutions to prepare robust policies. And, it is also possible to predict one's next course of action by real-time detection of emotions. This helps in the prevention of potential suicides or attacks and thus, is advantageous in saving human lives. Researchers face a difficult task when it comes to the detection of human emotions. Human sentiments are generally recognizable through facial expressions, but this is not the case all the time. Thus, parameters like a heartbeat, brain waves, pupil size, facial warmth, and others may be captured/measured for the determination of human emotions. Humans often produce distinctive facial gestures for a particular mood; the intensity may vary, and these can be easily ascertained. Certain human emotions, on the other hand, may have similar physical morphology but represent different moods and intensities (Singh, 2012). Detection of human emotions is a key area of research. The findings of the research are utilized by various industries for business purposes and by civic bodies for administration purposes.

A few areas, in which human emotion detection is utilized, are listed below:

- **Robotics:** To create intelligent and interactive playful toy robots which can behave in a particular way in response to a certain human gesture? An example will be the Sony AIBO Dog robot.
- **Marketing:** To add some dynamic and immersive effects to advertisement boards following the emotional state of a consumer to reach out to the consumer in a targeted manner.
- **Education:** To enhance the knowledge transfer and the teaching-learning process by assessing the learners 'perception from their emotions.
- **Entertainment:** To provide selected content to the audience based on their mood.
- **Surveillance:** To monitor suspicious activities and combat potential threats by reading the emotions of a crowd.
- **Suicide Prevention:** To prevent possible suicide attempts by assessing the state of mind of a person out in the public.

In most cases, detection of human emotions at a large scale is required. Hence, it is impractical to do the same manually. Therefore, automated systems for the detection of human emotions are required. Recent advancements in the automation industry have made it possible to build such automated systems with state-of-the-art sensors (Dzedzickis et al., 2020; Feidakis, et al., 2011) state that there are a total of 66 human emotions as per the fundamental taxonomy. Out of these, 10 emotions are deemed to be the fundamental ones and the rest are considered to be the secondary ones. Figure 1 depicts the fundamental emotions as described in (Feidakis et al., 2011) Detection of such a large number of human emotions is a difficult endeavor even with an automated system. Also, a captured/measured parameter is likely a result of mixed emotion, or the same physiological or facial parameter may point to more than one emotion. To avoid such ambiguities, a large number of emotion detection studies have been carried out with consideration of some other/further classification of human emotions (Feidakis et al., 2011). This explores the motional dimensions like activation and arousal, in which it is observed that whether a certain emotional element alleviates or aggravates one's mood (Russell, 1980; Csikszentmihaly, 2014).

Figure 1. Fundamental human emotions

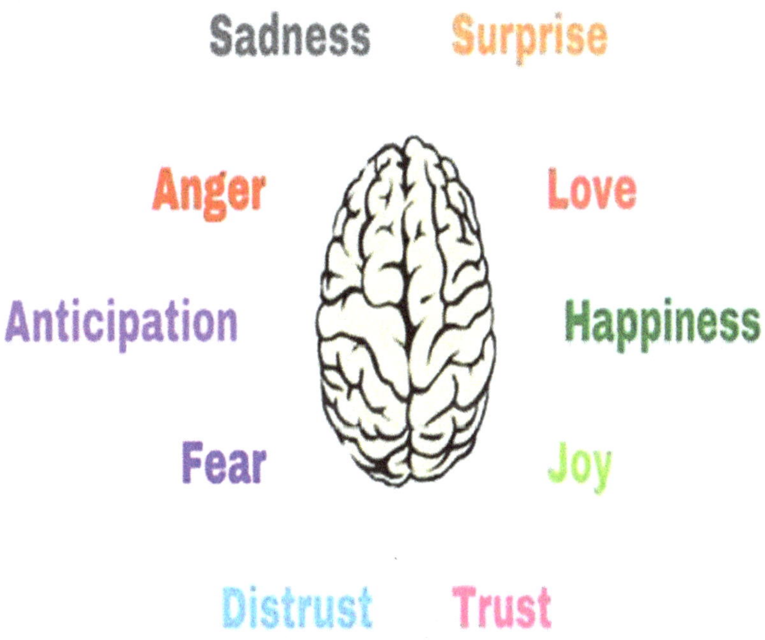

Several scholars based their research upon the findings of a model of emotions proposed by James Russell (Russell, 1980). This model comprehensively provides a perspective of various emotions and their dimensions distributed over a two-dimensional space as depicted in Figure 2. And now, with the advent of the Internet of Things (IoT), machine learning, and deep learning, it is becoming easier to adopt the latest sensor and computing capabilities for the detection of human emotions for rapid prototyping and building highly automated systems.

Figure 2. Model of emotions by James Russell

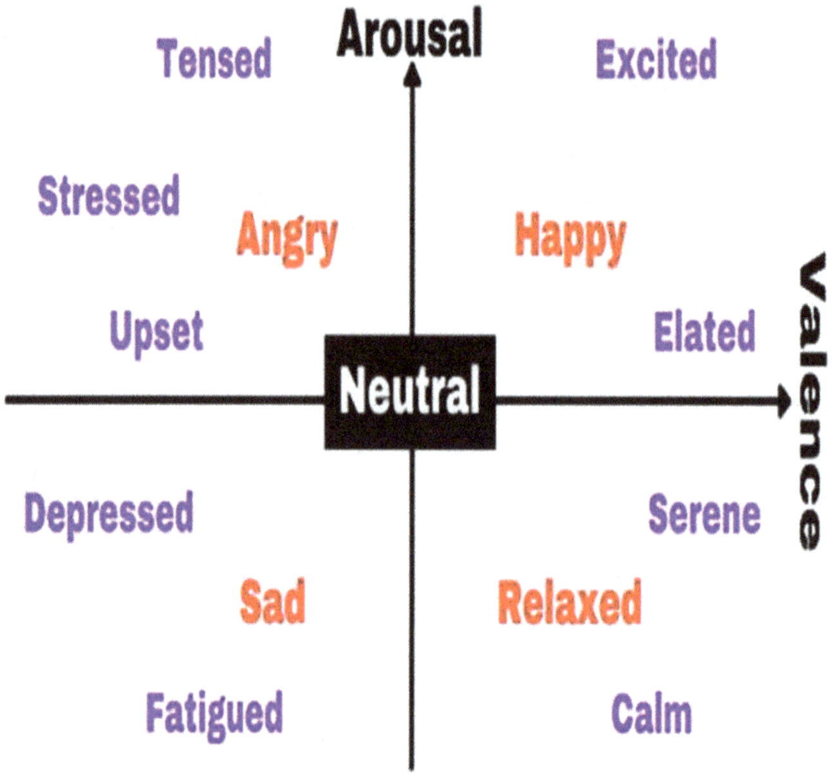

2. EXISTING METHODOLOGIES FOR DETECTION OF HUMAN EMOTIONS

The presented human emotions detection methods are categorized into two parts: one based on measurement of electrical parameters and the other based on the determination of non-electrical parameters of a human body. The non-electrical parameters can be determined either by contact onion-contact measurements. Human emotions are analyzed based on certain characteristics which include cognition, physiology, behavior, and others (Scherer, 2005; Gonçalves et al., 2017). Such an analysis can provide accurate data about the emotional state of a human. Automated systems for the detection of human emotions mainly analyze the nervous system of a human. These systems measure electrical impulses of the brain and can detect the changes in the impulses to analyze the mood of a person. The most popular techniques are ECG, EEG, blood pressure measurement, skin temperature measurement, eye movement tracking, respiratory rate measurement, heart rate measurement, and gesture analysis. Figure 3 enlists various methods of human emotions detection.

2.1 Methods Based on Measurement of Electrical Parameters of a Human Body

There are various methods for the measurement of electrical parameters of a human body which can be utilized for the detection of human emotions. The following methods are discussed in the presented work:

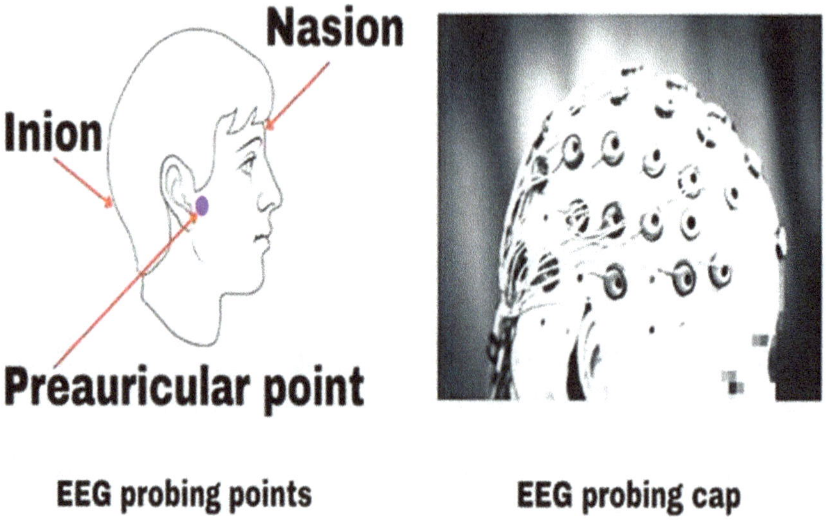

(i) Electroencephalography (EEG)
(ii) Electromyography (EMG)
(iii) Electrooculography (EOG)
(iv) Galvanic skin response (GSR)
(v) Electrocardiography (ECG)

Figure 3. Methods of detection of human emotions

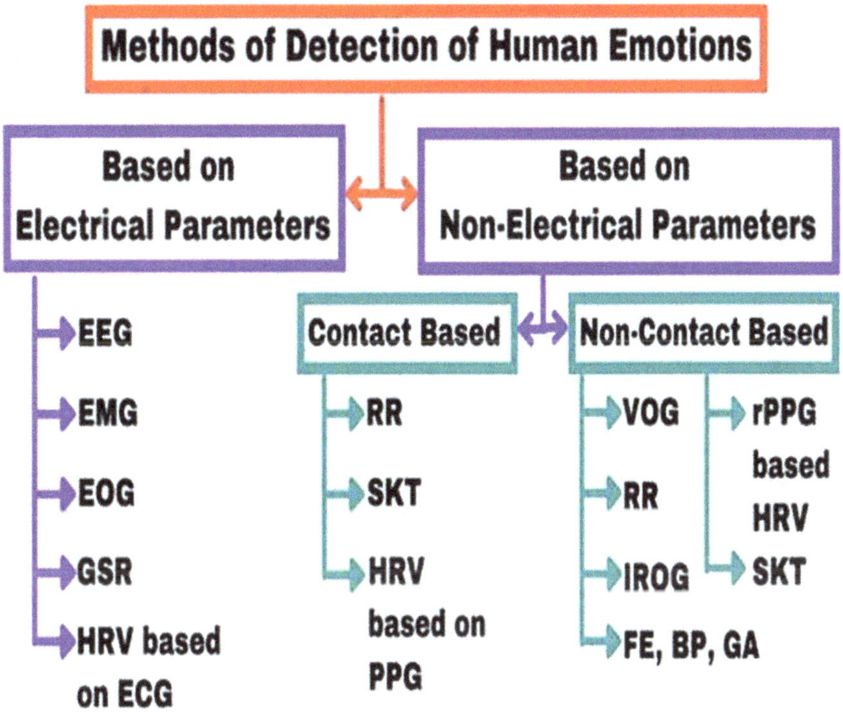

2.1.1 Electroencephalography (EEG)

EEG detects brain waves. Neurons in the human brain generate an electric potential during active mode. This potential can be measured from the outside of the human skull with the help of EEG. It is to be noted that some tissues and the skull lie in between the neurons and the electrodes, hence, it is not possible to get a precise and accurate location of the neuron activity. Therefore, several pairs of electrodes are placed on the head near the four strategic locations as depicted in Figure 4. These four positions on the human head are as follows:

(i) Nasion, the point where the top of the nose meets the ridge of the forehead.
(ii) Inion, the point at the rear lower part of the human skull
(iii) Left Preauricular point, the point on the cheekbone lying immediately to the left ear canal
(iv) Right Preauricular point, the point on the cheekbone lying immediately to the right ear canal

An EEG probing cap is also shown in Figure 4, the cap has a greater number of electrodes according to the widely accepted and standard international 10/20 testing method system.

Figure 4. EEG exam probing points and probing cap

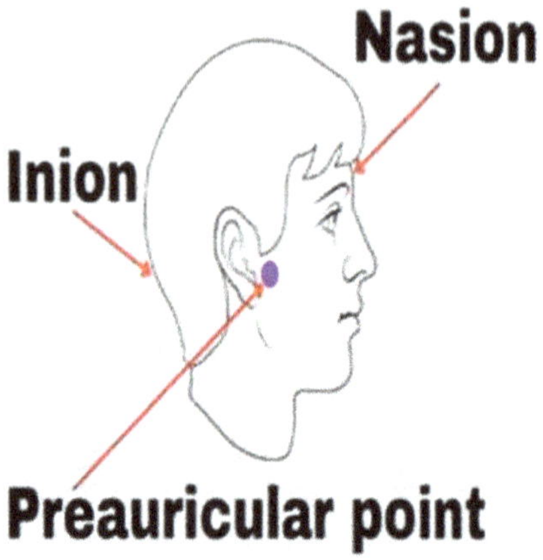

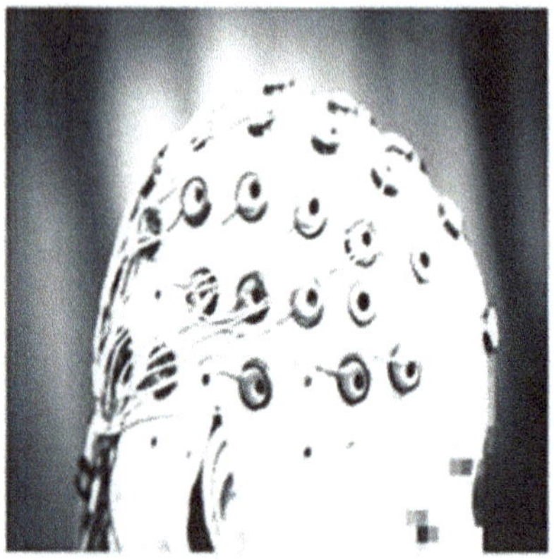

EEG probing points

EEG probing cap

The neurons in the human brain generate rhythmic and continuous signals. These signals are subdivided into four bands, according to their frequency, ranging from the most active to the least active. These bands are discussed below in Table 1.

Table 1. EEG wave bands

Band	Frequency	Amplitude	Description
Beta waves	15-35 Hz	lowest	the brain is in arousing mode; an extremely engaged mind generates beta waves
Alpha waves	8-14 Hz	more than beta	the brain is non-arousal mode; waves are generated when a person is resting
Theta waves	5-8 Hz	more than alpha	waves are generated when a person is napping
Delta waves	1-4 Hz	highest	waves are generated when a person is in deep sleep

No brain waves will be detected if a brain stops working completely i.e. when a person is dead. But, if a person is in deep dreamless sleep, then the frequency of the brain waves goes down to 2-3 Hz i.e., in the delta band. When a person lays down in rest before attempting to sleep, the brain waves are in the beta band. After that, when the person closes his eyes, the brainwaves fall into the alpha band, and after some time when the person falls asleep, the brain waves are in the theta band. Finally, when the person is in deep sleep, the brain waves are in the delta band. Various EEG analysis methods depend upon the object of interest. An efficient test to ascertain the level of valence and arousal is based on the fast Fourier transforms. Also, statistical methods can be used to detect a particular emotion and the strength of that emotion (Vijayan et al., 2015). Neural network-based online classification of EEG to build an emotion recognizer for patients who lost their ability to use their muscles and cannot speak or communicate in any other way found a success rate of more than 60% (Choppin, 20000). An emotion matrix was formed from the cross-correlation of EEG signals from different probe points for four different human moods (Musha, 2002). A study on only arousal was carried out, a comparison was made between only EEG measurement and EEG with physiological measurement and it was found that the latter case produced better results (Chanel, et al., 2006). An experiment on the determination of the power of EEG signals was conducted and tested at various probe points for synchronization, it was presented that the power corresponding to an emotion displayed similar values at all the points (Soleymani et al., 2012).The level of arousal and valence could also be ascertained by a three-layer technique based on EEG-ER which produced convincing results (Liu, et al., 2014). An automated system can be found in the literature that works on statistical methods of higher-order for the determination of human emotions (Zhang, et al., 2016). A study was carried out for recognition of human emotions based on relief channel selection and measurement of EEG (Mehmood and Lee, 2016). A smart system for human emotion detection was built and tested on special students for improving their learning process, the results were found to be highly satisfactory (Purnamasari, et al., 2017).

2.1.2 Electromyography (EMG)

To measure human emotions, electromyography (EMG) has been frequently employed. It's a test that determines the health of the nerve cells that regulate the muscles (motor neurons). Motor neurons generate electrical signals that are transmitted to the brain, causing muscles to contract. Electrodes are used to convert electric signals into graphs, numerical numbers, or aural signals, which researchers can then interpret. During diagnosis, a needle electrode has penetrated muscle to record the electrical activity in that muscle. As only a needle electrode is required it is a low risk and comparatively easy procedure. Electrodes other than needles can be used are surface electrodes to measure the intensity of the signal. Electromyography can easily identify human emotions even in cases where facial expressions are hidden or not much visible (Dimberg, 1982; Lundqvist, 1995). The EMG responses are also termed facial mimicry. The EMG response can be captured after 0.003 sec of application of external probe stimuli. It is proven in the literature that the corrugators, muscle which shows the negative effect of face and zygomatic, muscle which is linked with happiness are linked and affected by the states in the perceiver (JaninaKünecke, et al., 2014). The various EMG probe points are shown in Figure 5.

Facial mimicry is not required for the typical display of emotions. This requires a particular environment, where EMG signals are perceived to be emotional intents. Facial mimicry is better linked to hidden valence facial emotions (Hess and Fischer, 2013). A considerable relationship could be established between EMG and valence emotions in involuntary response to images, texts, and audio signals (Kappas and Thériault, 2000). A real-time system to extract human emotions using EMG and GSR found in literature produced appreciable results (Nakasone, et al., 2005). There is a mention in the literature of automated systems for data analysis and human emotion determination based on EMG, ECG, and GSR based on various bio-signals (Wagenar, et al., 2005; Katsis, et al., 2008).

Figure 5. EMG exam probing points

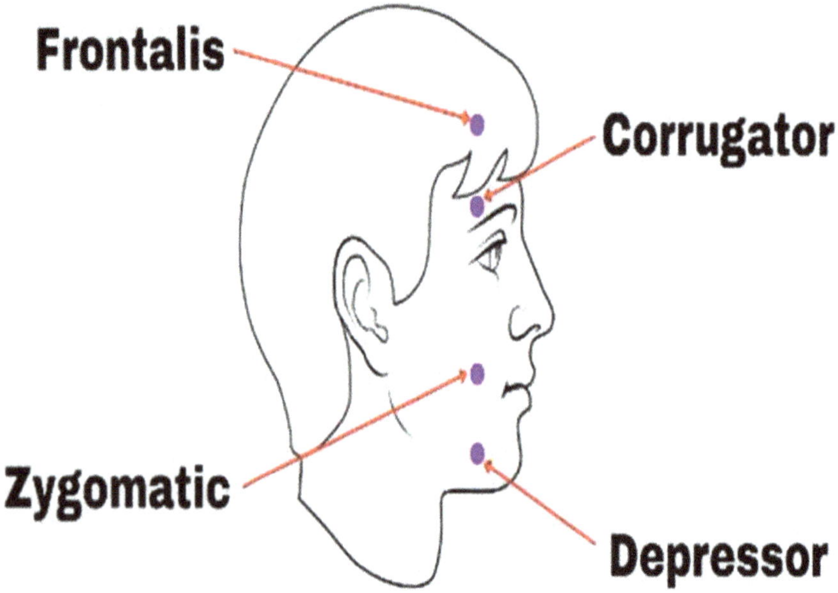

2.1.3 Electrooculography (EOG)

EOG is used to measure the potential of the eye. This cornea-retinal potential is measured between the front and back of the human eye. The signal generated by this technique is called an electrooculogram. EOG is used in the analysis of the movement of the eye. Whenever any emotion occurs in the human mind then eyes also start changing their size which can be measured by electrooculography. Horizontal EOG (HEOG) where the eye moves right and left and vertical EOG (VEOG) where the eye moves up and down, such movements result in Left/Up gaze: resulting in a positive peak in the recorded potential difference. Right/Down gaze: resulting in a negative peak in the recorded potential difference. Not only does eye movement have a distinctive electrical response, but also BLINKING can be detected as continuously rising and falling peaks. However, the main problem while recording the EOG is the head movement. To analyze the movement of the eye pair, electrodes are placed at the left or right of the eye or at up or down of the eye as shown in Figure 6.

Contact and non-contact measurement techniques can be used to apply EOG. EMG electrodes and the same apparatus are acceptable for contact measurements. Video oculography systems (VOG) or infrared camera infrared oculography (IROG) can be used to take non-contact measurements. Silver/Silver-Chloride electrodes can be used for the detection of human emotion by capturing EOG signals using a custom-built system for better measurement (Paul, et al, 2017). A system with a video-based eye tracker and EOG measurement has been tested to determine human emotions with substantial merits (Soundariya and Renuga, 2017). Most of the EOG measurement systems for recognizing human emotions and their classification as positive and negative are video-based systems. These video-based systems demonstrate better performance in finding the intensity of human emotions due to the availability of quality hardware (Chai, et al., 2017; Wang, et al., 2018).

Figure 6. EOG exam probing points

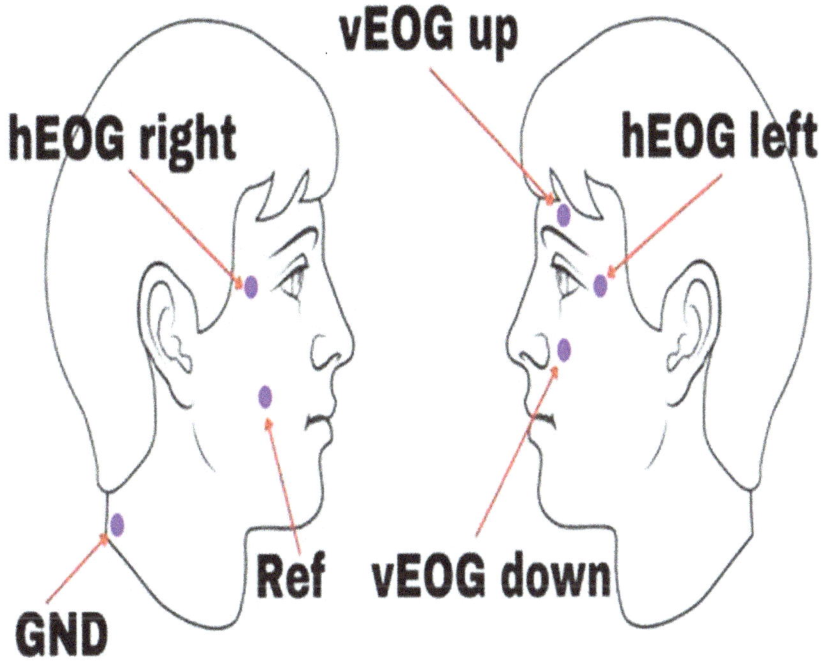

2.1.4 Galvanic Skin Response (GSR)

A variation in the electrical resistance due to changes in human emotion can be easily detected in the skin. A galvanometer can be used to measure this electrical pulse. The electrical resistance of the skin is measured using one or two sensors that contain silver/silver-chloride electrodes (Ayata, et al., 2017). These electrodes can be attached in a variety of ways, although the most common placement is on the fingers, wrist, or foot (Dooren, et al., 2012). A textile-based wearable electrode may also be used for the measurement of skin resistance (Greco, et al., 2016).Textile-based electrodes are also used to determine arousal and its level of intensity using exosomatic GSR. Similar work was done for emotions recognition in which a polar system to determine valence and arousal levels of emotions was used (Villon, et al., 2007). In another research work, another way for extracting data for human emotion measurement from the autonomous nervous system focused on high and low valance and arousal levels (Villon, et al., 2006). Research on human emotions using peripheral and EEG physiological signals over short periods with high neutral low valence and arousal levels. The Biosemi Active II system was employed, as well as a plethysmograph to assess blood pressure. In another paper, they use pattern recognition and classification approaches to measure human emotion from physiological information. The high and low levels were the focus of this study, and the Biosemi Active II device GSR sensing software and hardware were used (Chanel, et al., 2009). The probing measurement for GSR is shown in Figure 7.

Figure 7. GSR exam probing

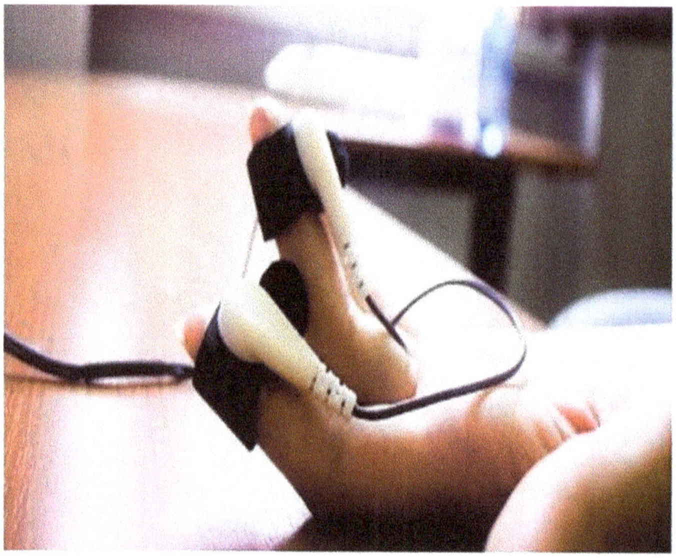

2.1.5 Electrocardiography (ECG)

An electrocardiography test is used to measure the electrical signals produced by the heartbeat. An electric signal is generated by the human heart at every beat. This signal is responsible for the working of the heart muscles, this causes the heart to contract and expand to pump blood. The upper chamber makes the P wave, as the impulse goes from upper to lower chamber a flat line is shown in ECG also called PR segment. Next, the bottom chamber makes the QRS complex wave. Lastly, a T wave is produced when the lower chamber is relaxed. The ECG wave at normal heart rate is shown in Figure 8. Any variability in heart rate can be obtained from ECG and emotion can be detected by analyzing this variability. This heart rate variability (HRV) is obtained by ECG. Every point on the ECG wave has its characteristics and is also related to heart activity (Subramanian, 2017; Mandala and Di, 2017).

Emotion detection is a complex procedure in HRV as compared to EEG. Because the heart rate variable changes with the movement of the object. Therefore, these signals are obtained when the person is in a calm state and not moving to avoid the noise signals. One more precaution taken during ECG is that space should not be affected by the change in the environment. (Cai et al., 2009) with the help of their research concluded that happiness cannot be recognized more precisely and easily than sadness. They also proposed a novel method for automatic feature recognition (Cai et al., 2009; Kumar, et al., 2017). Rattanyu with his co-worker (2010) proposed works on emotion recognition for robots working in the living area. Dissanayake et al. (2019) work on a machine learning program for 4 main emotions (Anger, sadness, pleasure, and joy).

Figure 8. Typical ECG signal

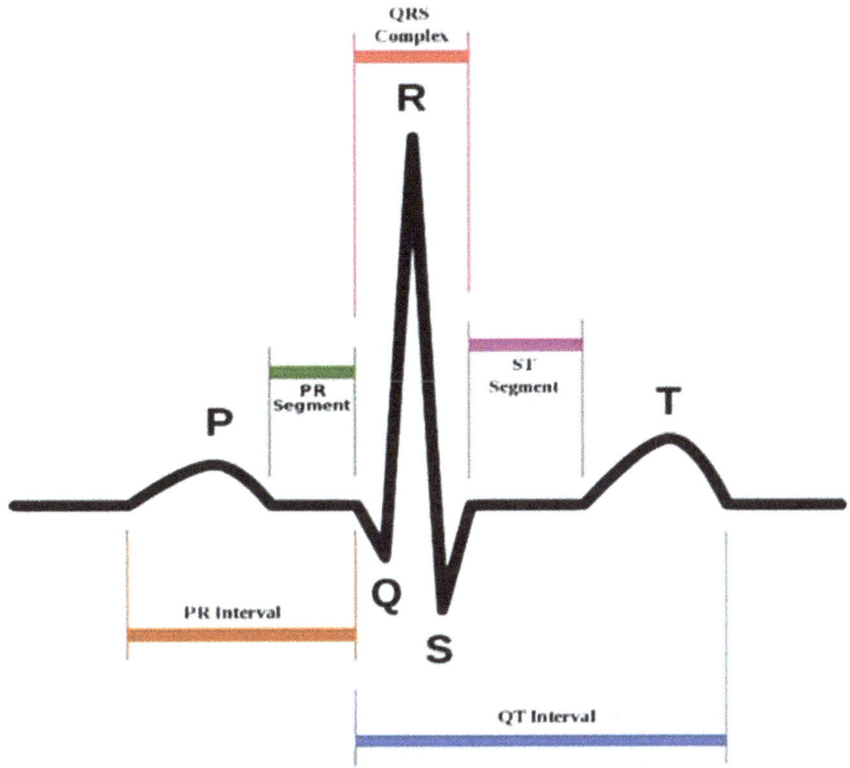

2.2 Methods Based on Measurement of Non-Electric Parameters

As we have seen in earlier literature, there are plenty of methods to measure human emotions which measure the electric parameters of the human body. There are other methods also that measure the non-electric parameters of the human body to detect human emotions. These non-electric parameters may be respiratory rate, skin temperature, BP, gesture, etc.

2.2.1 Respiratory Rate (RR)

The breath cycles completed in a minute by a person are called respiratory rate. This is normally measured when a person is in a static position. It may be affected by any abnormality in the body, for example- any illness, fever, or any other medical issues. During analyzing respiration rate, it should also be noted whether a person is breathing with any difficulty or not. The normal rate of respiration in adults is 12-16 per minute. The data collected from respiratory monitoring have very vital information regarding the emotional state of the human body. The speed and depth of respiratory rate of any human being normally change with the change in emotions. During excitement, one shows deep and rapid breathing, while tensed a person breath shallow and fast and people in relaxed emotion have deep and relaxed breathing. Also, a negative and calm state of emotion is shown by shallow and slow breathing. The respiratory rate can reach up to 40–50 per minute if a person is excited (Zhang, et al., 2017).There is various respiration rate measurement methods. These are based on principles like fluctuation in humidity, temperature, pressure, CO_2 concentration, O_2 concentration in breath going in and coming out (Ginsburg, et al., 2018). There are various ways that emotions and breathing patterns depend on each other.

(i) If a person is in anger, anxiety, or extremely distressed condition then the breathing becomes so rapid. Relationships between respiration i.e., breathing pattern and emotions are very relatable and can be easily noticed especially when we talk about the negative side of emotions, anger distress anxiety, or even rage. If any human being is in such a negative condition which makes perfect sense for the human body like stress or anxiety then the human body enters in an arousal state. Where increased respiration rate gives more oxygen to help fight the cause of the disturbance.

(ii) Breathing patterns can also alter human emotions. In 2006, a study published on Behavior Response & Therapy states that persons who had 15 minutes of slow and focused breathing exercises had more positivity than a group who had 15 minutes of unfocused breathing with low attention and worrying.

(iii) Breathing patterns affect the pain sensation in the human body. If respiration is slow then one would feel less pain sensation. Slow breathing goes beyond calm and peace into pain reduction, at least in some subjects.

(iv) Breathing also responds to odors, it isn't only about inhaling oxygen or exhaling carbon dioxide; it's also about receiving odors. Some studies have shown that our breathing patterns change according to the odor it receives. If one personnel counters the smell of garbage or rotten food that person breathes as shallowly and rapidly as possible, while good smells like perfumes or flowers one takes a long and slow breath. The important point about the breathing pattern in both the conditions is changing before the brain registers the type of smell i.e., a good or a bad smell.

(v) A very new study about emotions reveals that our emotional state also decides what we have exhaled and if we analyze chemically exhalations can identify the feeling of a person. According to research chemical composition of air in crowded stadiums. Every emotional state had its chemical composition.

2.2.2 Skin Temperature Measurement

For any automatic emotion detection, the most important part is a signal, which introduces the nervous system, which is not in human control. One such parameter is the temperature of the skin. Skin temperature depends upon the sweat and heart activity of any human. Thermal radiation of skin (outer part of the body also called cutaneously) depended on irrigation, this irrigation is controlled by the nervous system, and this automatic nervous system controls the vessels that irrigate the skin. There are mainly two types of skin temperature measurement techniques one is the contact method: In this method, various semiconductor sensors are implemented; the other method is a non-contact method which is mainly IR thermography. IR (Infrared) thermography is a method to measure radiations reflected by skin, these radiations further can be used to calculate the temperature. Functional Infrared Thermal Imaging is a proven non-invasive method of determination of human emotions based on skin temperature measurement (Malfaz and Salichs, 2004). In research on infants, it was concluded that their facial temperature decreases with joyful expressions (Nakanishi and Imai-Matsumura, 2008).Human emotions not only vary the temperature on the outer skin but also affect homeostasis (Bruno, et al., 2017). Sonkusare et al. (2019) proposed a novel automatic method for human emotion detection by measurement of temperature.

Lichtenbelt et al. (2006) evaluated the possibility of identification of human facial temperature without wires using temperature loggers (van MarkenLichtenbelt et al., 2007). Puri et al. (2005) proposed a non-contact measurement technique for the detection of human emotional states through thermal imaging. They present a novel Stress Cam method for the non-contact measurement. Said and Barr (2021) suggested a system based on FS-CNN for detecting faces on large scale images and predicting a person's emotional state. Minaee et al. (2021) propose a deep learning approach based on an attention convolutional network that can focus on essential areas of the face and improves significantly on many datasets, including the FER-2013, CK+, FERG, and JAFFE. Chowdhary et al. (2021) proposed using Resnet50, Vgg19, Inception V3, and Mobile Net. The model was trained and evaluated on the CK+ database, with a 96 percent accuracy (Minaee, et al., 2021). A thermal camera is used to take the temperature of the human face. It is used to measure the skin temperature with no contact as this camera takes temperature externally as shown in Figure 9. A thermal camera reads temperatures emitted by the human skin; it is not entered into the body, like traditional temperature detectors. This is the most emerging technique.

Figure 9. Image was taken by IR camera for temperature measurement of face

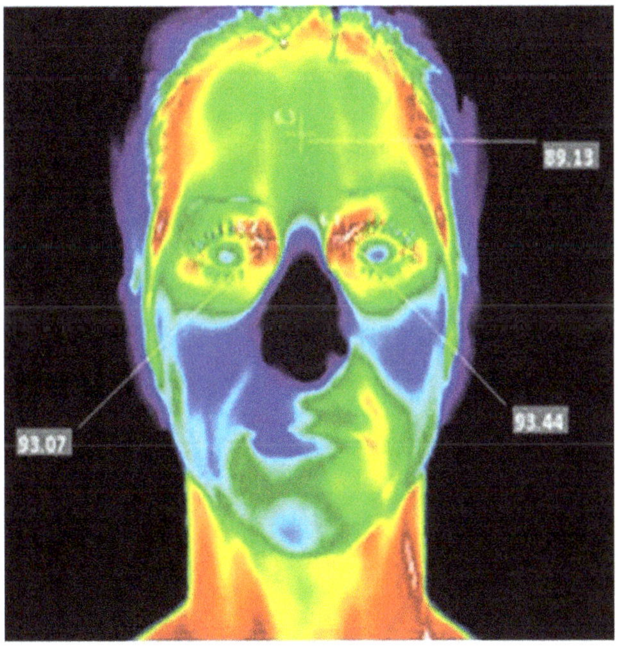

2.2.3 Heart Rate Variability (HRV)

It is a non-invasive procedure in which no electrode is inserted into the body. It's a precise and exact measurement of the Autonomic Nervous System (ANS), which reacts to a person's every action, including how he eats, sleep, dances/exercises, and manages stress. In the case of heart rate, the number of heartbeats is counted in a minute, while in the case of HRV, considerably closer and exact changes in time between any two consecutive heartbeats are noticed. Inter-beat intervals, RR intervals, NN intervals, and other terms for the time between two consecutive heartbeats are used. The period between two R-peaks of a basic ECG heart-beat waveform is defined as the RR-interval (Chowdary, et al., 2021). RR and NN intervals are the same with a different names.HRV can be measured by two methods:

(i) **ECG** is the traditional technique for the measurement of HRV (Shaffer, et al., 2016), ECG measures RR variation by detection of common peaks.
(ii) **PPG** (photoplethysmography) is the new method for the measurement of inter beat intervals, in this method one optical sensor is used. It is an optical way that identifies the variation of the volume of blood in the micro vascular tissue. It measures blood movement at the skin surface. A typical PPG device contains any light source for example LED device to emit light at affected tissue and one detector usually a photo detector to receive the reflected light. This is directly proportional to the blood volume changes same as ECG. The best thing about PPG is that no electrode is needed to connect to the body. It is noninvasive and as precise as ECG. In PPG only a touch is required i.e. only by touching the effective area for a small time does one get the readings? The other way of using PPGis rPPG (remote PPG) (Hsieh and Chin, 2011; Castaneda et l., 2018; Cañamero, 2005, 2019; Krasne et al., 2011). rPPG is a non-contact method. The typical waveform of ECG and PPG is shown in Figure 10.

Figure 10. ECG and PPG signals

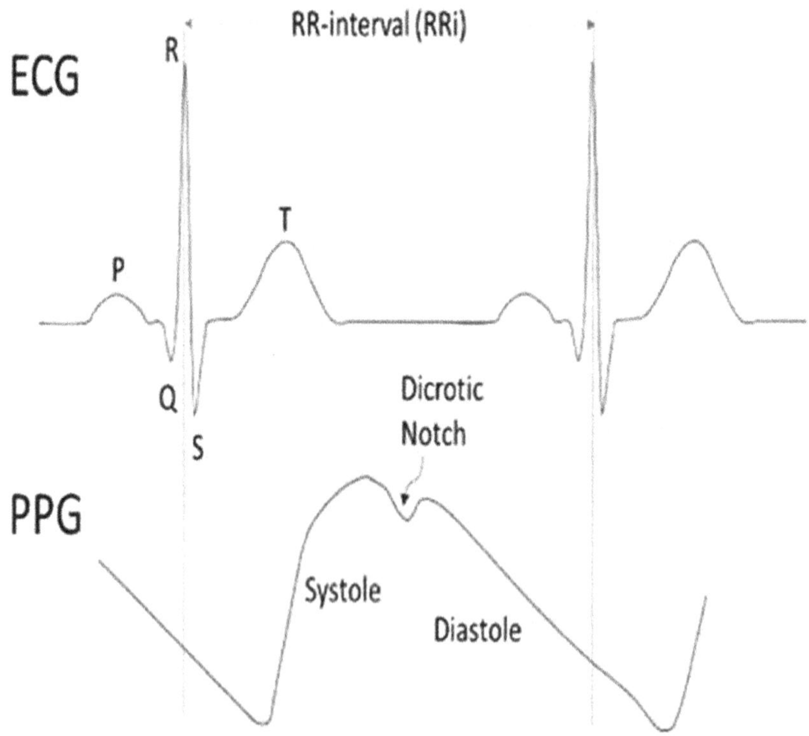

Many factors affect the recording of PPG. Some factors are heart-related i.e., cardiovascular activity, sensing i.e., the intensity of emitted light, and maybe biological factors. Thus, PPG reveals itself as a promising technology in daily activity assessments and as well as in health care, due to its cheap simple noninvasive portability and preciseness. Due to its non-invasiveness, low cost, and portability, AcPPG thus proposed itself as a potential technique for clinical and daily monitoring activity. It has the ability to equip healthcare providers with the instrument that will allow the early detection and diagnosis of cardiovascular problems, hence delivering deeper insight into a patient's health. However, more investigations using lower power consumption to identify even more critical health-related information can be performed.

3. DISCUSSION

Till now we have discussed many methods of emotion recognition and there are many more to go. In this paper, we came to know that human emotions are a very powerful tool for knowing about human health. As human emotions are directly proportional to human health and behavior. Human emotions are long known aspects but uncertainty in human behavior and emotions is a challenging thing to handle. These uncertainties in human emotions give a challenge for selecting accurate analysis and measurement techniques. There are mainly three types of measuring and analysis methods. Every method has its limitations, in electric parameter measurement, one needs direct contact to the particular i.e., we need a different type of electrodes it cannot be the non-contact type, for example, EEG, EMG, ECG, EOG. In the non-electric method it can be direct contact type or without contact. In the non-contact type we use optical sensors; these sensors are used for finding emotional recognition without touching the object. In addition, evaluation and recognition of humans are widely used in developing various interacting systems. These interaction systems are used to process various human behaviors.

4. CONCLUSION

Emotion recognition is one of the most crucial future components of human behavior. Emotion identification is vital for a variety of fields, including education, advertising, security, and engineering applications. Human emotion recognition paired with all of these technologies, as well as their implementation with machine learning and data analysis, will provide a big breakthrough to all sectors, beginning with education and marketing and ending with practically every industry. Also included is the normalization of the emotional state of a robot, which incorporates emotional aspects into the robots to enhance acceptability, credibility, and effectiveness. Also, in past year's robotics design mainly focused on human emotions which are based on neuro-computational models. Therefore, in future the robotics technology will also be used for the extraction of human emotions.

REFERENCES

Aminoff, M. J. (2012). Electroencephalography: General principles and clinical applications. In W. B. Saunders (Ed.), *Aminoff's Electro diagnosis in Clinical Neurology* (pp. 37–84). Elsevier B.V. doi:10.1016/B978-1-4557-0308-1.00003-0

Ayata, D., Yaslan, Y., & Kamasak, M. (2017). Emotion recognition via galvanic skin response: Comparison of machine learning algorithms and feature extraction methods. *Istanbul University-Journal of Electrical and Electronics Engineering*, *17*(1), 3129–3136.

Bruno, P., Melnyk, V., & Völckner, F. (2017). Temperature and emotions: Effects of physical temperature on responses to emotional advertising. *International Journal of Research in Marketing*, *34*(1), 302–320. doi:10.1016/j.ijresmar.2016.08.005

Cai, J., Liu, G., & Hao, M. (2009). The Research on Emotion Recognition from ECG Signal. *Proceedings of the 2009 International Conference on Information Technology and Computer Science*, 497–500.

Cañamero, L. (2005). Emotion understanding from the perspective of autonomous robots research. *Neural Network, 18*, 445–455. . doi:10.1016/j.neunet.2005.03.003

Cañamero, L. (2019). Embodied robot models for interdisciplinary emotion research. *IEEE Transactions on Affective Computing*, *1*. Advance online publication. doi:10.1109/TAFFC.2019.2908162

Castaneda, D., Esparza, A., Ghamari, M., Soltanpur, C., & Nazeran, H. (2018). A review on wearable photoplethysmography sensors and their potential future applications in health care. *International Journal of Biosensors & Bioelectronics*, *4*(4), 195–202. doi:10.15406/ijbsbe.2018.04.00125 PMID:30906922

Chai, X., Wang, Q., Zhao, Y., Li, Y., Liu, D., Liu, X., & Bai, O. (2017). A Fast, Efficient Domain Adaptation Technique for Cross-Domain Electroencephalography (EEG)-Based Emotion Recognition. *Sensors (Basel)*, *17*(5), 1014. doi:10.339017051014 PMID:28467371

Chanel, G., Kierkels, J. J. M., Soleymani, M., & Pun, T. (2009). Short-term emotion assessment in a recall paradigm. *International Journal of Human-Computer Studies*, *67*(8), 607–627. doi:10.1016/j.ijhcs.2009.03.005

Chanel, G., Kronegg, J., Grandjean, D., & Pun, T. (2006). Emotion assessment: Arousal evaluation using EEG's and peripheral physiological signals. Lecture Notes in Computer Science, 4105, 530.

Choppin, A. (2000). *EEG-based human interface for disabled individuals: Emotion expression with neural networks* [Ph.D. dissertation]. Tokyo Institute of Technology.

Chowdary, M.K., Nguyen, T.N. & Hemanth, D.J. (2021). Deep learning-based facial emotion recognition for human–computer interaction applications. *Neural Computing and Applications*. . doi:10.1007/s00521-021-06012-8

Csikszentmihalyi, M. (2014). *Flow and the Foundations of Positive Psychology: The collected works of MihalyCsikszentmihalyi; S.* Springer. doi:10.1007/978-94-017-9088-8

Dimberg, U. (1982). Facial Reactions to Facial Expressions. *Psychophysiology*, *9*(6), 643–647. doi:10.1111/j.1469-8986.1982.tb02516.x PMID:7178381

Dissanayake, T., Rajapaksha, Y., Ragel, R., & Nawinne, I. (2019). An Ensemble Learning Approach for Electrocardiogram Sensor Based Human Emotion Recognition. *Sensors (Basel)*, *19*(20), 4495. doi:10.339019204495 PMID:31623279

Dzedzickis, A., Kaklauskas, A., & Bucinskas, V. (2020). Human Emotion Recognition: Review of Sensors and Methods. *Sensors, 20*, 592. https://www.mdpi.com/1424-8220/20/3/592

EEG-Event Related Potentials. (n.d.). Available online: http://www.medicine.mcgill.ca/physio/vlab/biomed_signals/eeg_erp.htm

Emotion-Sensing Technology in the Internet of Things. (n.d.). Available online: https://onixsystems.com/blog/emotion-sensing-technology-in-the-internet-of-things

Feidakis, M., Daradoumis, T., & Caballe, S. (2011). Endowing e-Learning Systems with Emotion Awareness. *Proceedings of the 2011 Third International Conference on Intelligent Networking and Collaborative Systems,* 68–75.

Feidakis, M., Daradoumis, T., & Caballe, S. (2011). Emotion Measurement in Intelligent Tutoring Systems: What, When and How to Measure. *Proceedings of the 2011 Third International Conference on Intelligent Networking and Collaborative Systems.*

Ginsburg, A. S., Lenahan, J. L., Izadnegahdar, R., & Ansermino, J. M. (2018). A Systematic Review of Tools to Measure Respiratory Rate in Order to Identify Childhood Pneumonia. *American Journal of Respiratory and Critical Care Medicine*, *197*(9), 1116–1127. doi:10.1164/rccm.201711-2233CI PMID:29474107

Gonçalves, V. P., Giancristofaro, G. T., Filho, G. P. R., Johnson, T., Carvalho, V., Pessin, G., de Almeida Neris, V. P., & Ueyama, J. (2017). Assessing users' emotion at interaction time: A multimodal approach with multiple Sensors. *Soft Computing*, *21*(18), 5309–5323. doi:10.100700500 016 2115 0

Greco, A., Lanata, A., Citi, L., Vanello, N., Valenza, G., & Scilingo, E. (2016). Skin Admittance Measurement for Emotion Recognition: A Study over Frequency Sweep. *Electronics (Basel)*, *5*(4), 46. doi:10.3390/electronics5030046

Hess, U., & Fischer, A. (2013). Emotional Mimicry as Emotion Regulation. *Personality and Social Psychology Review*, *17*(2), 142–157. doi:10.1177/1088868312472607 PMID:23348982

Hsieh, P.-Y., & Chin, C.-L. (2011). The emotion recognition system with Heart Rate Variability and facial image features. *Proceedings of IEEE International Conference on Fuzzy Systems (FUZZ-IEEE 2011)*, 1933–1940. 10.1109/FUZZY.2011.6007734

Kappas, A., Bherer, F., & Thériault, M. (2000). Inhibiting Facial Expressions: Limitations to the voluntary control of facial expressions of emotions. *Motivation and Emotion*, *40*(4), 259–270. doi:10.1023/A:1010718815960

Katsis, C. D., Katertsidis, N., Ganiatsas, G., & Fotiadis, D. I. (2008). Toward Emotion Recognition in Car-Racing Drivers: A Biosignal Processing Approach. *IEEE Transactions on Systems, Man, and Cybernetics. Part A, Systems and Humans*, *38*(3), 502–512. doi:10.1109/TSMCA.2008.918624

Kim, W. J., Wagner, A. E., Kim, J., & Andre, E. (2005). From Physiological Signals to Emotions: Implementing and Comparing Selected Methods for Feature Extraction and Classification. *Proceedings of the 2005 IEEE International Conference on Multimedia and Expo*, 940–94.

Kumar, N., Alam, K., & Siddiqi, A. H. (2017). Wavelet Transform for Classification of EEG Signal using SVM and ANN. *Biomedical & Pharmacology Journal, 10*(4), 2061–2069. doi:10.13005/bpj/1328

Künecke, J., Hildebrandt, A., Recio, G., Sommer, W., & Wilhelm, O. (2014). Facial EMG Responses to Emotional Expressions Are Related to Emotion Perception Ability. *PLoS One*, *9*(1), e84053. Advance online publication. doi:10.1371/journal.pone.0084053 PMID:24489647

Larsen, J. T., Norris, C. J., & Cacioppo, J. T. (2003). Effects of positive and negative affect on electromyographic activity over zygomaticus major and corrugator supercilii. *Psychophysiology*, *40*(5), 776–785. doi:10.1111/1469-8986.00078 PMID:14696731

Liu, Y.-H., Wu, C.-T., Cheng, W.-T., Hsiao, Y.-T., Chen, P.-M., & Teng, J.-T. (2014). Emotion Recognition from SingleTrial EEG Based on Kernel Fisher's Emotion Pattern and Imbalanced Quasi-conformal Kernel Support Vector Machine. *Sensors (Basel)*, *14*(8), 13361–13388. doi:10.3390140813361 PMID:25061837

Lundqvist, L. O. (1995). Facial EMG reactions to facial expressions: A case of facial emotional contagion? *Scandinavian Journal of Psychology*, *36*(2), 130–141. doi:10.1111/j.1467-9450.1995.tb00974.x PMID:7644897

Malfaz, M., & Salichs, M. A. (2007). A new architecture for autonomous robots based on emotions. *IFAC Proceedings Volumes*, *37*, 805–809.

Mandala, S., & Di, T. C. (2017). ECG Parameters for Malignant Ventricular Arrhythmias: A Comprehensive Review. *Journal of Medical and Biological Engineering*, *37*(4), 441–453. doi:10.100740846-017-0281-x PMID:28867990

Mehmood, R., & Lee, H. (2017). Towards Building a Computer Aided Education System for Special Students Using Wearable Sensor Technologies. *Sensors (Basel)*, *17*(2), 317. doi:10.339017020317 PMID:28208734

Minaee, S., Minaei, M., & Abdolrashidi, A. (2021). Deep-Emotion: Facial Expression Recognition Using Attentional Convolutional Network. *Sensors (Basel)*, *21*(9), 3046. doi:10.339021093046 PMID:33925371

Musha, T., Asada, T., Yamashita, F., Kinoshita, T., Chen, Z., Matsuda, H., Masatake, U., & Shankle, W. R. (2002). A new EEG method for estimating cortical neuronal impairment that is sensitive to early-stage Alzheimer's disease. *Clinical Neurophysiology*, *113*(7), 1052–1058. doi:10.1016/S1388-2457(02)00128-1 PMID:12088699

Nakanishi, R., & Imai-Matsumura, K. (2008). Facial skin temperature decreases in infants with joyful expression. *Infant Behavior and Development*, *31*(1), 137–144. doi:10.1016/j.infbeh.2007.09.001 PMID:17983661

Nakasone, A., Prendinger, H., & Ishizuka, M. (2005). Infiniti Bio-signal Encoder. *Proceedings of the 5th International Workshop on Biosignal Interpretation*, 219–222.

Oxley, T. J., Opie, N. L., John, S. E., Rind, G. S., Ronayne, S. M., Wheeler, T. L., Judy, J. W., McDonald, A. J., Dornom, A., Lovell, T. J. H., Steward, C., Garrett, D. J., Moffat, B. A., Lui, E. H., Yassi, N., Campbell, B. C. V., Wong, Y. T., Fox, K. E., Nurse, E. S., ... O'Brien, T. J. (2016). Minimally invasive endovascular stent-electrode array for high-fidelity, chronic recording of cortical neural activity. *Nature Biotechnology*, *34*(3), 320–327. doi:10.1038/nbt.3428 PMID:26854476

Paul, S., Banerjee, A., & Tibarewala, D. N. (2017). Emotional eye movement analysis using electrooculography signal. *International Journal of Biomedical Engineering and Technology*, *23*(1), 59. doi:10.1504/IJBET.2017.082224

Puri, C., Olson, L., Pavlidis, I., Levine, J., & Stresscam, S. J. (2005). Non-contact measurement of users' emotional states through thermal imaging. *Proceedings of the Conference on Human Factors in Computing Systems (CHI EA 2005),* 1725–1728.

Purnamasari, P., Ratna, A., & Kusumoputro, B. (2017). Development of Filtered Bispectrum for EEG Signal Feature Extraction in Automatic Emotion Recognition Using Artificial Neural Networks. *Algorithms*, *10*(2), 63. doi:10.3390/a10020063

Rattanyu, K., Ohkura, M., & Mizukawa, M. (2010). Emotion Monitoring from Physiological Signals for Service Robots in the Living Space. Institute of Control, Robotics and Systems, 580–583.

Russell, J. A. (1980). A Circumplex Model of effect. *Journal of Personality and Social Psychology*, *39*(6), 1161–1178. doi:10.1037/h0077714

Said, Y., & Barr, M. (2021). Human emotion recognition based on facial expressions via deep learning on high-resolution images. *Multimedia Tools and Applications*, *80*(16), 25241–25253. doi:10.100711042-021-10918-9

Scherer, K. R. (2005). What are emotions? And how can they be measured? *Social Sciences Information. Information Sur les Sciences Sociales*, *44*(4), 695–729. doi:10.1177/0539018405058216

Shaffer, F., Shearman, F., Meehan, S., & Zachary. (2016). The Promise of Ultra-Short-Term (UST) Heart Rate Variability Measurements. *Psychology*. doi:10.5298/1081-5937-44.3.09

Singh, D. (2012). Human Emotion Recognition System. *International journal of Image. Graphics, and Signal Processing*, *8*(8), 50–56. doi:10.5815/ijigsp.2012.08.07

Soleymani, M., Lichtenauer, J., Pun, T., & Pantic, M. (2012). A Multimodal Database for Affect Recognition and Implicit Tagging. *IEEE Transactions on Affective Computing*, *3*(1), 42–55. doi:10.1109/T-AFFC.2011.25

Sonkusare, S., Ahmedt-Aristizabal, D., Aburn, M. J., Nguyen, V. T., Pang, T., Frydman, S., Denman, S., Fookes, C., Breakspear, M., & Guo, C. C. (2019). Detecting changes in facial temperature induced by a sudden auditory stimulus based on deep learning-assisted face tracking. *Scientific Reports*, *9*(1), 4729. doi:10.103841598-019-41172-7 PMID:30894584

Soundariya, R. S., & Renuga, R. (2017). Eye movement based emotion recognition using electrooculography. *Proceedings of the 2017 Innovations in Power and Advanced Computing Technologies (i-PACT).*

Subramanian, B. (2017). ECG signal classification and parameter estimation using multiwavelet transform. *Biomedical Research, 28*(7), 3187–3193.

Tjhjadi, H., & Ramli, K. (2020). Noninvasive Blood Pressure Classification Based on Photoplethysmography Using K-Nearest Neighbors Algorithm: A Feasibility Study. *Information (Basel), 11*(2), 93. doi:10.3390/info11020093

Van Dooren, M., de Vries, J.J. & Janssen, J.H. (2012). Emotional sweating across the body: Comparing 16 different skin conductance measurement locations. *Physiology & Behavior, 106*(2), 298-304.

Vanmarkenlichtenbelt, W., Daanen, H., Wouters, L., Fronczek, R., Raymann, R., Severens, N., & Vansomeren, E. (2006). Evaluation of wireless determination of skin temperature using iButtons. *Physiology & Behavior, 88*(4-5), 489–497. doi:10.1016/j.physbeh.2006.04.026 PMID:16797616

Vijayan, A. E., Sen, D., & Sudheer, A. P. (2015). EEG-Based Emotion Recognition Using Statistical Measures and Autoregressive Modeling. *Proceedings of the 2015 IEEE International Conference on Computational Intelligence & Communication Technology*, 587–591. 10.1109/CICT.2015.24

Villon, O., & Lisetti, C. (2006). A User-Modeling Approach to Build User's Psycho-Physiological Maps of Emotions using Bio-Sensors. *Proceedings of the ROMAN 2006–The 15th IEEE International Symposium on Robot and Human Interactive Communication*, 269–276.

Villon, O., & Lisetti, C. (2007). Toward Recognizing Individual's Subjective Emotion from Physiological Signals in Practical Application. *Proceedings of the Twentieth IEEE International Symposium on Computer-Based Medical Systems (CBMS'07)*, 357–362. 10.1109/CBMS.2007.112

Wang, Y., Lv, Z., & Zheng, Y. (2018). Automatic Emotion Perception Using Eye Movement Information for EHealthcare Systems. *Sensors (Basel), 18*(9), 2826. doi:10.339018092826

Zhang, J., Chen, M., Zhao, S., Hu, S., Shi, Z., & Cao, Y. (2016). Relief-Based EEG Sensor Selection Methods for Emotion Recognition. *Sensors (Basel), 16*(10), 1558. doi:10.339016101558

Zhang, Q., Chen, X., Zhan, Q., Yang, T., & Xia, S. (2017). Respiration-based emotion recognition with deep learning. *Computers in Industry, 92-93*, 84–90. doi:10.1016/j.compind.2017.04.005

Chapter 14
Transport Data Analytics With Selection of Tools and Techniques for Emergency Medical Services

Jayanthi Ganapathy
https://orcid.org/0000-0001-9701-6241
Sri Ramachandra Faculty of Engineering and Technology, India

Ramya M.
https://orcid.org/0000-0003-3084-3490
Sri Ramachandra Faculty of Engineering and Technology, India

Joselyn Diana C.
Sri Ramachandra Faculty of Engineering and Technology, India

ABSTRACT

Emergency medical services (EMS) are inevitable in urban transport. The sustainable transport services during emergency situations are inevitable. These emergency services and vehicle operations are influenced by traffic flow rate on highways. The objective of this chapter is to present the use of transport data analytics in sustainable mobility and transport. Travel time is a key factor in emergency vehicle operations as urban transport system is a time varying network. Temporal traffic information is a source for estimation of travel time on highways in emergency vehicle operations. The adverse traffic behavior during peak and non-peak hours of daily traffic profile hinders the operation of emergency vehicles during pandemic COVID-19 situations and so forth in evacuation planning when the situation arises. Hence, this chapter presents the modern techniques and tools used in estimation of traffic flow rate on highways to access the connectivity of road network for emergency vehicle operations.

DOI: 10.4018/978-1-6684-2508-4.ch014

INTRODUCTION

Urban transport system is a time varying network. Traffic congestion induces unpredicted delay in travel time. The traffic flow rate on highways at temporal scales contributes in travel time computation in successive time instances (Ermagun and Levinson, 2018; Huang et al. 2014; Jayanthi and Jothilakshmi, 2019; Jayanthi and Fausto, 2021). Formulation of Sequence Convolution based auto-encoder Long Short term Memory (SCAE-LSTM) network aims at sequencing the temporal traffic flow rate in preceding time instance to estimate the traffic flow in successive time instances. Given origin and destination (OD) pair, temporal traffic sequence helps in estimating traffic flow rate on highways. Hence, Spatial-TemporAl Reconnect (STAR) algorithm is proposed. The performance of STAR is investigated by conducting extensive experimentation on real traffic network of Chennai Metropolitan City.

The computational complexity of the algorithm is empirically analyzed. The proposed STAR algorithm is found to estimate traffic flow during peak hour traffic with reduced complexity in computation compared to other baseline methods in short term traffic flow predictions like LSTM, ConvLSTM and GRNN. Finally, conclusions on results are presented with directions for future research.

This chapter is organized to present the back ground on recent achievement followed by formulation of Sequence Convolution Auto-Encoder Long short term memory network with focus on time complexity measures. Finally, the chapter summarizes the work with directions for future research.

Background

Recent advancements in Intelligent Transport Systems (ITS) have revolved the transport industry nationwide across the globe to serve the public in better way. Traffic flow congestion estimation and management on highways is always in demand worldwide across all nations for safe and hassle free travel. Traffic congestion problem is inherent in travel time decisions and solving such problem is essential for travel guidance especially during peak hours of a journey. In early 1990's automated traffic controller was introduced (Bauer, 2009;Batz et.al, 2010, 2013) and the two broad spectrums of research in transportation that is everlasting in infrastructure planning are (i) Shortest path computation problem and (ii) Time series traffic forecasting. In spite of technology driven traffic management using IoV (Internet of Vehicles), monitoring and control of vehicular traffic remains a serious issue in real time thus, a fully automated traffic management system is not feasible. Therefore, it is essential to manage traffic flow congestion systematically as it cannot be avoided but can be mitigated (Chen et al. 2013, 2016). In this view, a speedup technique is necessary to bridge the gap between traffic flow estimation and path routing of vehicular traffic between origin and destination (OD). In a spatially connected network, it is essential to analyze spatial dependency of road segment with respect to upstream and downstream traffic flow thereby, road segments (a path) that are connecting the source and destination in preceding time instances are analyzed in successive time instances for re-establishing connectivity (Jayanthi and Fausto 2021, 2022). In this way, when traffic congestion is detected the path is reconnected based on spatial – temporal traffic information (Lingras, 2002; Ma, 2015, Nejad, 2017). In the interest of reducing travel delay, Spatial-TemporAl Re-connect (STAR) algorithm is proposed in which traffic flow is estimated by sequencing spatial and temporal traffic information. The traffic information in upstream and downstream road segments represents spatial traffic information, while traffic flow at each time instance forms temporal information (Wangyang et al, 2019; Zhao, 2017). The interest of this work is to formulate speedup technique by estimating traffic flow at each of arterial junctions between OD pair and re-establish path connectivity of road network based on spatial and temporal traffic sequences.

Research Challenges

Temporal variation in traffic flow essentially captures the recurring and non-recurring congestion in dynamics of physical traffic flow. However, temporal traffic information alone is not sufficient in travel decisions when there is a need for reliable path on a spatially connected road network. In route guidance, a path in a travel is said to be reliable when flow rate in successive time instance is made known (Jayanthi . This has motivated researchers to focus on influence of spatial characteristics in dynamics of traffic flow as flow rate from neighboring links contribute significant amount of traffic at current location. In this perspective, a fully automated traffic management system is not feasible. Therefore, it is essential to manage traffic flow congestion systematically as it cannot be avoided but can be mitigated. In this view, a speedup technique is necessary to bridge the gap between traffic flow estimation and path routing of vehicular traffic between origin and destination (OD). These challenges have motivated me in devising the research problem statement as discussed below:

Problem Statement

i. Statement – 1: Given travel time based traffic information sequence of uplink and downlink connecting the origin to destination, estimates the traffic flow at spatial intersection on highway.

In this work, both spatial and temporal information are essentially considered as they contribute significant information about traffic. In real road network, temporal variation in traffic volume has strong influence towards travel delay. Variation in travel time is the effect of congestion in time varying network. Traffic information at different time instances carry useful information about road network. Moreover, traffic information has to be analyzed at different time instances rather than arrival time and departure time alone. Edge weight augmented with temporal information would help in realizing real traffic conditions more effectively.

Identification of critical node (arterial junction) in the spatial network based on temporal variation of traffic with analysis on congestion patterns is required in real-time scenarios. Hence, temporal instances of traffic information are highly required in analyzing traffic at preceding instances. Traffic congestion incurred due to time varying travel time needs much consideration in solving path computation problem. Sequencing spatial and temporal traffic information in preceding time instance helps in estimating traffic flow in sequence in successive time instances by formalizing sequence convolution based auto-encoder Long Short term Memory (SCAE-LSTM) network. Thus, spatial-temporal traffic characteristics extracted using convolution of upstream and downstream traffic information sequence is fed externally to auto-encoder LSTM. LSTM predicts the traffic flow at target location in successive time instances.

ii. **Statement– 2:** Given origin and destination pair in a travel, augment the spatially connected network to reach destination considering the spatial – temporal dependence of traffic flow.

Given source and destination with start time of journey, path connecting the arterial intersections is checked for congestion in which speed of vehicle captured by sensors in upstream and downstream is sequenced in each time instance using sequence convolution. Auto-encoder is formalized to extract the characteristics of vehicle speed in adjacent links. Auto-encoder is integrated with LSTM to estimate traffic flow rate at arterial intersection. Path to destination is re-connected considering both distance and spatial dependence of adjacent links at each time instance until destination is reached.

In a spatially connected network, it is essential to analyze spatial dependency of road segment with respect to upstream and downstream traffic flow thereby, road segments (a path) that are connecting the source and destination in preceding time instances are analyzed in successive time instances for re-establishing connectivity. In this way, when traffic congestion is detected the path is reconnected based on spatial-temporal traffic information. In the interest of reducing travel delay, Spatial-TemporAl Re-connect (STAR) algorithm is proposed in which traffic flow is estimated by sequencing spatial and temporal traffic information. The traffic information in upstream and downstream road segments represents spatial traffic information, while traffic flow at each time instance forms temporal information. The interest of this work is to formulate speedup technique by estimating traffic flow at each of arterial junctions between OD pair and re-establish path connectivity of road network based on spatial and temporal traffic sequences.

Intelligent transport systems for Emergency vehicle operations

The performance of Spatial-TemporAl Re-connect (STAR) algorithm is analysed on time varying road traffic network. The computational complexity of any shortest path algorithm is dependent on number of nodes and arcs. The dependency of road segments connecting arterial junctions is analysed in re-establishing connectivity by formalising SCAE-LSTM network. The significance of STAR algorithm in managing traffic is reported with extensive experimentation under different traffic conditions in three different sites. The peak hour traffic is evaluated for each site during week days and weekends.

Study Area and Data Collection

Estimation of traffic speed using SCAE-LSTM and dynamic path connectivity using STAR algorithm is experimented on road network covering southern region of Chennai city located in Tamil Nadu state of India. The state highway SH-49 and SH-49A is chosen for this study as this highway experiences significant traffic on all working days and weekends. The length of study area considered in experimentation on state highway SH-49 (East Coast Road) is 690 Km. The length of the state highway SH-49A is 43.7 Km. This metropolitan transport network is a highly connected road network covering major arterial junctions connecting urban streets, motorways, and expressways.

The state highway of this southern region is facilitated with centralized toll collection center. Motor vehicle passing through this state highway connects three toll plazas namely (1) Perungudi Toll Plaza, which is entry to centralized toll collection center from northern region of Chennai city, (2) East Coast Road (ECR) and (3) Egattur toll plaza, which is exit of the toll collection center. Travel time during free flow is computed in early morning (5:00 AM – 6:00 AM), Afternoon (12:00 NOON – 02:00 PM) and post evening (10:00 PM-11:30 PM). The actual travel time is computed in morning peak hours (8:00 AM – 11:30 AM) and evening peak hours (05:00 PM – 9:00 PM) during week days while peak hour changes during weekends. The historical data set describing the vehicle speed in mile/ hr is used as training data set. Speed of vehicle in state highway SH-49 is captured by the sensor and stored in centralized server which is high end server located in Perungudi Toll Plaza. Estimation of vehicle speed is done by training auto-encoder LSTM with historical data set and validated by testing the model with actual speed of vehicle.

Table.1. Training and validation loss

Epoch	Phases	AE-LSTM	ConvLSTM	LSTM	GRNN
10	Train	0.6	0.61	0.625	0.678
	Test	0.79	0.79	0.81	0.86
20	Train	0.58	0.585	0.6	0.625
	Test	0.65	0.685	0.68	0.786
30	Train	0.556	0.547	0.57	0.6
	Test	0.73	0.62	0.6	0.75
40	Train	0.556	0.54	0.57	0.58
	Test	0.71	0.619	0.61	0.62
50	Train	0.524	0.54	0.6	0.572
	Test	0.65	0.61	0.602	0.6
60	Train	0.529	0.528	0.57	0.575
	Test	0.652	0.519	0.605	0.605
70	Train	0.423	0.528	0.512	0.55
	Test	0.49	0.598	0.575	0.6
80	Train	0.35	0.519	0.565	0.54
	Test	0.42	0.599	0.577	0.585
90	Train	0.31	0.52	0.56	0.525
	Test	0.389	0.589	0.58	0.575
100	Train	**0.25**	**0.5002**	**0.525**	**0.5**
	Test	**0.281**	**0.51**	**0.55**	**0.575**
110	Train	0.2499	0.5	0.5	0.5
	Test	0.279	0.5	0.5	0.5
120	Train	0.251	0.5	0.53	0.5
	Test	0.255	0.5	0.5	0.5

Vehicle miles travelled (VMT) recorded for 36 months between January 2017 and December 2020 is used for training the Auto-Encoder LSTM network, while VMT recorded for ten months between January 2021 and October 2021 is used as test data set in evaluating the system.

Performance of SCAE-LSTM

The training phase of LSTM requires computationally elaborate operational settings. The traffic data sets representing traffic speed, flow rate, and occupancy are voluminous and requires intensive computation methods. The potential issues concerned with the implementation of SCAE-LSTM in STAR are detailed as follows:

Given an origin and destination pair a matrix of LSTM nodes is formulated in which each LSTM node represents an arterial junction between origin and destination. During the training phase, the source of input to LSTM is the pre-trained auto-encoders whose primary function is to extract spatial-temporal traffic characteristics from upstream and downstream traffic flow in each hour of the day. Thus, extensive operational settings are required in initial training phase of LSTM nodes.

The core components operated in Algorithm I are extraction of spatial-temporal characteristics of physical traffic flow using frequent traffic sequences on upstream, downstream, and training auto-encoders using the extracted data sets. The training phase of LSTM requires computationally elaborate operational settings. The traffic data sets representing traffic speed, flow rate collected for 52 weeks is used in training auto-encoders with computationally intensive operational settings on arterial junctions. However, training and validation error does not vary in different operational settings considering the morning and evening peak hours of the day. The stability of the system is ensured even with traffic data collection at a temporal resolution of 15-minutes. Table 1 shows the training and validation loss in different epochs.

The issues concerned with implementing STAR are space complexity. Augmenting spatially connected road networks as described in Algorithm II requires the storage of spatial coordinates of the location on a Google Map. The location information and retrieval of spatial coordinates during the inclusion and exclusion of LSTM nodes incurs high space and memory utilization. The experimental setup was made for a maximum distance of 350 miles on state highway SH 49 and SH 49A for testing the performance of the STAR algorithm. However, other practical constraints have to be considered in the further investigation of routing vehicles, which is left to work in the future. The accuracy of models in the estimation of vehicle speed is evaluated both during training and testing phases. Models were trained to learn the behavior of traffic in the study area. Training accuracy best fits the model in learning the traffic behavior and it is validated using actual flow rate in the test data. The accuracy of models during training and validation is examined using mean relative error measure given in Equation (3). The error measure of base line models is compared with SCAE-LSTM. SCAE-LSTM fits well in learning the training data at epoch 100. Estimation of Vehicle miles is done at 15 minutes resolutions considering training and test accuracy at 100th epoch. The models descend with error rate gradually until epoch 100 and entropy log loss function for various epochs. The loss function is given in Equation (1),

$$Log\ loss = -\frac{1}{N}\sum_{i=1}^{N} Z_i logP + \left(1 - Z_i\right) log\left(1 - P\right) \quad (1)$$

where N is number of iterations; Z_i is the training data set; P is the joint probability of maximum likelihood estimates. The error rate of SCAE-LSTM is found to be less compared to ConvLSTM, while LSTM and GRNN are found to experience similar error rate. The speed of vehicle in miles per hour is estimated using Auto-Encoder LSTM. Congestion index is computed in proposed STAR using the estimated speed for managing traffic during peak hours.

$$RMSE(\lambda¢,\lambda) = \sqrt{\frac{\sum_{n=1}^{N}(-)^2}{N}} \tag{2}$$

$$MRE(\lambda¢,\lambda) = \frac{\left(\sum_{n=1}^{N}\frac{|-|}{}\right)}{N} \tag{3}$$

$$MAE(\lambda¢,\lambda) = \frac{\sum_{n=1}^{N}|-|}{N} \tag{4}$$

λ¢ is the predicted value, λ is the observed value, and N represents the number of data. The baseline models used in this evaluation are Convolution LSTM (ConvLSTM), LSTM, and Gated Recurrent Neural Network (GRNN). Auto-Encoder LSTM is formalized and implemented in Python 3.8 using tensor flow and keras packages which is available under GNU public license. Experimental analysis is conducted on 2.5GHz, 64-bit processor, 16GB RAM in Windows 10 environment. The performance of Auto-Encoder LSTM model is evaluated using Root Mean Square Error (RMSE), Mean Relative Error (MRE), and Mean Absolute Error (MAE) metrics shown in (2) through (4) and compared with baseline models. The accuracy of models in estimation of vehicle speed is evaluated both during training and testing phases. Models were trained to learn the behaviour of traffic in the study area. Training accuracy best fits the model in learning the traffic behaviour and it is validated using actual vehicle speed using test data. The model fits well in learning the training data at earlier epoch 100. Estimation of Vehicle miles is done at various temporal scales say less than or equal to 10 mins, 15 mins, and 30 mins resolutions considering training and test accuracy at 100th epoch.

The models descend with error rate gradually up to epoch 100 and entropy log loss function for various epochs. It is evident from Table 2 error rate of SCAE-LSTM is found to be less compared to ConvLSTM while, LSTM and GRNN are found to experience similar error rate. The proposed sequence convolution based Auto-Encoder LSTM is found to be stable in estimating speed of vehicle at different temporal resolutions compared to baseline models as Mean Relative Error (MRE) of the model does not vary and found to be in range in estimation of vehicle speed in different temporal resolutions. Thus, stability of the Auto-Encoder LSTM is ensured as spatial and temporal traffic information is sequenced at each time instance. The speed of vehicle is estimated from characteristic vehicle speed in sequence. In contrast, baseline models experiences variation in error rate which is due to inherent complexity of models in time series forecasting. Vehicles miles are estimated for various temporal scales, say less than or equal to 10 minutes, 15 minutes, and 30 minutes to check the stability of SCAE-LSTM.

Table 2. Error rate in estimation of vehicle miles/hr

Deep Learners	Facility	Temporal Resolution								
		£10 mins			£ 15 mins			£ 30 mins		
		RMSE	MRE	MAE	RMSE	MRE	MAE	RMSE	MRE	MAE
SCAE-LSTM	Expressways	3.45	0.05	0.20	3.79	0.05	0.32	5.78	0.05	0.40
	Arterials	4.73	0.04	0.25	4.88	0.04	0.35	5.04	0.04	0.45
	Freeways	3.23	0.05	0.11	3.11	0.05	0.41	4.35	0.05	0.11
ConvLSTM	Expressways	12.85	0.66	23.76	13.74	0.73	24.11	12.81	0.66	23.75
	Arterials	11.47	0.62	22.05	12.01	0.77	23.72	13.05	0.62	30.32
	Freeways	11.75	0.67	21.85	9.87	0.79	22.05	10.86	0.67	32.09
LSTM	Expressways	11.58	0.78	33.44	13.55	0.78	35.21	13.75	0.78	33.45
	Arterials	11.44	0.67	32.87	12.23	0.67	33.85	12.89	0.67	28.18
	Freeways	11.84	0.72	32.03	8.89	0.72	30.56	9.02	0.72	30.19
Gated RNN	Expressways	13.65	0.89	40.84	13.65	0.89	40.84	13.65	0.89	40.87
	Arterials	12.91	0.77	40.05	12.94	0.77	39.25	13.25	0.77	40.17
	Freeways	12.02	0.78	36.86	11.32	0.78	38.26	12.15	0.78	41.19

Time Complexity Analysis of STAR

In our previous research (Jayanthi and Jothilakshmi. 2019, 2020, and 2021) evaluation of traffic sequence patterns and rules for prediction of traffic volume on highways is reported in detail and used in upstream and downstream spatial traffic sequences, travel time based temporal traffic sequence pattern mining on this study. The evaluation of the proposed STAR algorithm targets two specific factors first, the time complexity in estimation of traffic flow using SCAE-LSTM for various distance measures. Second, the time complexity of speedup in path computation by augmenting arterial junctions between OD pair based on spatial-temporal traffic information sequence formulation during morning (MPHT) and evening peak hour traffic (EPHT).

The complexity of speedup technique STAR algorithm in path computation problem is analysed by experimenting the proposed spatial-temporal traffic information sequence formulation (SCAE-LSTM) on SH-49 and SH-49A for estimation of traffic flow in principle arterial junctions connecting OD pair. The proposed STAR algorithm is tested for (1) traffic flow estimation and (2) Augmentation of arterial junctions for OD pair based on spatial-temporal traffic information. The potential of SCAE-LSTM is compared with other baseline deep learner such as LSTM, ConvLSTM, and GRNN. Thus, the proposed speedup technique is evaluated for complexity in traffic flow estimation with SCAE-LSTM, LSTM, ConvLSTM and GRNN and results are compared. Average execution time of STAR algorithm is evaluated for various distance measures in miles. Experimental set up for evaluation of traffic flow with STAR algorithm started with minimum distance measure of 50 miles and extended to maximum distance measure of 300 miles on State Highway SH-49. The proposed STAR and baseline models are found to have the same complexity as the execution time of each model is found to be similar for less number of distance measure between 1 and 50 miles. But there is a gradual and significant reduction in complexity of STAR above 50 miles. A steep decrease in execution time is found with STAR for 50 miles and above while ConvLSTM exhibits the same behaviour only after 100 miles and LSTM and GRNN shows a gradual increase in complexity from 50 miles onward. Thus, STAR with SCAE-LSTM is found to have reduced complexity in computation time compared to STAR with other baseline models. This significance takes advantage of two principle elements (i) formulation of traffic information sequence at each time instance based on travel time (temporal traffic factor) and (ii) characteristic traffic sequence evaluated from both upstream and downstream road segments. The speedup of STAR in path computation is evaluated by the experimentation of the proposed formulation for different origin-destination (OD) pair. Experimental setup begins with the execution of STAR in augmenting arterial junction between OD pair based on traffic flow estimation using proposed SCAE-LSTM, LSTM, ConvLSTM and GRNN. A minimum number of 2 - 10 OD pair each with a distance measure of 200 miles is considered in this experimental setup. Mean execution time is evaluated for every 10 OD pair. This setup is extended to a maximum number of 200 OD pair of the same length. Each OD pair is located on the Google Map and arterial junctions connecting OD pair is extracted using Python Client library designed for Google Map API web services.

The proposed STAR exhibits identical characteristics in the evaluation of time complexity with respect to OD pair too. The significance of the proposed formulation of SCAE-LSTM is found to exhibit the same characteristics even when evaluated with respect to OD pairs. The proposed formulation is equivalently stable with baseline models too with respect to OD pairs. Hence, execution of the proposed formulation is found to be stable under different traffic conditions. However, average execution time in speedup evaluation of the proposed STAR for OD pair differs with execution time with respect to distance measure. This is due to the traffic behaviour during peak hours of day.

The speedup of the proposed STAR is evaluated during peak hours of the day both in the morning and evening. The speedup in augmenting arterial junctions for OD pair using STAR is found to be twice faster compared to ConvLSTM, 2.4 times that of LSTM, and three times faster compared to GRNN in both peak hours of the day. Nevertheless, the average execution time of STAR during peak hours in the evening is found to increase by 1.2 times compared to morning which is less significant compared to the stability of the model in different traffic conditions. The rate of execution of STAR is found to be stationary and identical with STAR (ConvLSTM) irrespective of peak hour of the day. These two models are found to be more stable beyond 100 OD pair compared to STAR (LSTM) and STAR (GRNN). However, STAR is faster compared to STAR (ConvLSTM) due to the formulation of spatial - temporal characteristic traffic sequence. Unlike the inherent complexity in the computation of hidden layers with LSTM and GRNN, STAR and STAR (ConvLSTM) are better speedup methods for path computation.

Sequence convolution based Auto-Encoder LSTM is found to be stable in estimating speed of vehicle at 15 minutes temporal resolutions compared to baseline models as mean relative error (MRE) of the model does not vary and found to be in range in estimation of vehicle speed in different temporal resolutions. Thus, stability of the Auto-Encoder LSTM is ensured as spatial and temporal traffic information is sequenced at each time instance. In the interest of reducing delay in travel, Spatial-TemporAl Reconnect (STAR) algorithm is proposed for traffic flow assessment on highways. The functional performance of the STAR algorithm is evaluated against other baseline deep leaners. Extensive experiments conducted on state highway SH-49 and SH-49A of Chennai metropolitan city in Tamil Nadu and evaluation results are reported. STAR is found to be twice faster compared to ConvLSTM, 2.4 times that of LSTM, and three times faster compared to GRNN in both peak hours of the day. Evaluation on functional performance of STAR when operated on travel time varying network has shown reduced complexity in computation.

The evaluation results of STAR thus, achieved have illustrated the significance of sequencing temporal and spatial factors and their logical analysis in augmenting arterial junction between OD pair.

FUTURE RESEARCH DIRECTIONS

In the interest of reducing travel time during peak hour, SCAE-LSTM network is formalised for estimating traffic flow in sequence in successive time instances. Accuracy and training performance of this model is compared with other baseline models LSTM, ConvLSTM, and GRNN. SCAE-LSTM is found to be stable in the estimation of vehicle speed at various temporal resolutions. Further, steps to evolve formulation of STAR for traffic management on connected vehicles have been taken to work in future.

CONCLUSION

Research on computational methods to reduce traffic congestion is the essential part of ITS infrastructure in the Urban Transportation system. Besides several speed up techniques in the computation of time dependent shortest paths found in literature, the logical analysis of spatial and temporal factors and their significance in traffic network was not the interest of transportation researchers over the past decade. This chapter presented the techniques and tools used in transport data analytics for emergency vehicle operations considering the traffic flow rate on highways. Further, the use of modern tools and techniques is illustrated with a case study on traffic flow rate estimation and augmentation of arterial junctions based on spatial-temporal traffic sequences.

REFERENCES

Batz, Geisberger, Sanders, & Vetter. (2013). Minimum time-dependent travel times with contraction hierarchies. *Journal of Experimental Algorithmics, 18*, 1.1–1.43.

Batz, R. (2010). *Time-dependent contraction hierarchies and approximation*. Experimental Algorithms.

Bauer, D. (2009). SHARC: 'Fast and Robust unidirectional routing. *ACM Journal of Experimental Algorithmics, 14*(2), 2-29.

Chen, & Lu, & Yang. (2016). Urban traffic flow prediction using a spatiotemporal random effects model. *Journal of Intelligent Transportation Systems, 20(3)*. doi:10.1080/15472450.2015.1072050

Chen, B. Y., Lam, W. H., Sumalee, A., Li, Q., & Tam, M. L. (2013). Reliable shortest path problems in stochastic time-dependent networks. *Journal of Intelligent Transport Systems, 18*(2), 177–189. doi:10.1080/15472450.2013.806851

Ermagun, A., & Levinson, D. (2018). Spatiotemporal traffic forecasting: Review and proposed directions. *Transport Reviews, 38*(6), 786–814. doi:10.1080/01441647.2018.1442887

Huang, W., Song, G., Hong, H., & Xie, K. (2014). Deep architecture for traffic flow prediction: Deep belief networks with multitask learning. *IEEE Transactions on Intelligent Transportation Systems*, *15*(5), 2191–2201. doi:10.1109/TITS.2014.2311123

Jayanthi & Márquez. (2021b). Travel Time Based Traffific Rerouting by Augmenting Traffic Flow Network with Temporal and Spatial Relations for Congestion Management. *Lecture Notes on Data Engineering and Communication Technologies, 78.*

Jayanthi, G. (2021). *Design of algorithms for IOT applications: a case study on intelligent transportation systems. In Internet of Things - Cases and Studies*. Springer.

Jayanthi, G. (2022). Multi Criteria Decision Making Analysis for sustainable Transport. In Sustainability - Cases And Studies in using Operations Research and Management Science Methods. Springer.

Jayanthi, G, & Jothilakshmi, P. (2019). Prediction of traffic volume by mining traffic sequences using travel time based PrefixSpan. *IET Intelligent Transport Systems, 13*(7), 1199-1210. doi:10.1049/iet-its.2018.5165

Jayanthi & Márquez. (2021a). Routing Vehicles on Highways by Augmenting Traffic Flow Network: A Review on Speed Up Techniques. Smart Innovation, Systems and Technologies.

Jayanthi & Márquez. (2021c). Data Mining and Information Technology in Transportation—A Review. In Lecture Notes on Data Engineering and Communications Technologies (Vol. 79). Springer. doi:10.1007/978-3-030-79206-0_64

Lingras, P., Sharma, S., & Zhong, M. (2002). Prediction of recreational travel using genetically designed regression and time-delay neural network models. *Transportation Research Record: Journal of the Transportation Research Board*, *13*(1), 435–446. doi:10.3141/1805-03

Ma, X., Tao, Z., Wang, Y., Yu, H., & Wang, Y. (2015). Long short-term memory neural network for traffic speed prediction using remote microwave sensor data. *Transport. Res. C Emerging Technol.*, *54*, 187–197. doi:10.1016/j.trc.2015.03.014

Nejad, L., Mashayekhy, L., Chinnam, R. B., & Phillips, A. (2017). Hierarchical time-dependent shortest path algorithms for vehicle routing under ITS. *IIE Transactions*, *48*(2), 158–169. doi:10.1080/0740817X.2015.1078523

Wangyang, W., Honghai, W., & Huadong, M. (2019). An AutoEncoder and LSTM-Based Traffic Flow Prediction Method. *Sensors (Basel)*, *19*(2946), 1–16. PMID:31277390

Zhao, Z., Chen, W., Wu, X., Chen, P. C. Y., & Liu, J. (2017). LSTM network: A deep learning approach for short-term traffic forecast. *IET Intelligent Transport Systems*, *11*(2), 68–75. doi:10.1049/iet-its.2016.0208

Chapter 15
Various Feature Selection Techniques Used for Predicting and Diagnosing Heart Disease

Dibakar Sinha
https://orcid.org/0000-0002-0053-6396
Shri Vaishnav Vidyapeeth Vishwavidyalaya, India

Ashish Sharma
GLA University, Mathura, India

ABSTRACT

To effectively treat cardiac patients before a heart attack occurs, a precise prognosis of heart disease is necessary. Recently, machine learning-based algorithms for predicting and diagnosing heart disease have been described. However, the lack of a sophisticated framework that can use several sources of data to forecast cardiac disease means that current algorithms cannot manage large datasets. These systems use standard methods for selecting data points and assigning weights to them according to their relevance. Heart disease diagnosis has also failed to benefit from the use of these techniques. A review of the various feature selection methods used in the detection of heart disease is provided in this chapter of the book. The data used in the trials comes from a UCI library and relates to heart disease. In order to test the biomedical system's efficiency, many well-known validation methods have been used. This allows doctors to recognize heart disease in patients at an early stage so that more treatment can be started.

INTRODUCTION

In machine learning (ML) the principal object of feature selection is to find the right feature combinations. The chapter is dedicated to a different implementation of the method of collection of features. Creating a ML model is basically a technique for extracting all the elements applicable to a query. A function must be declared vital because it is useful for creating a ML model of the issue under investigation (Zhang

DOI: 10.4018/978-1-6684-2508-4.ch015

et. al, 2021). The significance is considered in a general sense. One can ask why this purpose is at all relevant. Why should anyone be involved in the importance of this kind?

It is almost rare if all the data variables are useful for constructing a model when developing a ML model in real-life. Adding redundant variables decreases the model's generalization potential and can also reduce a classifier's overall accuracy. Besides, adding increased variables to a specification increases the model's total complexity.

Because relevant characteristics are often unknown for many real-world idea learning problems, we must add many candidate characteristics. Unfortunately, irrelevant features degrade both pace (due to high dimensionality) and predictive precision of idea learners' results (due to irrelevant information) (Alpaydin,2020). In positive induction, the condition is severe, as many candidate features are created to improve the power of the language of representation. The selection of parts is selecting a small features subset that is preferably proper and adequate to describe the definition of the target.

Choosing an good statistical method for a dataset while creating filter-based feature selection can be tedious for a ML developer.

The quantity of genomic data has increased with the advent of computing techniques, with a rapid pace making it impossible to use such data in the medical field without proper preprocessing, which in turn leads to more complexity and integrity problems, ultimately generating several difficulties such as storage, analysis, privacy and protection(Pavithra & Jayalakshmi,2020) . Therefore, in terms of its length, genomic data which appear simple to manage, yet because of the sophistication, variability and hybridist of its characteristics, it needs an overly complicated method. This is an information exploration method.

- Data recording specifications include a range of issues and tools about the capture and storing of data.
- "Pre-processing" is the first step before start doing research.
- Statistical research is the method of gathering and displaying evidence.
- It requires using the analysis and analysis of the data using various approaches to decide the meaning and value of the results.

In genomics, the key aim is to sequence all living species' genomes and obtain insights into the 'twinkle' of the human body. Now it is mainly about how you can get us out of the already sequenced results (Guo et al.,2021). The significant difficulties that genomic data poses show that the biological model must be healthy and prosperous in the preprocessing phase. It is essential to deal with these concerns to limit the specific features and pick only the most proper attributes. The preprocessing stage is necessary to ensure the efficiency of the analysis. Although with limited datasets, one cannot perform high-quality evaluations because of the sheer number of features and their complexity(Rao et al.,2021). Feature reduction is one of the aims of preprocessing phase. There are six significant types of feature selection algorithms.

The first three primary methods are (see Figure 1):

- **Filters** It is an individual step before other learning processes. The robots used independent standards to exclude contestants. The features are selected by comparing different forms of criterion's degree of significance to the target variable.
- **Wrappers** It's a function selection approach to improve a statistical algorithm by analyzing a particular subset of characteristics. The estimation of popularity is performed using a classifier that

calculates the relevancy of a given subset of features. This form of procedure is not quite common but has supplied proof of great strength and durability.

- **Embedded** It incorporates the general approaches of processor and wrapper processes. Multiple Filters and Wrapper methods are more efficient than conventional single Filters and Wrapper methods, but they have been very costly.

Figure 1. Basic feature selection methods
(Al-Tashi, 2020)

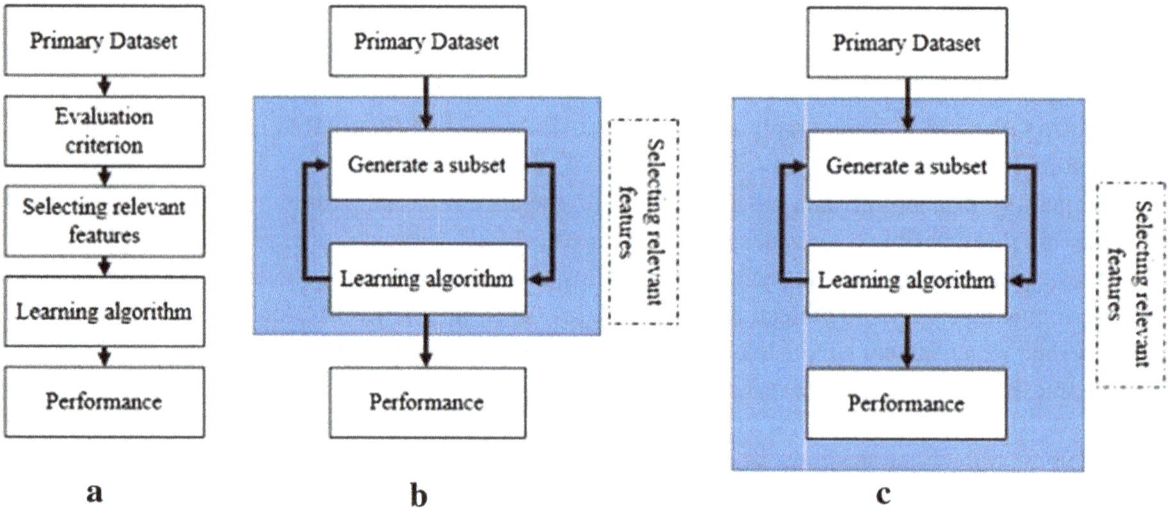

Other mathematical techniques of feature selection have been described and lauded in the literature. Some are generally based on the simple five styles of speech listed above(Rao et al., 2021).

- Hybrid strategies that can follow a set of conjunct main function collection approaches.
- It is using an aggregate of characteristics of diverse base classifiers. That is a separate function classification.
- Information can be combined for function selection.

LITERATURE SURVEY

Value of Feature Selection in ML

Top purpose to implement feature selection is:

- This helps speed up the training process of the machine learning algorithm.
- Simplifies a method.
- If subsets are selected correctly, a model is more reliable.
- Minimize over fitting

Our analysis examines the current feature selection approaches explicitly in the genomics to create a detailed feeling of the best-featured selection process.

Why Feature Selection?

Simple models are more comfortable to interpret: It's much easier to forecast a model's behavior with several variables.

- Shorter training time: Simplifying the model makes faster decisions, leading to decreased training costs and quicker model performance.
- Enhanced generalization by reducing over fitting: Some of the factors you are forecasting are only like noise. However, the ML model learns from the noise and sees over fitting while at the same time minimizing generalization. By cancelling these unrelated functions, we can significantly boost the generalization of ML models(Hopf & Reifenrath, 2021).
- Variable redundancy: Features of a given dataset are often highly correlated, and it is true that highly correlated features do include the same information. In this way, we can diminish the scale of contact without missing any information. Less noisy simulations imply that there is less risk of incorrect forecasts.

Feature selection strategies are meant to minimize the number of inputs considered most useful for the algorithm to forecast a particular variable(Yuan et al.,2020).

Feature collection strategies are either supervised or unsupervised.

The distinction between independent and dependent variable is based on whether the dependent variable is used or not. Unsupervised function selection does not consider the degree or distribution of the data, for example, approaches that end duplicate parameter implementing correlation. Feature filtering uses the goal variable, such as strategies that exclude unnecessary variables.

Different path to rationalizing the selection procedure for feature selection involves filter and wrapper approaches. Mentioned techniques are confirmed by using the holdout dataset mostly supervised.

Model selection approaches generate several configurations with various input parameter and pick those features that have the best value as per the metric(Pasha & Mohamed,2020). These methods don't include the variables forms, but they can be computationally costly. Bootstrap is an example of a wrapper function selection process.

Filter function selection algorithms use statistical methods to test the relationship between an input variable and the output variable and use these scores to provide (filter) the inputs for the mode

Feature selection types can be described as below.

- **Feature Selection**: Choose a module of input features from the dataset.
    - **Unsupervised**: Avoid target parameter (e.g., delete duplicate parameter).
        - Correlation
    - **Supervised**: Implement the target parameter (e.g., delete unrelated parameter).
        - **Wrapper**: Find useful subsets of features.
        - RFE
        - **Filter**: Choose features depending on the target parameter relationship .
        - Statistical Procedure

- § **Intrinsic**: Training phase automatic feature selection performing algorithm
- § Decision Trees
- **Dimensionality Reduction**: Project input data into a lower-dimensional feature space.

Filter Methods

Very commonly, the selection criterion is a correlation style statistic of input and output variables.

Choosing statistical measurements depends upon the kind of results(Lai et al.,2021). Most of the data may be of the numeric and categorical types. Popular data input variations as shown in figure 2 are:

- Number Variables
- Floating Point Variables.
- Integer Variables.
- Categorical Variables.
- Ordinal Variables.
- Boolean Variables
- Nominal Variables.

Figure 2. Different variable data types
(Zhang et al.,2021)

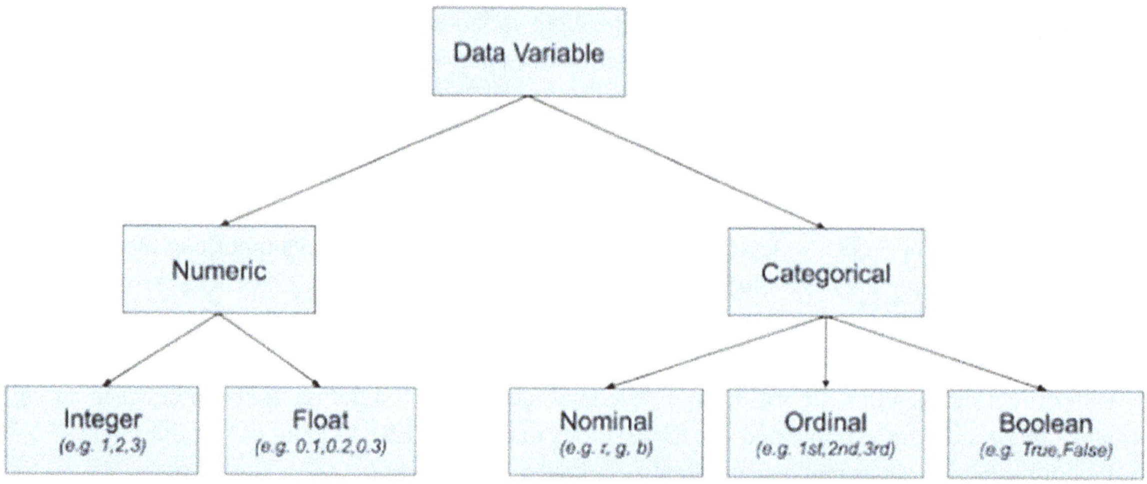

In this segment, we will analyze two kinds of parameters: numeric variables and categorical variables. We will also address two essential classes of parameters to concentrate on output and input.

Process parameters are those that are entered into a programming model. In function collection, we wish to disregard irrelevant functions. In this sense, the output variables those for which a template is supposed to diagnose, commonly known as the target variable(Wang et al.,2021).

Answer variables may reveal the type of computational modeling issue being done. For instance, a dependent variable implies a categorical output variable and a regression problem shows a problem of classification.

- **Numerical Output**: Predictive Regression modeling problem.
- **Categorical Output**: Predictive Classification modeling problem.

The methods used in calculating trends are measured one input variables for the target variable. In such instances, they are called Univariate statistical measures. This means that there is no communication in the filters.

Numerical Output, Numerical Input

This is a problem of regression predictor. The most basic methods are to apply a correlation coefficient as shown in figure 3, so as Pearson's as a linear correlation or rank-based techniques for a nonlinear correlation(Rustom et al., 2022).

- **Spearman's coefficient rank(nonlinear)**
- **Pearson's coefficient of correlation(linear).**

The filter methods use lower numerical requirements instead of cross-validation efficiency. This technique is much quicker and uses fewer CPU cycles than wrappers do. Using the filter approach over time series data is computationally cheaper.

Figure 3. Feature selection approaches
(Lazaar,2012)

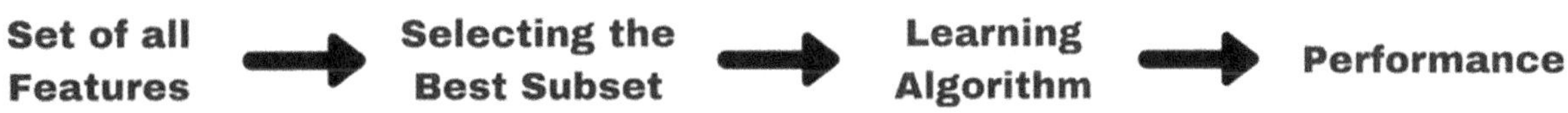

Filtering approaches are also used as a prior processing stage. The features selected are not based on any machine learning algorithms. The parts are chosen based on statistical interaction with the result. This is a subjective argument. We will see the details in following table 1 to grasp the correlation coefficient(Özyurt,2020).

Table 1. Correlation coefficient

Feature \ Response	Continuous	Categorical
Continuous	Pearson's Correlation	LDA
Categorical	Anova	Chi-Square

(Hoseini, 2020)

Information Gain

Information benefit decides the information that is lost during the transformation of the data. A decision tree can be used to classify proper functions for regression analysis. A graph and related code is shown in figure 4 below(Ghosh et al.,2021).

Figure 4. Information Gain Chart and python code for implementation
(Alpaydin, 2020)

```
from sklearn.feature_selection import mutual_info_classif
import matplotlib.pyplot as plt
%matplotlib inline

importances = mutual_info_classif(X, Y)
feat_importances = pd.Series(importances, dataframe.columns[0:len(dataframe.columns)-1])
feat_importances.plot(kind='barh', color = 'teal')
plt.show()
```

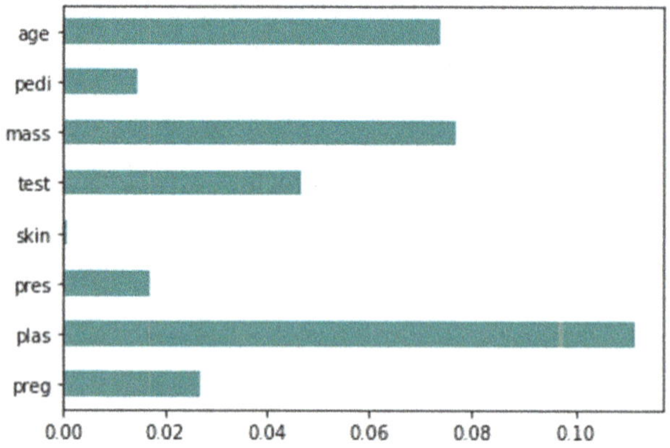

Pearson's Correlation

Correlation is implemented as a tool for quantifying the sum of the linear relationship among various continuous variables. Its result can be anywhere -1 to +1. Pearson's product was given as:

$$\rho X,Y = \frac{cov(X,Y)}{\sigma_x \sigma_Y}$$

Correlation is an assessment of the interaction between two variables. By inference, we can use one attribute to forecast the other. The correlation function is the best feature discovery tool because successful features are strongly correlated with the goal feature. Often, variables should be associated with the goal but should be uncorrelated with each other. A related code and heat map of a data set is shown in figure 5 using python(Lazar et al.,2012).

Figure 5. Heat map and python implementation of Pearson correlation
(Pavithra,2020)

```
import seaborn as sns
import matplotlib.pyplot as plt
%matplotlib inline

# Correlation matrix
cor = dataframe.corr()

# Plotting Heatmap
plt.figure(figsize = (10,6))
sns.heatmap(cor, annot = True)
<AxesSubplot:>
```

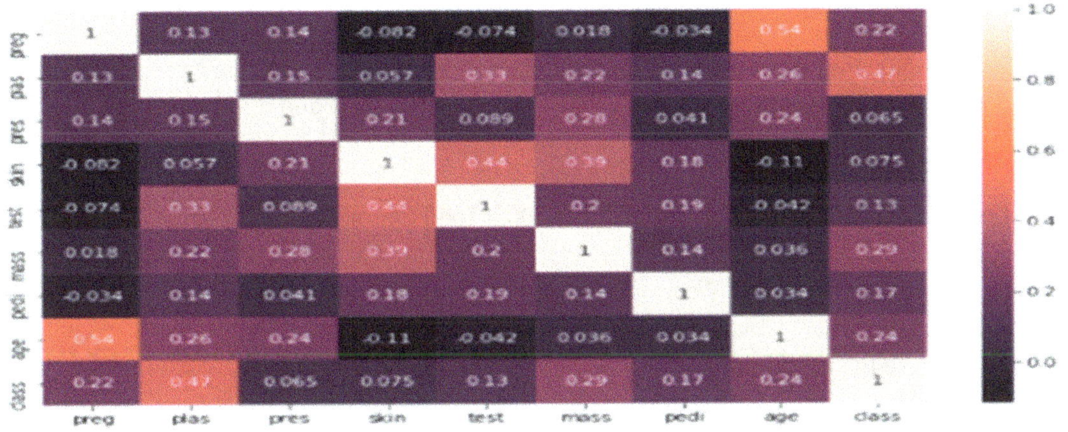

LDA

LDA is used to get features of linear combination that define a discrepancy between two or more stages.

ANOVA

ANOVA means the measurement of variation. In LDA, categorical independent variables are used, and there is a constant dependent variable. In this process, it checks equality of means of different classes.

Chi-Square

A statistical examination is conducted on a group of features to explore a specific theory about their interaction(Hosseini et al.,2020).

In this way, only the variable which carries the highest chi-square value will be considered.

Now let's construct a basic example to illustrate how we measure chi-squared for a sample.

So, let's assume there is a 25 Non-Right-Forwards and 75 Right-Forwards in the dataset. In the 100 places, 40 are good, and the other 55 are wrong. Can this mean that the player is more efficient on the flanks affect the team's overall performance? Below table 2 using Chi Square method is shown.

Table 2. Chi square feature selection method

	Good	Not Good			Good	Not Good	
Not RightForward	20	5	25	Not RightForward	15	10	25
RightForward	40	35	75	RightForward	45	25	75
	60	40	100		60	40	100

(Ghosh,2021)

The chi-squared value is measured as:

We need to decide the actual values of our variables of interest to determine our sample outcomes.

This is relatively easy. We add the sums of the values in every cell and divide it by the total number of observations.

So bucket is 25 (Row Sum) * 60 (Column Sum) / 100. (Total Observations)

Why should this be expected? We would predict one of the 25 players who are valuable in some statistics. Thus 15 players.

Then we will use the formula:

$$x_c^2 = \sum \frac{(O_i - E_i)^2}{E_i}$$

The chi-squared statistic is justified to be extended to non-negative numerical and categorical attributes.

Chi-squared valued analysis of our dataset as shown in figure 6 as:

Figure 6. Chi-squared valued analysis of our dataset
(Rao,2021)

```
from sklearn.feature_selection import SelectKBest
from sklearn.feature_selection import chi2

# Convert to categorical data by converting data to integers
X_cat = X.astype(int)

# Three features with highest chi-squared statistics are selected
chi2_features = SelectKBest(chi2, k = 3)
X_kbest_features = chi2_features.fit_transform(X_cat, Y)

# Reduced features
print('Original feature number:', X_cat.shape[1])
print('Reduced feature number:', X_kbest_features.shape[1])
```

```
Original feature number: 8
Reduced feature number: 3
```

Variance Threshold

The efficacy threshold is a primary baseline method for function choice. It excludes arbitrary features that are not at least "acceptable". Batch Normalization cuts all zero-variance functions. Even if we believe that characteristics with a higher variance supply more valuable knowledge, there is an issue here since we do not take the interaction between the features and target variables into account(Bhui et al.,2020).

Figure 7. Chi-squared valued analysis of our dataset
(Hopf,2021)

```
from sklearn.feature_selection import VarianceThreshold

# Resetting the value of X to make it non-categorical
X = array[:,0:8]

v_threshold = VarianceThreshold(threshold=0)
v_threshold.fit(X)  # fit finds the features with zero variance
v_threshold.get_support()
```

```
array([ True,  True,  True,  True,  True,  True,  True,  True])
```

Returns a Boolean vector, which may imply if a value has zero mean.

Fisher's Score:

Fisher's approach is a important feature selection techniques coming under supervised algorithm. Fisher' score return the ranks of the parameter depending on the scores in greater to lesser no order. Then variables are picked in conjunction with the scenario(Effrosynidis & Arampatzis,2021).

Filter method does not deal with reducing multi collinearity

Mean Absolute Difference (MAD)

"MAD" is the total variance in the mean value. The distinction between Insane and Variance tests is the lack of the standard deviation of the latter. The Insane, like the Variances, is indeed a discriminatory power calculation(Rustam et al.,2022).

Figure 8. Fisher Score
(Bekkerman,2003)

```
from skfeature.function.similarity_based import fisher_score
import matplotlib.pyplot as plt
%matplotlib inline

# Calculating scores
ranks = fisher_score.fisher_score(X, Y)

# Plotting the ranks
feat_importances = pd.Series(ranks, dataframe.columns[0:len(dataframe.columns)-1])
feat_importances.plot(kind='barh', color = 'teal')
plt.show()
```

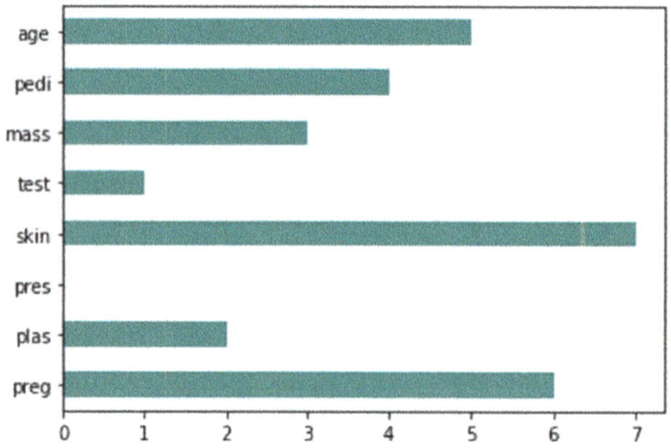

Figure 9. Graph for MAD
(Yuan,2020)

```
# Calculate MAD
mean_abs_diff = np.sum(np.abs(X -np.mean(X, axis =0 )), axis = 0)/X.shape[0]

# Plot the barchart
plt.bar(np.arange(X.shape[1]),mean_abs_diff, color = 'teal')
```

```
<BarContainer object of 8 artists>
```

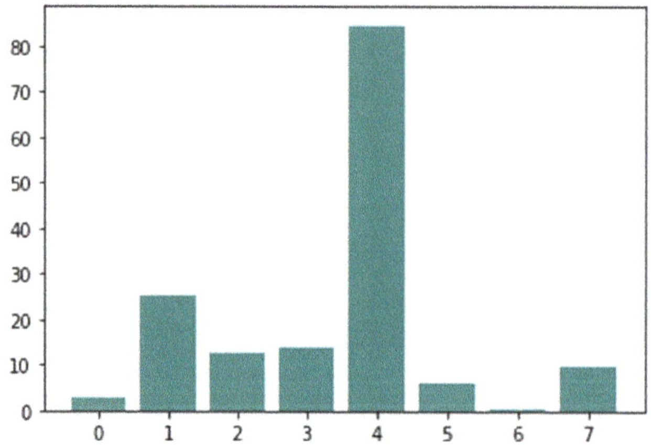

Dispersion Ratio

An alternative indicator of dispersion is the geometric mean (GM) and the arithmetic mean. For a set of points X's, it produces the AM or GM.

$$AM_i = \underline{X} = \frac{1}{n}\sum_{j=1}^{n} X_{ij},\quad GM_i = \left(\prod_{j=1}^{n} X_{ij}\right)^{\frac{1}{n}}$$

respectively, since equality is held if and only if, then the ratio can be used as a dispersion measure. Higher dispersion implies a higher value of Ri, thus a more relevant feature. Conversely, when all the feature samples have (roughly) the same value, Ri is close to 1, indicating a low relevance feature(Wang et al.,2021).

$$RM_i = \frac{AM_i}{GM_i} \epsilon \left[1, +\infty\right),$$

Figure 10. Graph for dispersion ration
(Effrosynidis & Arampatzis,2021)

```
X = X+1 # To avoid 0 for denominator
# Arithmetic Mean
am = np.mean(X, axis =0 )
#Geometric Mean
gm = np.power(np.prod(X, axis -0 ),1/X.shape[0])
# Ratio of Arithmetic Mean and Geometric Mean
disp_ratio = am/gm
# Plotting the bar chart
plt.bar(np.arange(X.shape[1]),disp_ratio, color = 'teal')
```

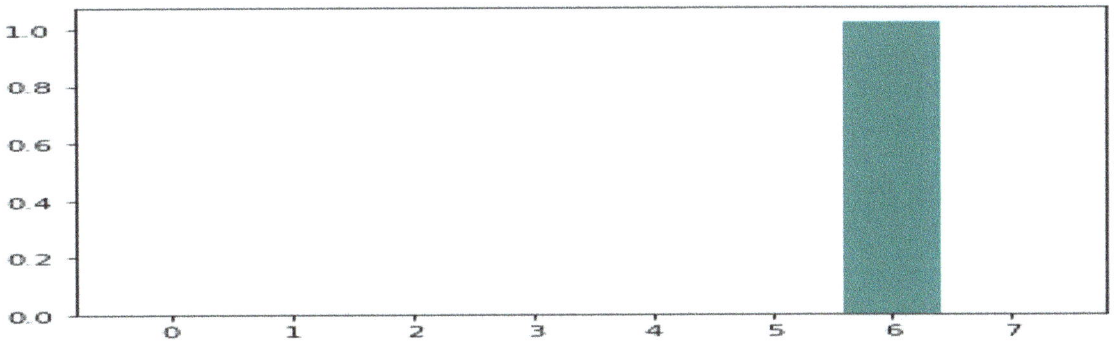

Tips and Tricks for Feature Selection

This chapter addresses some small concerns when using filters for feature collection.

Correlation Statistics

The scikit-learn library offers several statistics reports, including p-values.

For example:

- Pearson's Correlation Coefficient:
- ANOVA:
- Chi-Squared
- Mutual Information:

Moreover, the SciPy library gives an execution of various statistics, like Kendall's tau and Spearman's rank correlation

Selection Method

The library includes various filtering kinds until statistics have been decided for each input element for the output(Özyurt,2020).

Most people use these approaches.:

- Select the top k variables:
- Select the top percentile variables:

Transform Variables

Consider various mathematical techniques to get the correct result.

For example, it is also possible to turn a categorical variable into an ordinal to see if any exciting findings can come out.

There isa various approach to find discrete variables such as numbering, categorizing, rating…

Any statistical measures assume specific properties to the variables they are evaluating, such as taking a Gaussian probability distribution to the results and a linear relationship. You can convert data to satisfy the exam criteria, and you can test the data regardless of whether you try the test(Khan et al.,2020).

Wrapper Methods

We will use a small subset of features and train a model using them. By comparison with our earlier model, we decide to keep or remove functions from the subgroup. The issue is practically reduced to a search problem. Sees techniques are typically exceedingly tricky and time-consuming to be done.

Some popular types of wrapper methods are forward feature selection, backward feature elimination, recursive feature elimination, etc (Bommert,2020).

Figure 11. Wrapper Method
(Pasha et al.,2020)

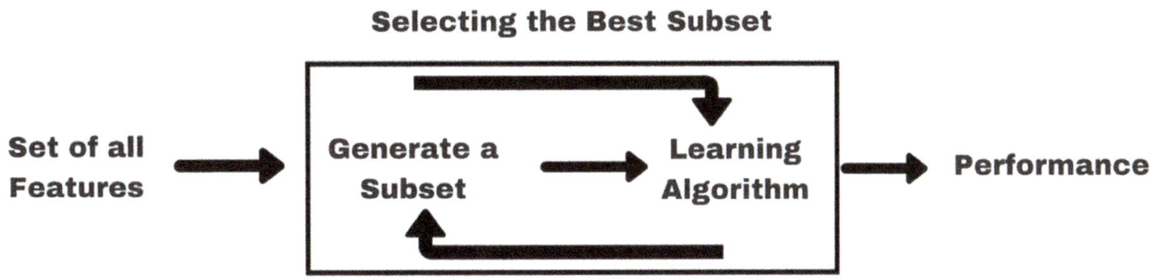

Forward Selection

The forward choice process begins with no functions. We continue adding each element until adding the new variable becomes redundant.

Figure 12. Python code for forward selection
(Pasha, 2020)

```
# Forward Feature Selection
from mlxtend.feature_selection import SequentialFeatureSelector
ffs = SequentialFeatureSelector(lr, k_features='best', forward = True, n_jobs=-1)
ffs.fit(X, Y)
features = list(ffs.k_feature_names_)
features = list(map(int, features))
lr.fit(x_train[features], y_train)
y_pred = lr.predict(x_train[features])
```

Backward Elimination

In backward elimination, we start with every function and then cut the least benefit features. We repeat this until there is no change in cutting functionality (Dhal,2021).

Figure 13. Python code for backward selection
(Pasha, 2020)

```
# Backward Feature Selection
from sklearn.linear_model import LogisticRegression
from mlxtend.feature_selection import SequentialFeatureSelector
lr = LogisticRegression(class_weight = 'balanced', solver = 'lbfgs', random_state=42, n_jobs=-1, max_iter=500)
lr.fit(X, Y)
bfs = SequentialFeatureSelector(lr, k_features='best', forward = False, n_jobs=-1)
bfs.fit(X, Y)
features = list(bfs.k_feature_names_)
features = list(map(int, features))
lr.fit(x_train[features], y_train)
y_pred = lr.predict(x_train[features])
```

Exhaustive Feature Selection

The best feature collection tool to-date is this. This is a sequence of assessments of each sub-set of functions. It measures any possible mix of factors and classifies outcomes into the best possible groupings.

Figure 14. Python code for exhaustive feature selection
(Pasha, 2020)

```
# Exhaustive Feature Selection
from mlxtend.feature_selection import ExhaustiveFeatureSelector

# import the algorithm you want to evaluate on your features.
from sklearn.ensemble import RandomForestClassifier

# create the ExhaustiveFeatureSelector object.
efs = ExhaustiveFeatureSelector(RandomForestClassifier(),
          min_features=4,
          max_features=8,
          scoring='roc_auc',
          cv=2)

# fit the object to the training data.
efs = efs.fit(X, Y)

# print the selected features.
selected_features = x_train.columns[list(efs.best_idx_)]
print(selected_features)

# print the final prediction score.
print(efs.best_score_)
```

```
Features: 163/163

Int64Index([0, 1, 2, 3, 4, 5, 6, 7], dtype='int64')
0.8252014925373135
```

Recursive Feature Elimination

It is a greedy algorithm to discover the best performing function subset. It constantly iterates on various theories, keeping the better or worst performing function until it reaches the desired goal. It continues to change the current model until the whole body is finished. The algorithm then lists the features based on how they cut the most (Hopf,2021).

Figure 15. Python code for recursive feature Selection
(Lai, 2021)

```
# Recursive Feature Selection
from sklearn.feature_selection import RFE
rfe = RFE(lr, n_features_to_select=7)
rfe.fit(x_train, y_train)
y_pred = rfe.predict(x_train)
```

One of the easiest ways to implement feature selection with wrappers is to use the Bora kit that incorporates feature selection and feature shadows.

It works in the following steps:

- Firstly, it offers unpredictability to a dataset by re-arranging the functions (shadow features).
- Thus, a random forest classifier is trained on the expanded collection of results. Each function's value is assessed using the Mean Decrease Accuracy measure to determine the most relevant features.
- At any iteration, it tests such that original characteristics have a higher value than the best of its surrounding features (i.e., with higher Z-score than the highest Z-score of its surrounding features) and continuously excludes features which are considered not to be useful.
- The procedure stops when the outcomes of the features all get accepted or denied, or because the random forest runs have been completed.

Difference between Filter and Wrapper Methods

The main differences between the filter and wrapper methods for feature selection are:

- Filter methods are used to measure the importance of features, while wrapper methods are used to calculate the utility of a subset of features.
- Filter approaches are comparatively more effective in operation since they need little preparation for it to function. Computational tools for wrapper methods are often very costly.
- Filter methods use mathematical methods for comparing unique features. Cross-validation is used in wrapper methods to reach a subset of features.
- Filter methods might skip the excellent collection of features in several instances ; however, wrapper methods often do the best job choosing parts in any case.
- The additional features used by the wrapper methods, the more vulnerable the model would be to overfitting as opposed to using fewer characteristics from the filter methods.

Embedded Methods

Much as how wrapper methods consider the relationship between functions and templates, embedded methods do the same. They use feature selection as part of their model building process, and less computation is needed.

This approach aims to incorporate the utility of all the earlier policies and conducts the collection of variables during preparation. This approach uses the highest precision by integrating all sides of the model (Wang,2021).

Figure 16. Embedded Methods
(Chen,2020)

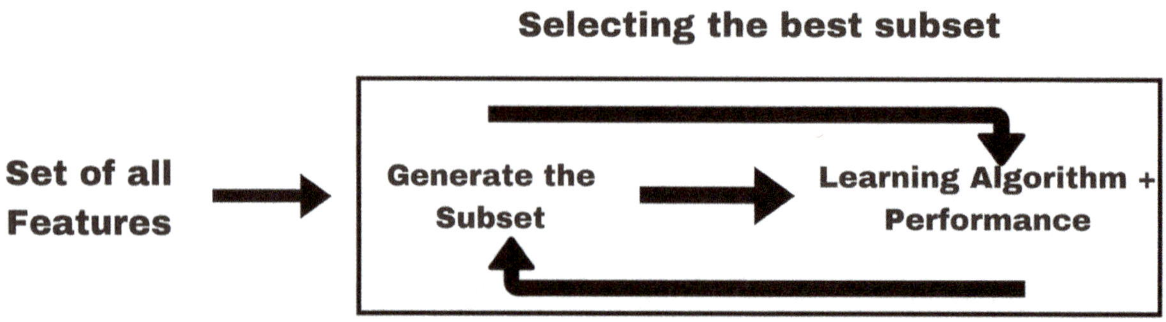

To use this process, people should mix filter and wrapper methods. It's implemented via algorithms that feature pick via their built-in function.

To minimize overfitting, many machines learning approaches such as LASSO and RIDGE have built-in penalization functions that remove overfitting.

Lasso Regression

Big L1 regularization that adds a penalty equal to the total sum of all coefficients. This is needed to change how much freedom the machine learning model has, i.e., not overfitting the results. In linear model regularization, there is an extra penalty for coefficients which multiply predictors. L1 regularization can reduce the size of a few of the coefficients and makes it scale well. Thus, the function may be excised from the model (Chen,2020).

Figure 17. Python Code for Lasso Regression
(Bommert,2021)

```
from sklearn.linear_model import LogisticRegression
from sklearn.feature_selection import SelectFromModel

# Set the regularization parameter C=1
logistic = LogisticRegression(C=1, penalty="l1", solver='liblinear', random_state=7).fit(X, Y)
model = SelectFromModel(logistic, prefit=True)

X_new = model.transform(X)

# Dropped columns have values of all 0s, keep other columns
selected_columns = selected_features.columns[selected_features.var() != 0]
selected_columns
```

```
Int64Index([0, 1, 2, 3, 4, 5, 6, 7], dtype='int64')
```

Ridge Regression

The L2 regularization approach applies “penalty” (i.e., a cost) equal to the square of the coefficients’ size.

Random Forest Importance

Random Forests is somewhat of Bagging Algorithms that yields the output by using a given number of trees. The tree-based techniques used by random forests generally rank based on their ability to minimize impurity or in some terms a reduction in the impurity (Gini impurity) over all trees. Nodes with the highest reduction in impurity exist at the beginning of the branches, while the nodes with the smallest decrease in impurity are found at the trees’ end. By trimming trees so that the lowest rising components are removed, we can separate the most noteworthy features (Masmoudi,2020).

Figure 18. Python Code for Random Forrest
(Bommert,2021)

```
from sklearn.ensemble import RandomForestClassifier

# create the random forest with your hyperparameters.
model = RandomForestClassifier(n_estimators=340)

# fit the model to start training.
model.fit(X, Y)

# get the importance of the resulting features.
importances = model.feature_importances_

# create a data frame for visualization.
final_df = pd.DataFrame({"Features": pd.DataFrame(X).columns, "Importances":importances})
final_df.set_index('Importances')

# sort in ascending order to better visualization.
final_df = final_df.sort_values('Importances')

# plot the feature importances in bars.
final_df.plot.bar(color = 'teal')
```

```
<AxesSubplot:>
```

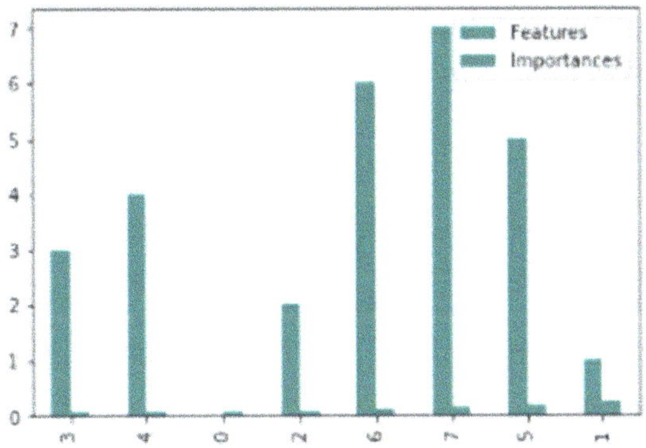

CONCLUSION

Few approaches related to feature selection are presented. These strategies help minimize the data's dimensionality or reduce the number of variables while retaining the volatility of the data.

There are also other feature selection techniques, aside from the methods discussed above. There are also dual approaches that use both methods of filtering and wrapping. The literature on the specification of feature selection techniques covering the uses of machine learning and pattern recognition are very comprehensive.

In most of the cases only a single dataset can be used to pick feature selection algorithms, as each underlying algorithm behaves differently.

Feature selection approaches illustrate that in machine learning systems, more data is not necessarily healthy. A function selection algorithm can be chosen for the application at hand, based on the considerations like: simplicity, reliability, number of reduced functions, precision of classification, specifications for storage and computation.

Overall, the collection of features will often have advantages, such as providing insight into the results, better classification model, boost generalization of irrelevant variables and recognition. In addition, feature architecture and the option of functionality are essential components of any machine learning pipeline. In this article, some of the most used function selection methods and the workflow when it comes to feature selection are clarified. In addition, some intuition was attempted in these approaches, but more is needed to integrate this methodology in day-to-day practice.

REFERENCES

Al-Tashi, Q., Abdulkadir, S. J., Rais, H. M., Mirjalili, S., & Alhussian, H. (2020). Approaches to multi-objective feature selection: A systematic literature review. *IEEE Access: Practical Innovations, Open Solutions*, *8*, 125076–125096. doi:10.1109/ACCESS.2020.3007291

Alpaydin, E. (2020). *Introduction to machine learning*. MIT Press.

Bekkerman, R., El-Yaniv, R., Tishby, N., & Winter, Y. (2003). Distributional word clusters vs. words for text categorization. *Journal of Machine Learning Research*, *3*(Mar), 1183–1208.

Bhui, N., Ram, P. K., & Kuila, P. (2020, July). Feature selection from microarray data based on deep learning approach. In *2020 11th International Conference on Computing, Communication and Networking Technologies (ICCCNT)* (pp. 1-5). IEEE.

Bommert, A., Sun, X., Bischl, B., Rahnenführer, J., & Lang, M. (2020). Benchmark for filter methods for feature selection in high-dimensional classification data. *Computational Statistics & Data Analysis*, *143*, 106839.

Chen, J., Zeng, Y., Li, Y., & Huang, G. B. (2020). Unsupervised feature selection based extreme learning machine for clustering. *Neurocomputing*, *386*, 198–207.

Dhal, P., & Azad, C. (2021). A comprehensive survey on feature selection in the various fields of machine learning. *Applied Intelligence*, 1–39.

Effrosynidis, D., & Arampatzis, A. (2021). An evaluation of feature selection methods for environmental data. *Ecological Informatics*, *61*, 101224.

Ghosh, P., Azam, S., Jonkman, M., Karim, A., Shamrat, F. J. M., Ignatious, E., Shultana, S., Beeravolu, A. R., & De Boer, F. (2021). Efficient prediction of cardiovascular disease using machine learning algorithms with relief and LASSO feature selection techniques. *IEEE Access: Practical Innovations, Open Solutions*, *9*, 19304–19326. doi:10.1109/ACCESS.2021.3053759

Guo, Y., Zhang, B., Sun, Y., Jiang, K., & Wu, K. (2021). Machine learning based feature selection and knowledge reasoning for CBR system under big data. *Pattern Recognition*, *112*, 107805.

Hopf, K., & Reifenrath, S. (2021). *Filter Methods for Feature Selection in Supervised Machine Learning Applications--Review and Benchmark.* arXiv preprint arXiv:2111.12140.

Hosseini, F. S., Choubin, B., Mosavi, A., Nabipour, N., Shamshirband, S., Darabi, H., & Haghighi, A. T. (2020). Flash-flood hazard assessment using ensembles and Bayesian-based machine l earning models: Application of the simulated annealing feature selection method. *The Science of the Total Environment*, *711*, 135161.

Khan, M. A., Ashraf, I., Alhaisoni, M., Damaševičius, R., Scherer, R., Rehman, A., & Bukhari, S. A. C. (2020). Multimodal brain tumor classification using deep learning and robust feature selection: A machine learning application for radiologists. *Diagnostics (Basel)*, *10*(8), 565.

Lai, P. K., Fernando, A., Cloutier, T. K., Kingsbury, J. S., Gokarn, Y., Halloran, K. T., ... Trout, B. L. (2021). Machine learning feature selection for predicting high concentration therapeutic antibody aggregation. *Journal of Pharmaceutical Sciences*, *110*(4), 1583–1591.

Lazar, C., Taminau, J., Meganck, S., Steenhoff, D., Coletta, A., Molter, C., de Schaetzen, V., Duque, R., Bersini, H., & Nowe, A. (2012). A survey on filter techniques for feature selection in gene expression microarray analysis. *IEEE/ACM Transactions on Computational Biology and Bioinformatics*, *9*(4), 1106–1119. doi:10.1109/TCBB.2012.33 PMID:22350210

Masmoudi, S., Elghazel, H., Taieb, D., Yazar, O., & Kallel, A. (2020). A machine-learning framework for predicting multiple air pollutants' concentrations via multi-target regression and feature selection. *The Science of the Total Environment*, *715*, 136991.

Özyurt, F. (2020). Efficient deep feature selection for remote sensing image recognition with fused deep learning architectures. *The Journal of Supercomputing*, *76*(11), 8413–8431.

Pasha, S. J., & Mohamed, E. S. (2020, February). Ensemble gain ratio feature selection (EGFS) model with machine learning and data mining algorithms for disease risk prediction. In *2020 International Conference on Inventive Computation Technologies (ICICT)* (pp. 590-596). IEEE.

Pavithra, V., & Jayalakshmi, V. (2020, June). Review of feature selection techniques for predicting diseases. In *2020 5th International Conference on Communication and Electronics Systems (ICCES)* (pp. 1213-1217). IEEE.

Rao, P. S., Kumar, A. S., Niyaz, Q., Sidike, P., & Devabhaktuni, V. K. (2021). Binary chemical reaction optimization based feature selection techniques for machine learning classification problems. *Expert Systems with Applications*, *167*, 114169.

Rustam, F., Reshi, A. A., Aljedaani, W., Alhossan, A., Ishaq, A., Shafi, S., ... Rupapara, V. (2022). Vector mosquito image classification using novel RIFS feature selection and machine learning models for disease epidemiology. *Saudi Journal of Biological Sciences*, *29*(1), 583–594.

Sivaranjani, S., Ananya, S., Aravinth, J., & Karthika, R. (2021, March). Diabetes prediction using machine learning algorithms with feature selection and dimensionality reduction. In *2021 7th International Conference on Advanced Computing and Communication Systems (ICACCS)* (Vol. 1, pp. 141-146). IEEE.

Upadhyay, D., Manero, J., Zaman, M., & Sampalli, S. (2020). Gradient boosting feature selection with machine learning classifiers for intrusion detection on power grids. *IEEE eTransactions on Network and Service Management*, *18*(1), 1104–1116.

Wang, Z., Nie, F., Zhang, C., Wang, R., & Li, X. (2021). Joint nonlinear feature selection and continuous values regression network. *Pattern Recognition Letters*, *150*, 197–206.

Yuan, X., Yuan, J., Jiang, T., & Ain, Q. U. (2020). Integrated long-term stock selection models based on feature selection and machine learning algorithms for China stock market. *IEEE Access: Practical Innovations, Open Solutions*, *8*, 22672–22685.

Zhang, N., Gupta, A., Chen, Z., & Ong, Y. S. (2021). Evolutionary machine learning with minions: A case study in feature selection. *IEEE Transactions on Evolutionary Computation*, *26*(1), 130–144. doi:10.1109/TEVC.2021.3099289

Compilation of References

3playmedia. (n.d.). https://www.3playmedia.com/blog/growing-population-hearing-loss/

Abdullah, A., Abdul-Kadir, N. A., & Che, H. F. K. (2020). An Optimization of IMU Sensors-Based Approach for Malaysian Sign Language Recognition. In *2020 6th International Conference on Computing Engineering and Design (ICCED). 2020 6th International Conference on Computing Engineering and Design (ICCED).* IEEE. 10.1109/ICCED51276.2020.9415838

Afif, M. H., Hedar, A.-R., Abdel Hamid, T. H., & Mahdy, Y. B. (2013). SS-SVM (3SVM): A new classification method for hepatitis disease diagnosis. *International Journal of Advanced Computer Science and Applications*, *4*(2), 53–58.

Ahn, B. G., Noh, Y. H., & Jeong, D. U. (2015). *Smart chair based on multi heart rate detection system.* IEEE Sensors.

Ak, M. F. (2020, June). A comparative analysis of breast cancer detection and diagnosis using data visualization and machine learning applications. In Healthcare (Vol. 8, No. 2, p. 111). Multidisciplinary Digital Publishing Institute. doi:10.3390/healthcare8020111

Akselrod-Ballin, A., Karlinsky, L., Alpert, S., Hashoul, S., Ben-Ari, R., & Barkan, E. (2016). *A Region Based Convolutional Network for Tumor Detection and Classification in Breast Mammography.* . doi:10.1007/978-3-319-46976-8_21

Al Ghayab, H. R., Li, Y., Siuly, S., & Abdulla, S. (2019). Epileptic seizures detection in EEGs blending frequency domain with information gain technique. *Soft Computing*, *23*(1), 227–239. doi:10.100700500-018-3487-0

Alarabeyyat, A., & Alhanahnah, M. (2016, August). Breast cancer detection using k-nearest neighbor machine learning algorithm. In *2016 9th International Conference on Developments in eSystems Engineering (DeSE)* (pp. 35-39). IEEE.

Alfian, G., Rhee, J., Ahn, H., Lee, J., Farooq, U., Ijaz, M. F., & Syaekhoni, M. A. (2017). Integration of RFID, wireless sensor networks, and data mining in an e-pedigree food traceability system. *Journal of Food Engineering*, *212*, 65–75. doi:10.1016/j.jfoodeng.2017.05.008

Al-Hagery, Alfaiz, & Alorinim, & Althunayan. (2015). Knowledge discovery in the data sets of hepatitis disease for diagnosis and prediction to support and serve community. *International Journal of Computer and Electronics Research*, *4*(6), 118–125.

Almeida, I., & Barros, P. (2020). *Denoising Autoencoder - Deep Learning*. Academic Press.

Almotiri, S. H., Khan, M. A., & Alghamdi, M. A. (2016). Mobile health (m-health) system in the context of iot. *2016 IEEE 4th International Conference on Future Internet of Things and Cloud Workshops (FiCloudW)*, 39–42.

Alpaydin, E. (2020). *Introduction to machine learning*. MIT Press.

Al-Tashi, Q., Abdulkadir, S. J., Rais, H. M., Mirjalili, S., & Alhussian, H. (2020). Approaches to multi-objective feature selection: A systematic literature review. *IEEE Access: Practical Innovations, Open Solutions*, *8*, 125076–125096. doi:10.1109/ACCESS.2020.3007291

Aminikhanghahi, S., Shin, S., Wang, W., Jeon, S. I., Son, S. H., & Pack, C. (2015, April). Study of wireless mammography image transmission impacts on robust cyber-aided diagnosis systems. In *Proceedings of the 30th Annual ACM Symposium on Applied Computing* (pp. 2252-2256). 10.1145/2695664.2695832

Aminoff, M. J. (2012). Electroencephalography: General principles and clinical applications. In W. B. Saunders (Ed.), *Aminoff's Electro diagnosis in Clinical Neurology* (pp. 37–84). Elsevier B.V. doi:10.1016/B978-1-4557-0308-1.00003-0

Anastasopoulos, C., Weikert, T., Yang, S., Abdulkadir, A., Schmülling, L., Bühler, C., Paciolla, F., Sexauer, R., Cyriac, J., Nesic, I., Twerenbold, R., Bremerich, J., Stieltjes, B., Sauter, A. W., & Sommer, G. (2020). Development and clinical implementation of tailored image analysis tools for COVID-19 amid the pandemic: The synergetic effect of an open, clinically embedded software development platform and machine learning. *European Journal of Radiology*, *131*, 109233. doi:10.1016/j.ejrad.2020.109233 PMID:32927416

Anderson, G. H. (1999). Effect of age on hypertension: Analysis of over 4,800 referred hypertensive patients. *Saudi Journal of Kidney Diseases and Transplantation*, *10*(3), 286. PMID:18212439

Apache. (2016). *SystemML (incubating)*. http://systemml.apache.org

Arevalo, J., González, F., Ramos, R., Oliveira, J., Lopez, G., & Angel, M. (2015). Representation learning for mammography mass lesion classification with convolutional neural networks. *Computer Methods and Programs in Biomedicine*, *127*, 248–257. Advance online publication. doi:10.1016/j.cmpb.2015.12.014 PMID:26826901

Armaly, Z., Assady, S., & Abassi, Z. (2013). Corin: A new player in the regulation of salt–water balance and blood pressure. *Current Opinion in Nephrology and Hypertension*, *22*(6), 713–722. doi:10.1097/01.mnh.0000435609.35789.32 PMID:24100222

Arunachalam, A. R., & Michael, G. (2018). An efficient system for posture recognition based fall detection system and health monitoring. *International Journal of Pure and Applied Mathematics*, *118*(18), 1019–1027.

Aruna, S., Rajagopalan, S. P., & Nandakishore, L. V. (2011). Knowledge based analysis of various statistical tools in detecting breast cancer. *Computer Science and Information Technology*, *2*, 37–45.

Ashari, A. (2015). On Optimizing Machine Learning Workloads via Kernel Fusion. PPoPP. doi:10.1145/2688500.2688521

Asri, H., Mousannif, H., Al Moatassime, H., & Noel, T. (2016). Using machine learning algorithms for breast cancer risk prediction and diagnosis. *Procedia Computer Science*, *83*, 1064–1069. doi:10.1016/j.procs.2016.04.224

Averina, V. A., Othmer, H. G., Fink, G. D., & Osborn, J. W. (2012). A new conceptual paradigm for the haemodynamics of salt-sensitive hypertension: A mathematical modelling approach. *The Journal of Physiology*, *590*(23), 5975–5992. doi:10.1113/jphysiol.2012.228619 PMID:22890716

Ayata, D., Yaslan, Y., & Kamasak, M. (2017). Emotion recognition via galvanic skin response: Comparison of machine learning algorithms and feature extraction methods. *Istanbul University-Journal of Electrical and Electronics Engineering*, *17*(1), 3129–3136.

Ba-Alwi, F. M., & Hintaya, H. M. (2013). Comparative study for analysis the prognostic in hepatitis data: Data mining approach. *International Journal of Scientific and Engineering Research*, *4*(8), 680–685.

Bantupalli, K., & Xie, Y. (2018). American Sign Language Recognition using Deep Learning and Computer Vision. In *2018 IEEE International Conference on Big Data (Big Data). 2018 IEEE International Conference on Big Data (Big Data).* IEEE. 10.1109/BigData.2018.8622141

Barbado, R., Araque, O., & Iglesias, C. A. (2019). A framework for fake review detection in online consumer electronics retailers. *Information Processing & Management, 56*(4), 1234–1244. doi:10.1016/j.ipm.2019.03.002

Barger, T. S., Brown, D. E., & Alwan, M. (2005). Health-status monitoring through analysis of behavioral patterns. *IEEE Transactions on Systems, Man, and Cybernetics. Part A, Systems and Humans, 5*(1), 22–27. doi:10.1109/TSMCA.2004.838474

Barioul, R., Ghribi, S. F., Ben Jmaa Derbel, H., & Kanoun, O. (2020). Four Sensors Bracelet for American Sign Language Recognition based on Wrist Force Myography. In *2020 IEEE International Conference on Computational Intelligence and Virtual Environments for Measurement Systems and Applications (CIVEMSA).* IEEE. 10.1109/CIVEMSA48639.2020.9132742

Baronzio, G., Parmar, G., & Baronzio, M. (2015). Overview of methods for overcoming hindrance to drug delivery to tumors, with special attention to tumor interstitial fluid. *Frontiers in Oncology, 5.* Advance online publication. doi:10.3389/fonc.2015.00165 PMID:26258072

Bashir, L. Z. (2015). Solve simple linear equation using evolutionary algorithm. *World Scientific News, 19,* 148–167.

Bassey, P. (2019, September 19). Logistic Regression Vs Support Vector Machines (SVM). *Medium.*

Batz, Geisberger, Sanders, & Vetter. (2013). Minimum time-dependent travel times with contraction hierarchies. *Journal of Experimental Algorithmics, 18,* 1.1–1.43.

Batz, R. (2010). *Time-dependent contraction hierarchies and approximation.* Experimental Algorithms.

Bauer, D. (2009). SHARC: 'Fast and Robust unidirectional routing. *ACM Journal of Experimental Algorithmics, 14*(2), 2-29.

Beeraka, S. M., Kumar, A., Sameer, M., Ghosh, S., & Gupta, B. (2022). Accuracy Enhancement of Epileptic Seizure Detection: A Deep Learning Approach with Hardware Realization of STFT. *Circuits, Systems, and Signal Processing, 41*(1), 461–484. doi:10.100700034-021-01789-4

Beevers, G., Lip, G. Y., & O'Brien, E. (2001, April 14). The pathophysiology of hypertension. *British Medical Journal, 322*(7291), 912–916. doi:10.1136/bmj.322.7291.912 PMID:11302910

Bekkerman, R., El-Yaniv, R., Tishby, N., & Winter, Y. (2003). Distributional word clusters vs. words for text categorization. *Journal of Machine Learning Research, 3*(Mar), 1183–1208.

Bengio, Y., Courville, A., & Vincent, P. (2013, August). Representation learning: A review and new perspectives. *IEEE Transactions on Pattern Analysis and Machine Intelligence, 35*(8), 17981828. doi:10.1109/TPAMI.2013.50 PMID:23787338

Bhoi, A., & Joshi, S. (2018). *Various Approaches to Aspect-based Sentiment Analysis.* Retrieved from https://arxiv.org/abs/1805.01984

Bhui, N., Ram, P. K., & Kuila, P. (2020, July). Feature selection from microarray data based on deep learning approach. In *2020 11th International Conference on Computing, Communication and Networking Technologies (ICCCNT)* (pp. 1-5). IEEE.

Bin Othman, M. F., & Yau, T. M. S. (2007). Comparison of different classification techniques using WEKA for breast cancer. In *3rd Kuala Lumpur international conference on biomedical engineering 2006* (pp. 520-523). Springer. 10.1007/978-3-540-68017-8_131

Blair, S. N. (1984). Physical fitness and incidence of hypertension in healthy normotensive men and women. *Journal of the American Medical Association*, *252*(4), 487–490. doi:10.1001/jama.1984.03350040017014 PMID:6737638

Bobade, P., & Vani, M. (2020). Stress Detection with Machine Learning and Deep Learning using Multimodal Physiological Data. *Proceedings of the 2nd International Conference on Inventive Research in Computing Applications, ICIRCA 2020*, 51–57. 10.1109/ICIRCA48905.2020.9183244

Boehm, Dusenberry, Eriksson, Evfimievski, Manshadi, Pansare, Reinwald, Reiss, Sen, Surve, & Tatikonda. (n.d.). *SystemML: Declarative Machine Learning on Spark*. IBM Research.

Boehm. (2014). Hybrid Parallelization Strategies for Large-Scale Machine Learning in SystemML. *PVLDB*, *7*(7).

Boehm. (2014). SystemML's Optimizer: Plan Generation for Large-Scale Machine Learning Programs. *IEEE Data Eng. Bull.*, *37*(3).

Boehm. (2016). *Declarative Machine Learning - A Classification of Basic Properties and Types*. CoRR, abs/1605.05826.

Bolívar, J. J. (2013). Essential Hypertension: An approach to its etiology and neurogenic pathophysiology. *International Journal of Hypertension*, *2013*, 1–11. doi:10.1155/2013/547809 PMID:24386559

Bommert, A., Sun, X., Bischl, B., Rahnenführer, J., & Lang, M. (2020). Benchmark for filter methods for feature selection in high-dimensional classification data. *Computational Statistics & Data Analysis*, *143*, 106839.

Borges, L. R. (1989). Analysis of the Wisconsin breast cancer dataset and machine learning for breast cancer detection. *Group*, *1*(369), 15–19.

Bray, F., Ren, J. S., Masuyer, E., & Ferlay, J. (2013). *Estimates of global cancer prevalence for 27 sites in the adult*. Academic Press.

Bray, F., Ferlay, J., Soerjomataram, I., Siegel, R. L., Torre, L. A., & Jemal, A. (2018). Global cancer statistics 2018: GLOBOCAN estimates of incidence and mortality worldwide for 36 cancers in 185 countries. *CA: a Cancer Journal for Clinicians*, *68*(6), 394–424. doi:10.3322/caac.21492 PMID:30207593

Breiman, L. (2001). Random forests. *Machine Learning*, *45*(1), 5–32. doi:10.1023/A:1010933404324

Brinkmann, B. H., Patterson, E. E., Vite, C., Vasoli, V. M., Crepeau, D., Stead, M., Howbert, J. J., Cherkassky, V., Wagenaar, J. B., Litt, B., & Worrell, G. A. (2015). Forecasting seizures using intracranial eeg measures and svm in naturally occurring canine epilepsy. *PLoS One*, *10*(8), e0133900. doi:10.1371/journal.pone.0133900 PMID:26241907

Bruno, P., Melnyk, V., & Völckner, F. (2017). Temperature and emotions: Effects of physical temperature on responses to emotional advertising. *International Journal of Research in Marketing*, *34*(1), 302–320. doi:10.1016/j.ijresmar.2016.08.005

Byun, H., & Lee, S. W. (2003). A survey on pattern recognition applications of support vector machines. *International Journal of Pattern Recognition and Artificial Intelligence*, *17*(03), 459–486. doi:10.1142/S0218001403002460

Cai, J., Liu, G., & Hao, M. (2009). The Research on Emotion Recognition from ECG Signal. *Proceedings of the 2009 International Conference on Information Technology and Computer Science*, 497–500.

Cañamero, L. (2005). Emotion understanding from the perspective of autonomous robots research. *Neural Network*, *18*, 445–455. . doi:10.1016/j.neunet.2005.03.003

Cañamero, L. (2019). Embodied robot models for interdisciplinary emotion research. *IEEE Transactions on Affective Computing*, *1*. Advance online publication. doi:10.1109/TAFFC.2019.2908162

Castaneda, D., Esparza, A., Ghamari, M., Soltanpur, C., & Nazeran, H. (2018). A review on wearable photoplethysmography sensors and their potential future applications in health care. *International Journal of Biosensors & Bioelectronics*, *4*(4), 195–202. doi:10.15406/ijbsbe.2018.04.00125 PMID:30906922

Chai, X., Wang, Q., Zhao, Y., Li, Y., Liu, D., Liu, X., & Bai, O. (2017). A Fast, Efficient Domain Adaptation Technique for Cross-Domain Electroencephalography (EEG)-Based Emotion Recognition. *Sensors (Basel)*, *17*(5), 1014. doi:10.339017051014 PMID:28467371

Chanel, G., Kronegg, J., Grandjean, D., & Pun, T. (2006). Emotion assessment: Arousal evaluation using EEG's and peripheral physiological signals. Lecture Notes in Computer Science, 4105, 530.

Chanel, G., Kierkels, J. J. M., Soleymani, M., & Pun, T. (2009). Short-term emotion assessment in a recall paradigm. *International Journal of Human-Computer Studies*, *67*(8), 607–627. doi:10.1016/j.ijhcs.2009.03.005

Chaovalitwongse, W. A., Fan, Y.-J., & Sachdeo, R. C. (2007). On the time series k-nearest neighbor classification of abnormal brain activity. *IEEE Transactions on Systems, Man, and Cybernetics. Part A, Systems and Humans*, *37*(6), 1005–1016. doi:10.1109/TSMCA.2007.897589

Charkoudian, N., & Rabbitts, J. A. (2009). Sympathetic neural mechanisms in human cardiovascular health and disease. *Mayo Clinic Proceedings*, *84*(9), 822–830. doi:10.4065/84.9.822

Charles, L., Triscott, J., & Dobbs, B. (2017). Secondary hypertension: Discovering the underlying cause. *American Family Physician*, *96*(7), 453–461. PMID:29094913

Chatterjee, A. N., & Roy, P. K. (2020). *Smoking habit: A bio mathematical study*. Communications in Mathematical Biology and Neuroscience. doi:10.28919/cmbn/4319

Chaurasia, V., & Pal, S. (2014). Data mining techniques: To predict and resolve breast cancer survivability. *International Journal of Computer Science and Mobile Computing IJCSMC*, *3*(1), 10–22.

Chehal, D., Gupta, P., & Gulati, P. (2020). Implementation and comparison of topic modeling techniques based on user reviews in e-commerce recommendations. *Journal of Ambient Intelligence and Humanized Computing*, (0123456789). Advance online publication. doi:10.100712652-020-01956-6

Chen, T., He, T., Benesty, M., Khotilovich, V., Tang, Y., & Cho, H. (2015). Xgboost: extreme gradient boosting. *R package version 0.4-2*, *1*(4), 1-4.

Chen, B. Y., Lam, W. H., Sumalee, A., Li, Q., & Tam, M. L. (2013). Reliable shortest path problems in stochastic time-dependent networks. *Journal of Intelligent Transport Systems*, *18*(2), 177–189. doi:10.1080/15472450.2013.806851

Chen, H., Engkvist, O., Wang, Y., Olivecrona, M., & Blaschke, T. (2018). The rise of deep learning in drug discovery. *Drug Discovery Today*, *23*(6), 1241–1250. Advance online publication. doi:10.1016/j.drudis.2018.01.039 PMID:29366762

Chen, J., Zeng, Y., Li, Y., & Huang, G. B. (2020). Unsupervised feature selection based extreme learning machine for clustering. *Neurocomputing*, *386*, 198–207.

Chen, & Lu, & Yang. (2016). Urban traffic flow prediction using a spatiotemporal random effects model. *Journal of Intelligent Transportation Systems, 20(3).* doi:10.1080/15472450.2015.1072050

Chen, M., Hao, Y., Hwang, K., Wang, L., & Wang, L. (2017). Disease Prediction by Machine Learning over Big Data from Healthcare Communities. *IEEE Access: Practical Innovations, Open Solutions*, *5*, 8869–8879. doi:10.1109/ACCESS.2017.2694446

Chen, S., Zhang, Z., Yang, J., Wang, J., Zhai, X., Bärnighausen, T., & Wang, C. (2020). Fangcang shelter hospitals: A novel concept for responding to public health emergencies. *Lancet, 395*(10232), 1305–1314. doi:10.1016/S0140-6736(20)30744-3 PMID:32247320

Chen, T., & Guestrin, C. (2016, August). Xgboost: A scalable tree boosting system. In *Proceedings of the 22nd acm sigkdd international conference on knowledge discovery and data mining* (pp. 785-794). 10.1145/2939672.2939785

Ching, T., Himmelstein, D. S., Beaulieu-Jones, B. K., Kalinin, A. A., Do, B. T., Way, G. P., Ferrero, E., Agapow, P. M., Zietz, M., Hoffman, M. M., Xie, W., Rosen, G. L., Lengerich, B. J., Israeli, J., Lanchantin, J., Woloszynek, S., Carpenter, A. E., Shrikumar, A., Xu, J., ... Greene, C. S. (2018). Opportunities and obstacles for deep learning in biology and medicine. *Journal of the Royal Society, Interface, 15*(141), 20170387. doi:10.1098/rsif.2017.0387 PMID:29618526

Chiuchisan, I., Costin, H. N., & Geman, O. (2014). Adopting the internet of things technologies in health care systems. *2014 International Conference and Exposition on Electrical and Power Engineering (EPE)*, 532–535. 10.1109/ICEPE.2014.6969965

Choppin, A. (2000). *EEG-based human interface for disabled individuals: Emotion expression with neural networks* [Ph.D. dissertation]. Tokyo Institute of Technology.

Chowdary, M.K., Nguyen, T.N. & Hemanth, D.J. (2021). Deep learning-based facial emotion recognition for human–computer interaction applications. *Neural Computing and Applications.* . doi:10.1007/s00521-021-06012-8

Christopher, T., & Jamera Banu, J. (2016). Study of Classification Algorithm for Lung Cancer Prediction. *International Journal of Innovative Science, Engineering & Technology, 3*(2), 42–49.

Chugh, A., & Panda, S. P. (2022). Improved MEDC Protocol through Relay Nodes in Wireless Sensor Networks. In *Futuristic Sustainable Energy & Technology: Proceedings of the International Conference on Futuristic Sustainable Energy &Technology (ICFSE, 2021)* (p. 259). CRC Press. 10.1201/9781003272328-30

Chugh, A., & Panda, S. (2018). Strengthening clustering through relay nodes in sensor networks. *Procedia Computer Science, 132*, 689–695. doi:10.1016/j.procs.2018.05.072

Chugh, A., & Panda, S. (2019). Energy efficient techniques in wireless sensor networks. *Recent Patents on Engineering, 13*(1), 13–19. doi:10.2174/1872212112666180731114046

Chugh, A., & Panda, S. (2020). Relay Node Employment for Performance Enhancement of MEDC in Wireless Sensor Network. *International Journal of Innovative Technology and Exploring Engineering, 9*(6), 835–839. doi:10.35940/ijitee.F3943.049620

Cismondi, F., Fialho, A. S., Vieira, S. M., Reti, S. R., Sousa, J. M. C., & Finkelstein, S. N. (2013). Missing data in medical databases: Impute, delete or classify? *Artificial Intelligence in Medicine, 58*(1), 63–72. doi:10.1016/j.artmed.2013.01.003 PMID:23428358

Clauberg, R. (2004). RFID and sensor networks. *Proc. RFID Workshop.*

Clemmer, J. S., Pruett, W. A., Coleman, T. G., Hall, J. E., & Hester, R. L. (2017). Mechanisms of blood pressure salt sensitivity: New insights from mathematical modeling. *American Journal of Physiology. Regulatory, Integrative and Comparative Physiology, 312*(4), R451–R466.

Consolidated F. D. I. Policy, Press Information Bureau (PIB), Media Reports, Pharmaceuticals Export Promotion Council, AIOCD-AWACS, IQVIA. (n.d.). https://www.ibef.org/industry/pharmaceutical-india.aspx

Coorevits, P., Sundgren, M., Klein, G. O., Bahr, A., Claerhout, B., Daniel, C., Dugas, M., Dupont, D., Schmidt, A., Singleton, P., De Moor, G., & Kalra, D. (2013). Electronic health records: New opportunities for clinical research. *Journal of Internal Medicine*, *274*(6), 547–560. doi:10.1111/joim.12119 PMID:23952476

Csikszentmihalyi, M. (2014). *Flow and the Foundations of Positive Psychology: The collected works of MihalyCsikszentmihalyi; S.* Springer. doi:10.1007/978-94-017-9088-8

Cuno, A., Condori-Fernandez, N., Mendoza, A., & Lovon, W. R. (2020). A FAIR evaluation of public datasets for stress detection systems. *Proceedings - International Conference of the Chilean Computer Science Society, SCCC*. 10.1109/SCCC51225.2020.9281274

Cuzzo, B., Padala, S. A., & Lappin, S. L. (2020). *Vasopressin (Antidiuretic Hormone, ADH)*. StatPearls.

Dalmış, M., Gubern-Mérida, A., Vreemann, S., Karssemeijer, N., Mann, R., & Platel, B. (2016). A computer-aided diagnosis system for breast DCE-MRI at high spatiotemporal resolution. *Medical Physics*, *43*(1), 84–94. doi:10.1118/1.4937787 PMID:26745902

Das, A. (2020). Challenges faced by healthcare-related sectors in India during COVID-19 pandemic: A review. *International Journal of Advanced Research*, *8*(8), 639–641. doi:10.21474/IJAR01/11536

Davenport, T., & Kalakota, R. (2019). The potential for artificial intelligence in healthcare. *Future Healthcare Journal*, *6*(2), 94–98. doi:10.7861/futurehosp.6-2-94 PMID:31363513

de Giorgio, A. (2015). *A study on the similarities of Deep Belief Networks and Stacked Autoencoders.* . doi:10.13140/RG.2.1.3502.8883

De Souza, A. M. A., West, C. A., de Abreu, A. R. R., Pai, A. V., Mesquita, L. B. T., Ji, H., & Sandberg, K. (2018). Role of the renin angiotensin system in blood pressure allostasis-induced by severe food restriction in female fischer rats. *Scientific Reports*, *8*(1), 10327. Advance online publication. doi:10.103841598-018-28593-6 PMID:29985423

Delen, D., Walker, G., & Kadam, A. (2005). Predicting breast cancer survivability: A comparison of three data mining methods. *Artificial Intelligence in Medicine*, *34*(2), 113–127. doi:10.1016/j.artmed.2004.07.002 PMID:15894176

Dey, D., & Kumar, P. (2019). A novel approach to identify the determinants of online review helpfulness and predict the helpfulness score across product categories. In Lecture Notes in Computer Science (including subseries Lecture Notes in Artificial Intelligence and Lecture Notes in Bioinformatics) (Vol. 11932, pp. 365–388). Springer. doi:10.1007/978-3-030-37188-3_21

Dhal, P., & Azad, C. (2021). A comprehensive survey on feature selection in the various fields of machine learning. *Applied Intelligence*, 1–39.

Dhungel, N., Carneiro, G., & Bradley, A. (2015). Deep Learning and Structured Prediction for the Segmentation of Mass in Mammograms. *Deep Learning and Structured Prediction for the Segmentation of Mass in Mammograms.*, *9349*, 605–612. Advance online publication. doi:10.1007/978-3-319-24553-9_74

Dimberg, U. (1982). Facial Reactions to Facial Expressions. *Psychophysiology*, *9*(6), 643–647. doi:10.1111/j.1469-8986.1982.tb02516.x PMID:7178381

Dissanayake, T., Rajapaksha, Y., Ragel, R., & Nawinne, I. (2019). An Ensemble Learning Approach for Electrocardiogram Sensor Based Human Emotion Recognition. *Sensors (Basel)*, *19*(20), 4495. doi:10.339019204495 PMID:31623279

Duch, W., Swaminathan, K., & Meller, J. (2007). Artificial Intelligence Approaches for Rational Drug Design and Discovery. *Current Pharmaceutical Design*, *13*(14), 1497–1508. Advance online publication. doi:10.2174/138161207780765954 PMID:17504169

Durai, S. G., Ganesh, S. H., & Christy, A. J. (2017, February). Novel linear regressive classifier for the diagnosis of breast cancer. In *2017 World Congress on Computing and Communication Technologies (WCCCT)* (pp. 136-139). IEEE. 10.1109/WCCCT.2016.40

Durga & Karuppiah. (2017). Lung disease prediction system using data mining techniques. *Journal of Advanced Research in Dynamical and Control Systems, 9*(5), 62-66.

Dwivedi, A., Bali, R. K., Belsis, M. A., Naguib, R. N. G., Every, P., & Nassar, N. S. (2003). Towards a practical healthcare information security model for healthcare institutions. *4th International IEEE EMBS Special Topic Conference on Information Technology Applications in Biomedicine*, 114–117. 10.1109/ITAB.2003.1222486

Dzedzickis, A., Kaklauskas, A., & Bucinskas, V. (2020). Human Emotion Recognition: Review of Sensors and Methods. *Sensors, 20*, 592. https://www.mdpi.com/1424-8220/20/3/592

EEG-Event Related Potentials. (n.d.). Available online: http://www.medicine.mcgill.ca/physio/vlab/biomed_signals/eeg_erp.htm

Effrosynidis, D., & Arampatzis, A. (2021). An evaluation of feature selection methods for environmental data. *Ecological Informatics, 61*, 101224.

Elearning Providers. (2006). https://www.tutorialspoint.com/machine_learning_with_python/machine_learning_with_python_classification_algorithms_support_vector_machine.htm

Elger, C. E. (2001). Future trends in epileptology. *Current Opinion in Neurology, 14*(2), 185186. doi:10.1097/00019052-200104000-00008 PMID:11262733

Elliott, W. J. (2009). Trends in hypertension prevalence, awareness, treatment, and control rates in United States adults between 1988–1994 and 1999–2004. *Yearbook of Cardiology, 5-7*, 5–7. Advance online publication. doi:10.1016/S0145-4145(08)79400-0

Elmogy, A. M., Tariq, U., Ibrahim, A., & Mohammed, A. (2021). Fake Reviews Detection using Supervised Machine Learning. *International Journal of Advanced Computer Science and Applications, 12*(1), 601–606. doi:10.14569/IJACSA.2021.0120169

Emmanuel, T., Maupong, T., Mpoeleng, D., Semong, T., Mphago, B., & Tabona, O. (2021). A survey on missing data in machine learning. *Journal of Big Data, 8*(1), 1–37. doi:10.1186/s40537-021-00516-9

Emotion-Sensing Technology in the Internet of Things. (n.d.). Available online: https://onixsystems.com/blog/emotion-sensing-technology-in-the-internet-of-things

Enriko, Suryanegara, & Gunawan. (2016). Heart Disease Prediction System using k-Nearest Neighbor Algorithm with Simplified Patient's Health Parameters. *Journal of Telecommunication, Electronic and Computer Engineering, 8*(12).

Erlay, J., Ervik, M., Dikshit, R., Eser, S., & Mathers, C. (2012). Cancer incidence and mortality worldwide: IARC CancerBase No. 11. *GLOBOCAN, 1*.

Ermagun, A., & Levinson, D. (2018). Spatiotemporal traffic forecasting: Review and proposed directions. *Transport Reviews, 38*(6), 786–814. doi:10.1080/01441647.2018.1442887

Everett, B., & Zajacova, A. (2015). Gender differences in hypertension and hypertension awareness among young adults. *Biodemography and Social Biology, 61*(1), 1–17. doi:10.1080/19485565.2014.929488 PMID:25879259

Evers, L. (2007). Sensorscheme: Supply chain management automation using wireless sensor networks. In *2007 IEEE Conference on Emerging Technologies and Factory Automation (EFTA 2007)*. IEEE. 10.1109/EFTA.2007.4416802

Evers, L., & Havinga, P. (2007). Supply chain management automation using wireless sensor networks. In *2007 IEEE International Conference on Mobile Adhoc and Sensor Systems*. IEEE. 10.1109/MOBHOC.2007.4428689

Fagard, R. H. (1995). The role of exercise in blood pressure control: Supportive evidence. *Journal of Hypertension, 13*(11), 1223–1227. doi:10.1097/00004872-199511000-00001 PMID:8984117

Fang, M., Chen, Y., Xue, R., Wang, H., Chakraborty, N., Su, T., & Dai, Y. (2021). A hybrid machine learning approach for hypertension risk prediction. *Neural Computing & Applications, 0*. Advance online publication. doi:10.100700521-021-06060-0

Fan, M., & Chou, C. (2019, March). Detecting Abnormal Pattern of Epileptic Seizures via Temporal Synchronization of EEG Signals. *IEEE Transactions on Biomedical Engineering, 66*(3), 601–608. doi:10.1109/TBME.2018.2850959 PMID:29993518

Feidakis, M., Daradoumis, T., & Caballe, S. (2011). Emotion Measurement in Intelligent Tutoring Systems: What, When and How to Measure. *Proceedings of the 2011 Third International Conference on Intelligent Networking and Collaborative Systems.*

Feidakis, M., Daradoumis, T., & Caballe, S. (2011). Endowing e-Learning Systems with Emotion Awareness. *Proceedings of the 2011 Third International Conference on Intelligent Networking and Collaborative Systems,* 68–75.

Filipp, F. V. (2019). Opportunities for Artificial Intelligence in Advancing Precision Medicine. *Current Genetic Medicine Reports, 7*(4), 208–213. doi:10.100740142-019-00177-4 PMID:31871830

Finset, A. (2021). Challenges for healthcare communication during the COVID-19 pandemic. *Patient Education and Counseling, 104*(2), 215–216. doi:10.1016/j.pec.2021.01.006 PMID:33518199

Fischer, A., & Igel, C. (2014). Training restricted Boltzmann machines: An introduction. *Pattern Recognition, 47*(1), 25–39. doi:10.1016/j.patcog.2013.05.025

Foëx, P., & Sear, J. W. (2004). Hypertension: Pathophysiology and treatment. *Continuing Education in Anaesthesia, Critical Care & Pain, 4*(3), 71–75. doi:10.1093/bjaceaccp/mkh020

Földiák, P., & Endres, D. (2008). Sparse coding. *Scholarpedia., 3*(1), 2984. doi:10.4249cholarpedia.2984

Fonseca, P., Mendoza, J., Wainer, J., Ferrer, J., Pinto, J., Guerrero, J., & Castaneda, B. (2015). *Automatic breast density classification using a convolutional neural network architecture search procedure*. doi:10.1117/12.2081576

Fotin, S., Yin, Y., Haldankar, H., Hoffmeister, J., & Periaswamy, S. (2016). *Detection of soft tissue densities from digital breast tomosynthesis: comparison of conventional and deep learning approaches.* . doi:10.1117/12.2217045

Galaz, V., Centeno, M., Callahan, P., Causevic, A., Patterson, T., Brass, I., Baum, S., Farber, D., Fischer, J., Garcia, D., McPhearson, T., Jiménez, D., King, B., Larcey, P., & Levy, K. (2021). Artificial intelligence, systemic risks, and sustainability. *Technology in Society, 67*, 101741. doi:10.1016/j.techsoc.2021.101741

Gao, S., Tsang, I., & Chia, L.-T. (2012). Laplacian Sparse Coding, Hypergraph Laplacian Sparse Coding, and Applications. *IEEE Transactions on Pattern Analysis and Machine Intelligence, 35*(1), 92–104. Advance online publication. doi:10.1109/TPAMI.2012.63 PMID:22392702

Gayathri, B. M., & Sumathi, C. P. (2015, December). Mamdani fuzzy inference system for breast cancer risk detection. In *2015 IEEE International Conference on Computational Intelligence and Computing Research (ICCIC)* (pp. 1-6). IEEE. 10.1109/ICCIC.2015.7435670

Gayathri, B. M., & Sumathi, C. P. (2016, December). Comparative study of relevance vector machine with various machine learning techniques used for detecting breast cancer. In *2016 IEEE International Conference on Computational Intelligence and Computing Research (ICCIC)* (pp. 1-5). IEEE. 10.1109/ICCIC.2016.7919576

Gc, S., Kasaudhan, R., Heo, T. K., & Choi, H. D. (2015, October). Variability measurement for breast cancer classification of mammographic masses. In *Proceedings of the 2015 Conference on research in adaptive and convergent systems* (pp. 177-182). 10.1145/2811411.2811505

Gerage, A. M., Benedetti, T. R. B., Farah, B. Q., Santana, F. da S., Ohara, D., Andersen, L. B., & Ritti-Dias, R. M. (2015). Sedentary behavior and light physical activity are associated with brachial and central blood pressure in hypertensive patients. *PLoS One, 10*(12), e0146078. doi:10.1371/journal.pone.0146078 PMID:26717310

Ghosh, P., Azam, S., Jonkman, M., Karim, A., Shamrat, F. J. M., Ignatious, E., Shultana, S., Beeravolu, A. R., & De Boer, F. (2021). Efficient prediction of cardiovascular disease using machine learning algorithms with relief and LASSO feature selection techniques. *IEEE Access: Practical Innovations, Open Solutions, 9*, 19304–19326. doi:10.1109/ACCESS.2021.3053759

Ghumbre & Ghatol (2009). Hepatitis B Diagnosis Using Logical Inference AndGeneralized Regression Neural Networks. *Proceedings of IEEE International Advance Computing Conference (IACC 2009).*

Giannakakis, G., Pediaditis, M., Manousos, D., Kazantzaki, E., Chiarugi, F., Simos, P. G., Marias, K., & Tsiknakis, M. (2017). Stress and anxiety detection using facial cues from videos. *Biomedical Signal Processing and Control, 31*, 89–101. doi:10.1016/j.bspc.2016.06.020

Gillman-Wells, C. C., Sankar, T. K., & Vadodaria, S. (2021). COVID-19 Reducing the Risks: Telemedicine is the New Norm for Surgical Consultations and Communications. *Aesthetic Plastic Surgery, 45*(1), 343–348. doi:10.100700266-020-01907-8 PMID:32885319

Ginsburg, A. S., Lenahan, J. L., Izadnegahdar, R., & Ansermino, J. M. (2018). A Systematic Review of Tools to Measure Respiratory Rate in Order to Identify Childhood Pneumonia. *American Journal of Respiratory and Critical Care Medicine, 197*(9), 1116–1127. doi:10.1164/rccm.201711-2233CI PMID:29474107

Golmohammadi, M., Ziyabari, S., Shah, V., de Diego, S. L., Obeid, I., & Picone, J. (2017). Deep architectures for automated seizure detection in scalp EEGs. https://arxiv.org/abs/1712.09776

Gomez, Laurent, & El Moustaine. (2012). Risk assessment along supply chain: A RFID and wireless sensor network integration approach. *Sensors & Transducers, 14*(2), 269.

Gonçalves, V. P., Giancristofaro, G. T., Filho, G. P. R., Johnson, T., Carvalho, V., Pessin, G., de Almeida Neris, V. P., & Ueyama, J. (2017). Assessing users' emotion at interaction time: A multimodal approach with multiple Sensors. *Soft Computing, 21*(18), 5309–5323. doi:10.100700500-016-2115-0

Greco, A., Lanata, A., Citi, L., Vanello, N., Valenza, G., & Scilingo, E. (2016). Skin Admittance Measurement for Emotion Recognition: A Study over Frequency Sweep. *Electronics (Basel), 5*(4), 46. doi:10.3390/electronics5030046

Guo, X., Lin, W., Li, Y., Liu, Z., Yang, L., Zhao, S., & Zhu, Z. (2020). DKEN: Deep knowledge-enhanced network for recommender systems. *Information Sciences, 540*, 263–277. doi:10.1016/j.ins.2020.06.041

Guo, Y., Liu, Y., Oerlemans, A., Lao, S.-Y., Wu, S., & Lew, M. (2015). Deep learning for visual understanding: A review. *Neurocomputing, 187*, 27–48. Advance online publication. doi:10.1016/j.neucom.2015.09.116

Guo, Y., Zhang, B., Sun, Y., Jiang, K., & Wu, K. (2021). Machine learning based feature selection and knowledge reasoning for CBR system under big data. *Pattern Recognition, 112*, 107805.

Gupta, M. S. D., Patchava, V., & Menezes, V. (2015). Healthcare based on iot using raspberry pi. *2015 International Conference on Green Computing and Internet of Things (ICGCIoT)*, 796–799. 10.1109/ICGCIoT.2015.7380571

Gupta, R., Gaur, K., & Ram, C. V. (2018). Emerging trends in hypertension epidemiology in India. *Journal of Human Hypertension*, *33*(8), 575–587. doi:10.103841371-018-0117-3 PMID:30254382

Hajek, P., & Barushka, A. (2019). A Comparative Study of Machine Learning Methods for Detection of Fake Online Consumer Reviews. *ACM International Conference Proceeding Series*, 18–22. 10.1145/3383902.3383909

Han, J., Pei, J., & Kamber, M. (2011). *Data mining: concepts and techniques*. Elsevier.

Hazra, A., Mandal, S. K., & Gupta, A. (2016). Study and analysis of breast cancer cell detection using Naïve Bayes, SVM and ensemble algorithms. *International Journal of Computers and Applications*, *145*(2), 39–45. doi:10.5120/ijca2016910595

He, C., Fan, X., & Li, Y. (2013). Toward Ubiquitous Healthcare Services With a Novel Efficient Cloud Platform. *IEEE Transactions on Biomedical Engineering*, *60*(1), 230–234. doi:10.1109/TBME.2012.2222404 PMID:23060318

He, K., Zhang, X., Ren, S., & Sun, J. (2014). Spatial Pyramid Pooling in Deep Convolutional Networks for Visual Recognition. *IEEE Transactions on Pattern Analysis and Machine Intelligence*, *37*(9), 1904–1916. Advance online publication. doi:10.1109/TPAMI.2015.2389824 PMID:26353135

He, K., Zhang, X., Ren, S., & Sun, J. (2016). Deep Residual Learning for Image Recognition. *2016 IEEE Conference on Computer Vision and Pattern Recognition (CVPR)*, 770-778. 10.1109/CVPR.2016.90

He, L., Hu, D., Wan, M., Wen, Y., von Deneen, K. M., & Zhou, M. (2016). Common bayesian network for classification of eeg-based multiclass motor imagery bci. *IEEE Transactions on Systems, Man, and Cybernetics. Systems*, *46*(6), 843–854. doi:10.1109/TSMC.2015.2450680

Hess, U., & Fischer, A. (2013). Emotional Mimicry as Emotion Regulation. *Personality and Social Psychology Review*, *17*(2), 142–157. doi:10.1177/1088868312472607 PMID:23348982

Hindustan Times. (n.d.). https://www.hindustantimes.com/analysis/breach-the-wall-of-silence-give-state-recognition-to-indian-sign-language/story-hg7lj7LTWzfKgYB19prOhP.html

Hinton, G., Srivastava, N., Krizhevsky, A., Sutskever, I., & Salakhutdinov, R. (2012). *Improving neural networks by preventing co-adaptation of feature detectors*. arXiv preprint. arXiv.

Hinton, G. E., & Salakhutdinov, R. R. (2006). Reducing the dimensionality of data with neural networks. *Science*, *313*(5786), 504507. doi:10.1126cience.1127647 PMID:16873662

Holovatyy, A., Teslyuk, A. V., Iwaniec, M., & Mashevska, M. (2017). Development of the system for monitoring vibration accelerations based on the RaspberryPi microcontroller and the ADXL345 Accelerometer. *Eastern-European Journal of Enterprise Technologies*, *6*(9), 52–61. doi:10.15587/1729-4061.2017.116082

Hopf, K., & Reifenrath, S. (2021). *Filter Methods for Feature Selection in Supervised Machine Learning Applications--Review and Benchmark*. arXiv preprint arXiv:2111.12140.

Hosseini asl, E., Gimel'farb, G., & El-Baz, A. (2016). Alzheimer's Disease Diagnostics by a Deeply Supervised Adaptable 3D Convolutional Network. *Computational and Mathematical Methods in Medicine*.

Hosseini, F. S., Choubin, B., Mosavi, A., Nabipour, N., Shamshirband, S., Darabi, H., & Haghighi, A. T. (2020). Flash-flood hazard assessment using ensembles and Bayesian-based machine l earning models: Application of the simulated annealing feature selection method. *The Science of the Total Environment*, *711*, 135161.

Hsieh, P.-Y., & Chin, C.-L. (2011). The emotion recognition system with Heart Rate Variability and facial image features. *Proceedings of IEEE International Conference on Fuzzy Systems (FUZZ-IEEE 2011)*, 1933–1940. 10.1109/FUZZY.2011.6007734

Huang, G., Liu, Z., & Weinberger, K. Q. (2017). Densely Connected Convolutional Networks. *2017 IEEE Conference on Computer Vision and Pattern Recognition (CVPR)*, 2261-2269. 10.1109/CVPR.2017.243

Huang, W., Song, G., Hong, H., & Xie, K. (2014). Deep architecture for traffic flow prediction: Deep belief networks with multitask learning. *IEEE Transactions on Intelligent Transportation Systems, 15*(5), 2191–2201. doi:10.1109/TITS.2014.2311123

Hunter, J. D. (2007). Matplotlib: A 2D graphics environment. *Computing in Science Engineering, 9*(3), 90-95.

Hussein, R., Palangi, H., & Ward, R. K. Z. (2019). Optimized deep neural network architecture for robust detection of epileptic seizures using EEG signals. *Clinical Neurophysiology, 130*(1), 25-37. doi:10.1016/j.clinph.2018.10.010

Indian Sign Language. (n.d.). https://indiansignlanguage.org/

Istepanaian, R. S. H., & Zhang, Y.-T. (2012). Guest editorial introduction to the special section: 4 G health—The long-term evolution of m-health. *IEEE Transactions on Information Technology in Biomedicine, 16*(1), 1–5. doi:10.1109/TITB.2012.2183269 PMID:22271836

Jaiswal. (2021). https://www.javatpoint.com/machine-learning-naive-bayes-classifier

Jamieson, A., Drukker, K., & Giger, M. (2012). Breast Image Feature Learning with Adaptive Deconvolutional Networks. *Proc SPIE, 8315.* . doi:10.1117/12.910710

Jayanthi & Márquez. (2021a). Routing Vehicles on Highways by Augmenting Traffic Flow Network: A Review on Speed Up Techniques. Smart Innovation, Systems and Technologies.

Jayanthi & Márquez. (2021b). Travel Time Based Traffific Rerouting by Augmenting Traffic Flow Network with Temporal and Spatial Relations for Congestion Management. *Lecture Notes on Data Engineering and Communication Technologies, 78.*

Jayanthi & Márquez. (2021c). Data Mining and Information Technology in Transportation—A Review. In Lecture Notes on Data Engineering and Communications Technologies (Vol. 79). Springer. doi:10.1007/978-3-030-79206-0_64

Jayanthi, G, & Jothilakshmi, P. (2019). Prediction of traffic volume by mining traffic sequences using travel time based PrefixSpan. *IET Intelligent Transport Systems, 13*(7), 1199-1210. doi:10.1049/iet-its.2018.5165

Jayanthi, G. (2022). Multi Criteria Decision Making Analysis for sustainable Transport. In Sustainability - Cases And Studies in using Operations Research and Management Science Methods. Springer.

Jayanthi, G. (2021). *Design of algorithms for IOT applications: a case study on intelligent transportation systems. In Internet of Things - Cases and Studies.* Springer.

Jiang, Z., Xu, W., & Chen, S. (2017, September). Classification of benign and malignant breast cancer based on DWI texture features. In *Proceedings of the International Conference on Bioinformatics and Computational Intelligence* (pp. 11-15). 10.1145/3135954.3135964

Jirachanchaisiri, P., Kitsupapaisan, J., & Maneeroj, S. (2019). Bayesian flexible mixture model with rating conversion on multi-criteria recommender system. *International Journal of Web Information Systems, 15*(4), 402–419. doi:10.1108/IJWIS-10-2018-0074

John, S., Krege, J., Oliver, P., Hagaman, J. R., Hodgin, J. B., Pang, S. C., Flynn, T. G., & Smithies, O. (1995). Genetic decreases in atrial natriuretic peptide and salt-sensitive hypertension. *Science*, *267*(5198), 679–681. doi:10.1126cience.7839143 PMID:7839143

Joyner, M. J., Charkoudian, N., & Wallin, B. G. (2008). A sympathetic view of the sympathetic nervous system and human blood pressure regulation. *Experimental Physiology*, *93*(6), 715–724. doi:10.1113/expphysiol.2007.039545 PMID:18326553

Joyner, M. J., Charkoudian, N., & Wallin, B. G. (2010). Sympathetic nnervous ssystem and blood pressure in humans. *Hypertension*, *56*(1), 10–16. doi:10.1161/HYPERTENSIONAHA.109.140186 PMID:20497993

Kadhim, A. I. (2019). Survey on supervised machine learning techniques for automatic text classification. *Artificial Intelligence Review*, *52*(1), 273–292. doi:10.100710462-018-09677-1

Kakousis, K., Paspallis, N., & Papadopoulos, G. A. (2010). A survey of software adaptation in mobile and ubiquitous computing. *Enterprise Information Systems*, *4*(4), 355–389. doi:10.1080/17517575.2010.509814

Kang, W., Kapitanova, K., & Son, S. H. (2012). RDDS: A real-time data distribution service for cyber-physical systems. *IEEE Transactions on Industrial Informatics*, *8*(2), 393–405. doi:10.1109/TII.2012.2183878

Kaplan, A., Cao, H., FitzGerald, J. M., Vogelmeier, C. F., Pfister, P., & Mastoridis, P. (2021). Artificial Intelligence/Machine Learning in Respiratory Medicine and Potential Role in Asthma and COPD Diagnosis. *The Journal of Allergy and Clinical Immunology*, *9*(6), 2255–2261. PMID:33618053

Kappas, A., Bherer, F., & Thériault, M. (2000). Inhibiting Facial Expressions: Limitations to the voluntary control of facial expressions of emotions. *Motivation and Emotion*, *40*(4), 259–270. doi:10.1023/A:1010718815960

Karthikeyan & Thangaraju. (2013). Analysis of classification algorithms applied to hepatitis patients. *International Journal of Computer Applications*, *62*(15), 25-30.

Katsis, C. D., Katertsidis, N., Ganiatsas, G., & Fotiadis, D. I. (2008). Toward Emotion Recognition in Car-Racing Drivers: A Biosignal Processing Approach. *IEEE Transactions on Systems, Man, and Cybernetics. Part A, Systems and Humans*, *38*(3), 502–512. doi:10.1109/TSMCA.2008.918624

Ker, J., Wang, L., Rao, J., & Lim, T. (2017). Deep Learning Applications in Medical Image Analysis. *IEEE Access*. . doi:10.1109/ACCESS.2017.2788044

Khan, M. A., Ashraf, I., Alhaisoni, M., Damaševičius, R., Scherer, R., Rehman, A., & Bukhari, S. A. C. (2020). Multimodal brain tumor classification using deep learning and robust feature selection: A machine learning application for radiologists. *Diagnostics (Basel)*, *10*(8), 565.

Kharya, S., & Soni, S. (2016). Weighted naive bayes classifier: A predictive model for breast cancer detection. *International Journal of Computers and Applications*, *133*(9), 32–37. doi:10.5120/ijca2016908023

Khateeb & Usman. (2017). Efficient Heart Disease Prediction System using K-Nearest Neighbor Classification Technique. *Proceedings of the International Conference on Big Data and Internet of Thing.* 10.1145/3175684.3175703

Khojasteh, S., Villar, J., Chira, C., González, V., & de la Cal, E. (2018). Improving fall detection using an On-wrist Wearable Accelerometer. *Sensors (Basel)*, *18*(5), 1350. doi:10.339018051350 PMID:29701721

Khorashadizade, N., & Rezaei, H. (2015). New method for rapid diagnosis of hepatitis disease based on reduction feature and machine learning. *Journal of Advanced Computer Science & Technology*, *4*(1), 148–155. doi:10.14419/jacst.v4i1.4353

Kim, W. J., Wagner, A. E., Kim, J., & Andre, E. (2005). From Physiological Signals to Emotions: Implementing and Comparing Selected Methods for Feature Extraction and Classification. *Proceedings of the 2005 IEEE International Conference on Multimedia and Expo*, 940–94.

Kisilev, P., Sason, E., Barkan, E., & Hashoul, S. (2016). *Medical Image Description Using Multi-task-loss CNN*. . doi:10.1007/978-3-319-46976-8_13

Kojuri, J., Boostani, R., Dehghani, P., Nowroozipour, F., & Saki, N. (2015). Prediction of acute myocardial infarction with artificial neural networks in patients with non-diagnostic electrocardiogram. *Journal of Cardiovascular Disease Research*, *6*(2), 51-19.

Kokubo, Y., Iwashima, Y., & Kamide, K. (2015). Hypertension: Introduction, Types, Causes, and Complications. *Pathophysiology and Pharmacotherapy of Cardiovascular Disease*, 635–653. doi:10.1007/978-3-319-15961-4_30

Koldijk, S., Sappelli, M., Verberne, S., Neerincx, M. A., & Kraaij, W. (2014). The Swell knowledge work dataset for stress and user modeling research. *ICMI 2014 - Proceedings of the 2014 International Conference on Multimodal Interaction*, 291–298. 10.1145/2663204.2663257

Koldijk, S., Neerincx, M. A., & Kraaij, W. (2018). Detecting Work Stress in Offices by Combining Unobtrusive Sensors. *IEEE Transactions on Affective Computing*, *9*(2), 227–239. doi:10.1109/TAFFC.2016.2610975

Kooi, T., Litjens, G., Ginneken, B., Gubern-Mérida, A., Sánchez, C., Mann, R., Heeten, G., & Karssemeijer, N. (2016). Large Scale Deep Learning for Computer Aided Detection of Mammographic Lesions. *Medical Image Analysis*, *35*, 303–312. Advance online publication. doi:10.1016/j.media.2016.07.007 PMID:27497072

Kou, G., Yang, P., Peng, Y., Xiao, F., Chen, Y., & Alsaadi, F. E. (2020). Evaluation of feature selection methods for text classification with small datasets using multiple criteria decision-making methods. *Applied Soft Computing*, *86*, 105836. doi:10.1016/j.asoc.2019.105836

Kourou, K., Exarchos, T. P., Exarchos, K. P., Karamouzis, M. V., & Fotiadis, D. I. (2015). Machine learning applications in cancer prognosis and prediction. *Computational and Structural Biotechnology Journal*, *13*, 8–17. doi:10.1016/j.csbj.2014.11.005 PMID:25750696

Krizhevsky, A., Sutskever, I., & Hinton, G. (2012). ImageNet Classification with Deep Convolutional Neural Networks. *Neural Information Processing Systems.*, *25*. Advance online publication. doi:10.1145/3065386

Kulkarni, S., O'Farrell, I., Erasi, M., & Kochar, M. S. (1998). Stress and hypertension. *WMJ: Official Publication of the State Medical Society of Wisconsin*, *97*(11), 34. PMID:9894438

Kumanyika, S. K., & Cutler, J. A. (1997). Dietary sodium reduction: Is there cause for concern? *Journal of the American College of Nutrition*, *16*(3), 192–203. doi:10.1080/07315724.1997.10718674 PMID:9176824

Kumar Gupta, V., & Singh Rana, P. (2020). Ensemble Technique for Toxicity Prediction of Small Drug Molecules of the Antioxidant Response Element Signalling Pathway. *The Computer Journal*, *00*(0). Advance online publication. doi:10.1093/comjnl/bxaa001

Kumar, N., Alam, K., & Siddiqi, A. H. (2017). Wavelet Transform for Classification of EEG Signal using SVM and ANN. *Biomedical & Pharmacology Journal*, *10*(4), 2061–2069. doi:10.13005/bpj/1328

Kumar, R., Pannu, H. S., & Malhi, A. K. (2020). Aspect-based sentiment analysis using deep networks and stochastic optimization. *Neural Computing & Applications*, *32*(8), 3221–3235. doi:10.100700521-019-04105-z

Künecke, J., Hildebrandt, A., Recio, G., Sommer, W., & Wilhelm, O. (2014). Facial EMG Responses to Emotional Expressions Are Related to Emotion Perception Ability. *PLoS One*, *9*(1), e84053. Advance online publication. doi:10.1371/journal.pone.0084053 PMID:24489647

Kyusakov, R., Eliasson, J., Delsing, J., Deventer, J. V., & Gustafsson, J. (2013). Integration of wireless sensor and actuator nodes with IT infrastructure using service-oriented architecture. *IEEE Transactions on Industrial Informatics*, *9*(1), 43–51. doi:10.1109/TII.2012.2198655

Lai, P. K., Fernando, A., Cloutier, T. K., Kingsbury, J. S., Gokarn, Y., Halloran, K. T., ... Trout, B. L. (2021). Machine learning feature selection for predicting high concentration therapeutic antibody aggregation. *Journal of Pharmaceutical Sciences*, *110*(4), 1583–1591.

Larsen, J. T., Norris, C. J., & Cacioppo, J. T. (2003). Effects of positive and negative affect on electromyographic activity over zygomaticus major and corrugator supercilii. *Psychophysiology*, *40*(5), 776–785. doi:10.1111/1469-8986.00078 PMID:14696731

Lazar, C., Taminau, J., Meganck, S., Steenhoff, D., Coletta, A., Molter, C., de Schaetzen, V., Duque, R., Bersini, H., & Nowe, A. (2012). A survey on filter techniques for feature selection in gene expression microarray analysis. *IEEE/ACM Transactions on Computational Biology and Bioinformatics*, *9*(4), 1106–1119. doi:10.1109/TCBB.2012.33 PMID:22350210

Lee, C. Y. W., & Burnett, J. C. Jr. (2007). Natriuretic peptides and therapeutic applications. *Heart Failure Reviews*, *12*(2), 131. Advance online publication. doi:10.100710741-007-9016-3 PMID:17440808

Li, Z., Shen, H., & Alsaify, B. (2008). Integrating RFID with wireless sensor networks for inhabitant, environment and health monitoring. In *2008 14th IEEE International Conference on Parallel and Distributed Systems*. IEEE. 10.1109/ICPADS.2008.66

Lichman, M. (2013). *UCI machine learning repository*. http://archive. ics. uci. edu/ml

Li, G., & Shi, J. (2010). Wireless sensor network technology and its application potentials for service innovation in supply chain management. *International Journal of Applied Logistics*, *1*(4), 30–51. doi:10.4018/jal.2010100103

Linardatos, P., Papastefanopoulos, V., & Kotsiantis, S. (2020). Explainable AI: A Review of Machine Learning Interpretability Methods. *Entropy (Basel, Switzerland)*, *23*, 18. doi:10.3390/e23010018

Lin, D., & Jingtao, S. (2015). A recommender system based on contextual information of click and purchase data to items for e-commerce. *Third International Conference on Cyberspace Technology (CCT 2015)*, 1–6. 10.1049/cp.2015.0823

Lingras, P., Sharma, S., & Zhong, M. (2002). Prediction of recreational travel using genetically designed regression and time-delay neural network models. *Transportation Research Record: Journal of the Transportation Research Board*, *13*(1), 435–446. doi:10.3141/1805-03

Lin, L.-C., Chen, S. C.-J., Chiang, C.-T., Wu, H.-C., Yang, R.-C., & Ouyang, C.-S. (2016). Classification preictal and interictal stages via integrating interchannel and time-domain analysis of eeg features. *Clinical EEG and Neuroscience*. PMID:27177554

Li, R., Zhang, W., Suk, H.-I., Wang, L., Li, J., Shen, D., & Ji, S. (2014). *Deep Learning Based Imaging Data Completion for Improved Brain Disease Diagnosis*. doi:10.1007/978-3-319-10443-0_39

Li, S., Xu, L., Wang, X., & Wang, J. (2012). Integration of hybrid wireless networks in cloud services oriented enterprise information systems. *Enterprise Information Systems*, *6*(2), 165–187. doi:10.1080/17517575.2011.654266

Litt, B., & Echauz, J. (2002). Prediction of epileptic seizures. *The Lancet Neurology*, *1*(1), 22-30. doi:10.1016/S1474-4422(02)00003-0

Liu, S., & Xiao, Q. (2015). A Signer-Independent Sign Language Recognition System Based on the Weighted KNN/HMM. In *2015 7th International Conference on Intelligent Human-Machine Systems and Cybernetics. 2015 7th International Conference on Intelligent Human-Machine Systems and Cybernetics (IHMSC)*. IEEE. 10.1109/IHMSC.2015.71

Liu, Y.-H., Wu, C.-T., Cheng, W.-T., Hsiao, Y.-T., Chen, P.-M., & Teng, J.-T. (2014). Emotion Recognition from Single-Trial EEG Based on Kernel Fisher's Emotion Pattern and Imbalanced Quasi-conformal Kernel Support Vector Machine. *Sensors (Basel), 14*(8), 13361–13388. doi:10.3390140813361 PMID:25061837

Liu, Y., Lee, J. M., & Lee, C. (2020). The challenges and opportunities of a global health crisis: The management and business implications of COVID-19 from an Asian perspective. *Asian Business & Management, 19*(3), 277–297. doi:10.105741291-020-00119-x

Lopes, N., & Ribeiro, B. (2015). *Deep Belief Networks (DBNs)*. doi:10.1007/978-3-319-06938-8_8

López-Ludeña, V., San-Segundo, R., González Morcillo, C., López, J. C., & Pardo Muñoz, J. M. (2013). Increasing adaptability of a speech into sign language translation system. In Expert Systems with Applications (Vol. 40, Issue 4, pp. 1312–1322). Elsevier BV. doi:10.1016/j.eswa.2012.08.059

Lundqvist, L. O. (1995). Facial EMG reactions to facial expressions: A case of facial emotional contagion? *Scandinavian Journal of Psychology, 36*(2), 130–141. doi:10.1111/j.1467-9450.1995.tb00974.x PMID:7644897

Mahajan, Lavhate, Waghmare, & Pingale. (2017). A Survey on Women's Security System Using GPS and GSM. *International Journal of Innovative Research in Computer and Communication Engineering, 5*(2), 1560–1563.

Mak, K. K., & Pichika, M. R. (2019). Artificial intelligence in drug development: Present status and future prospects. *Drug Discovery Today, 24*(3), 773–780. Advance online publication. doi:10.1016/j.drudis.2018.11.014 PMID:30472429

Malfaz, M., & Salichs, M. A. (2007). A new architecture for autonomous robots based on emotions. *IFAC Proceedings Volumes, 37*, 805–809.

Mallick, B., & Patro, A. K. (2016). Heart rate monitoring system using finger tip through arduino and processing software. *International Journal of Science Engineering and Technology Research, 5*(1), 84–89.

Mandala, S., & Di, T. C. (2017). ECG Parameters for Malignant Ventricular Arrhythmias: A Comprehensive Review. *Journal of Medical and Biological Engineering, 37*(4), 441–453. doi:10.100740846-017-0281-x PMID:28867990

Mandel, J. S. P. (2015). A Comparison of Six Methods for Missing Data Imputation. *Journal of Biometrics & Biostatistics, 06*(01), 1–6. doi:10.4172/2155-6180.1000224

Manocha, A., Kumar, G., Bhatia, M., & Sharma, A. (2021). IoT-inspired machine learning-assisted sedentary behavior analysis in smart healthcare industry. *Journal of Ambient Intelligence and Humanized Computing*, (0123456789). Advance online publication. doi:10.100712652-021-03371-x

Mao, Ma, He, & Luo. (2017). Highly Portable, Sensor-Based System for Human Fall Monitoring. *Sensors, 17*(9). . doi:10.3390/s17092096

Masmoudi, S., Elghazel, H., Taieb, D., Yazar, O., & Kallel, A. (2020). A machine-learning framework for predicting multiple air pollutants' concentrations via multi-target regression and feature selection. *The Science of the Total Environment, 715*, 136991.

Ma, X., Tao, Z., Wang, Y., Yu, H., & Wang, Y. (2015). Long short-term memory neural network for traffic speed prediction using remote microwave sensor data. *Transport. Res. C Emerging Technol., 54*, 187–197. doi:10.1016/j.trc.2015.03.014

McCall, J. (2005). Genetic algorithms for modelling and optimisation. *Journal of Computational and Applied Mathematics, 184*(1), 205–222. doi:10.1016/j.cam.2004.07.034

McGrath, M. F., de Bold, M. L. K., & Adolfo, J. (2005). The endocrine function of the heart. *Trends in Endocrinology and Metabolism, 16*(10), 469–477. doi:10.1016/j.tem.2005.10.007 PMID:16269246

McLoone, V. (2014). *Modelling of Long and Short Term Blood Pressure Control Systems* (Doctoral dissertation). National University of Ireland, Maynooth, Ireland.

McLoone, V. I. (2014). *Modelling of long and short term blood pressure control systems* (Doctoral dissertation). National University of Ireland Maynooth.

Meelab, S., Bunupuradah, I., Suttiruang, J., Sakulrojanawong, S., Thongkua, N., Chantawiboonchai, C., & Sakboonyarat, B. (2019). Prevalence and associated factors of uncontrolled blood pressure among hypertensive patients in the rural communities in the central areas in Thailand: A cross-sectional study. *PLoS One, 14*(2), e0212572. doi:10.1371/journal.pone.0212572 PMID:30779818

Mehmood, R., & Lee, H. (2017). Towards Building a Computer Aided Education System for Special Students Using Wearable Sensor Technologies. *Sensors (Basel), 17*(2), 317. doi:10.339017020317 PMID:28208734

Melder, A., Burns, P., Mcloughlin, I., & Teede, H. (2018). Examining 'institutional entrepreneurship' in healthcare redesign and improvement through comparative case study research: A study protocol. *BMJ Open, 8*(8), e020807. doi:10.1136/bmjopen-2017-020807 PMID:30082347

Minaee, S., Minaei, M., & Abdolrashidi, A. (2021). Deep-Emotion: Facial Expression Recognition Using Attentional Convolutional Network. *Sensors (Basel), 21*(9), 3046. doi:10.339021093046 PMID:33925371

Min, S., Lee, B., & Yoon, S. (2016). Deep learning in bioinformatics. *Briefings in Bioinformatics, 18*(5), 851869. PMID:27473064

Moeskops, P., Wolterink, J., Van der Velden, B., Gilhuijs, K., Leiner, T., Viergever, M., & Išgum, I. (2016). Deep Learning for Multi-Task Medical Image Segmentation in Multiple Modalities. *LNCS, 9901*, 478–486. doi:10.1007/978-3-319-46723-8_55

Moh'd Rasoul, A., Al-Gawagzeh, M. Y., & Alsaaidah, B. A. (2012). Solving mammography problems of breast cancer detection using artificial neural networks and image processing techniques. *Indian Journal of Science and Technology, 5*(4), 2520–2528.

Mohammed, M., Khan, M. B., & Bashier, E. B. M. (2016). *Machine learning: algorithms and applications*. CRC Press. doi:10.1201/9781315371658

Moise, N., Schwartz, J., Bring, R., Shimbo, D., & Kronish, I. M. (2014). Antihypertensive drug class and adherence: An electronic monitoring study. *American Journal of Hypertension, 28*(6), 717–721. doi:10.1093/ajh/hpu199 PMID:25344354

Molka-Danielsen, J., Engelseth, P., & Wang, H. (2018). Large scale integration of wireless sensor network technologies for air quality monitoring at a logistics shipping base. *Journal of Industrial Information Integration, 10*, 20–28. doi:10.1016/j.jii.2018.02.001

Monisha, D. G., Monisha, M., Pavithra, G., & Subhashini, R. (2016). Women Safety Device andApplication-FEMME. *Indian Journal of Science and Technology, 9*(10), 1–6. doi:10.17485/ijst/2016/v9i10/88898

Mormann, F., Andrzejak, R. G., Elger, C. E., & Lehnertz, K. (2006). Seizure prediction: The long and winding road. *Brain, 130*(2), 314333. PMID:17008335

Muduli, L., Mishra, D. P., & Jana, P. K. (2018). Application of wireless sensor network for environmental monitoring in underground coal mines: A systematic review. *Journal of Network and Computer Applications*, *106*, 48–67. doi:10.1016/j.jnca.2017.12.022

Muhammad, A. N., Aseere, A. M., Chiroma, H., Shah, H., Gital, A. Y., & Hashem, I. A. T. (2021). Deep learning application in smart cities: Recent development, taxonomy, challenges and research prospects. In *Neural Computing and Applications* (Vol. 33). Springer London. doi:10.1007/s00521-020-05151-8

Musha, T., Asada, T., Yamashita, F., Kinoshita, T., Chen, Z., Matsuda, H., Masatake, U., & Shankle, W. R. (2002). A new EEG method for estimating cortical neuronal impairment that is sensitive to early-stage Alzheimer's disease. *Clinical Neurophysiology*, *113*(7), 1052–1058. doi:10.1016/S1388-2457(02)00128-1 PMID:12088699

Nair, V., & Hinton, G. E. (2010). *Rectified linear units improve restricted boltzmann machines*. Available https://dl.acm.org/citation.cfm

Nakanishi, R., & Imai-Matsumura, K. (2008). Facial skin temperature decreases in infants with joyful expression. *Infant Behavior and Development*, *31*(1), 137–144. doi:10.1016/j.infbeh.2007.09.001 PMID:17983661

Nakasone, A., Prendinger, H., & Ishizuka, M. (2005). Infiniti Bio-signal Encoder. *Proceedings of the 5th International Workshop on Biosignal Interpretation*, 219–222.

Nechuta, S. J., Caan, B. J., Chen, W. Y., Flatt, S. W., Lu, W., Patterson, R. E., Poole, E. M., Kwan, M. L., Chen, Z., Weltzien, E., Pierce, J. P., & Shu, X. O. (2011). The After Breast Cancer Pooling Project: Rationale, methodology, and breast cancer survivor characteristics. *Cancer Causes & Control*, *22*(9), 1319–1331. doi:10.100710552-011-9805-9 PMID:21710192

Nejad, L., Mashayekhy, L., Chinnam, R. B., & Phillips, A. (2017). Hierarchical time-dependent shortest path algorithms for vehicle routing under ITS. *IIE Transactions*, *48*(2), 158–169. doi:10.1080/0740817X.2015.1078523

Ngadi, M., Amine, A., & Nassih, B. (2016, November). A robust approach for mammographic image classification using NSVC algorithm. In *Proceedings of the Mediterranean Conference on Pattern Recognition and Artificial Intelligence* (pp. 44-49). 10.1145/3038884.3038892

Nguyen, C., Wang, Y., & Nguyen, H. N. (2013). *Random forest classifier combined with feature selection for breast cancer diagnosis and prognostic*. Academic Press.

Nguyen, G., Dlugolinsky, S., Bobák, M., Tran, V., López García, Á., Heredia, I., Malík, P., & Hluchý, L. (2019). Machine Learning and Deep Learning frameworks and libraries for large-scale data mining: A survey. *Artificial Intelligence Review*, *52*(1), 77–124. doi:10.100710462-018-09679-z

Niang, M., Dupéré, S., Alami, H., & Gagnon, M. P. (2021). Why is repositioning public health innovation towards a social paradigm necessary? A reflection on the field of public health through the examples of Ebola and Covid-19. *Globalization and Health*, *17*(1), 46. doi:10.118612992-021-00695-3 PMID:33853631

Niarchos, A. P., Pickering, T. G., Case, D. B., Sullivan, P., & Laragh, J. H. (1979). Role of the renin-angiotensin system in blood pressure regulation. The cardiovascular effects of converting enzyme inhibition in normotensive subjects. *Circulation Research*, *45*(6), 829–837. doi:10.1161/01.RES.45.6.829 PMID:498446

Ogwumu, O., Amoo, S., Eguda, F., Adeyefa, E., & Abubakar, S. (2015). A mathematical model for estimating the weight of human beings using some anthropometric parameters (A Case Study of Taraba State of Nigerias Community). *British Journal of Mathematics and Computer Science*, *8*(2), 147–158. doi:10.9734/BJMCS/2015/10987

Olanow, C. W., Watts, R. L., & Koller, W. C. (2001). An algorithm (decision tree) for the management of Parkinson's disease (2001): Treatment Guidelines. *Neurology*, *56*(suppl 5), S1–S88. doi:10.1212/WNL.56.suppl_5.S1 PMID:11402154

Ouichka, O., Echtioui, A., & Hamam, H. (2022). Deep Learning Models for Predicting Epileptic Seizures Using iEEG Signals. *Electronics (Basel)*, *11*(4), 605. doi:10.3390/electronics11040605

Oxley, T. J., Opie, N. L., John, S. E., Rind, G. S., Ronayne, S. M., Wheeler, T. L., Judy, J. W., McDonald, A. J., Dornom, A., Lovell, T. J. H., Steward, C., Garrett, D. J., Moffat, B. A., Lui, E. H., Yassi, N., Campbell, B. C. V., Wong, Y. T., Fox, K. E., Nurse, E. S., ... O'Brien, T. J. (2016). Minimally invasive endovascular stent-electrode array for high-fidelity, chronic recording of cortical neural activity. *Nature Biotechnology*, *34*(3), 320–327. doi:10.1038/nbt.3428 PMID:26854476

Ozdemir, M. A., Cura, O. K., & Akan, A. (2021). Epileptic EEG classification by using time-frequency images for deep learning. *International Journal of Neural Systems*, *31*(8), 2150026. doi:10.1142/S012906572150026X PMID:34039254

Özyurt, F. (2020). Efficient deep feature selection for remote sensing image recognition with fused deep learning architectures. *The Journal of Supercomputing*, *76*(11), 8413–8431.

Panchal, D., & Shah, S. (2011). Artificial intelligence based expert system for Hepatitis B diagnosis. *International Journal of Modeling and Optimization*, *1*(4), 362–366. doi:10.7763/IJMO.2011.V1.61

Pandya, R., & Pandya, J. (2015). C5. 0 algorithm to improved decision tree with feature selection and reduced error pruning. *International Journal of Computers and Applications*, *117*(16), 18–21. doi:10.5120/20639-3318

Pant, A. (2019, January 22). Introduction to Logistic Regression. *Towardsdatascience.*

Paradkar, A., & Sharma, D. (2015). All in one Intelligent Safety System for Women Security. *International Journal of Computers and Applications*, *130*(11), 33–40. doi:10.5120/ijca2015907144

Parashar, J., & Rai, M. (2020). Breast cancer images classification by clustering of ROI and mapping of features by CNN with XGBOOST learning. *Materials Today: Proceedings*. Advance online publication. doi:10.1016/j.matpr.2020.09.650

Park, Y. S., Cosgrove, G. R., Madsen, J. R., Eskandar, E. N., Hochberg, L. R., Cash, S. S., & Truccolo, W. (2020, March). Early Detection of Human Epileptic Seizures Based on Intracortical Microelectrode Array Signals. *IEEE Transactions on Biomedical Engineering*, *67*(3), 817–831. doi:10.1109/TBME.2019.2921448 PMID:31180831

Parlikar, A. S., & Dahe, P. D. (2019). Application of linear programming-genetic algorithm combination for Urmodi reservoir operation. In *International Conference on Reliability, Risk Maintenance and Engineering Management* (pp. 98-103). Springer.

Pasha, S. J., & Mohamed, E. S. (2020, February). Ensemble gain ratio feature selection (EGFS) model with machine learning and data mining algorithms for disease risk prediction. In *2020 International Conference on Inventive Computation Technologies (ICICT)* (pp. 590-596). IEEE.

Paul, D. (2020). *'Artificial intelligence in drug discovery and development', Drug Discovery Today*. Elsevier Ltd. doi:10.1016/j.drudis.2020.10.010

Paul, S., Banerjee, A., & Tibarewala, D. N. (2017). Emotional eye movement analysis using electrooculography signal. *International Journal of Biomedical Engineering and Technology*, *23*(1), 59. doi:10.1504/IJBET.2017.082224

Pavithra, V., & Jayalakshmi, V. (2020, June). Review of feature selection techniques for predicting diseases. In *2020 5th International Conference on Communication and Electronics Systems (ICCES)* (pp. 1213-1217). IEEE.

Payan, A., & Montana, G. (2015). Predicting Alzheimer's disease: a neuroimaging study with 3D convolutional neural networks. *ICPRAM 2015 - 4th International Conference on Pattern Recognition Applications and Methods, Proceedings, 2.*

Pedregosa, F., Varoquaux, G., Gramfort, A., Michel, V., Thirion, B., Grisel, O., ... Duchesnay, E. (2011). Scikit-learn: Machine learning in Python. *The Journal of Machine Learning Research, 12*, 2825-2830.

Pereira, N., Andersson, B., & Tovar, E. (2007). WiDom:Adominance protocol for wireless medium access. *IEEE Transactions on Industrial Informatics*, *3*(2), 120–130. doi:10.1109/TII.2007.898461

Perez, V., & Chang, E. T. (2014). Sodium-to-potassium ratio and blood pressure, hypertension, and related factors. *Advances in Nutrition*, *5*(6), 712–741. doi:10.3945/an.114.006783 PMID:25398734

Philip Schmidt, A., Reiss, R., & Duerichen, K. V. L. (2018). Introducing WESAD, a multimodal dataset for wearable Stress and Affect Detection. *International Conference on Multimodal Interaction 2018.*

Pinto, E. (2007). Blood pressure and ageing. *Postgraduate Medical Journal*, *83*(976), 109–114. doi:10.1136/pgmj.2006.048371 PMID:17308214

Podder, K. K., Tabassum, S., Khan, L. E., Salam, K. M. A., Maruf, R. I., & Ahmed, A. (2021). *Design of a Sign Language Transformer to Enable the Participation of Persons with Disabilities in Remote Healthcare Systems for Ensuring Universal Healthcare Coverage. In 2021 IEEE Technology & Engineering Management Conference - Europe (TEMSCON-EUR).* IEEE. doi:10.1109/TEMSCON-EUR52034.2021.9488605

Portnoy, J., Waller, M., & Elliott, T. (2020). Telemedicine in the Era of COVID-19. *The Journal of Allergy and Clinical Immunology. In Practice*, *8*(5), 1489–1491. doi:10.1016/j.jaip.2020.03.008 PMID:32220575

Potter, L. R., Abbey-Hosch, S., & Dickey, D. M. (2006). Natriuretic peptides, their receptors, and cyclic guanosine monophosphate-dependent signaling functions. *Endocrine Reviews*, *27*(1), 47–72. doi:10.1210/er.2005-0014 PMID:16291870

Pouliot, M.-C., Després, J.-P., Lemieux, S., Moorjani, S., Bouchard, C., Tremblay, A., & Lupien, P. J. (1994). Waist circumference and abdominal sagittal diameter: Best simple anthropometric indexes of abdominal visceral adipose tissue accumulation and related cardiovascular risk in men and women. *The American Journal of Cardiology*, *73*(7), 460–468. doi:10.1016/0002-9149(94)90676-9

Puddey, I. B., Beilin, L. J., & Vandongen, R. (1987). Regular alcohol use raises blood pressure in treated hypertensive subjects. *Lancet*, *329*(8534), 647–651. doi:10.1016/S0140-6736(87)90413-2 PMID:2882082

Puri, C., Olson, L., Pavlidis, I., Levine, J., & Stresscam, S. J. (2005). Non-contact measurement of users' emotional states through thermal imaging. *Proceedings of the Conference on Human Factors in Computing Systems (CHI EA 2005),* 1725–1728.

Purnamasari, P., Ratna, A., & Kusumoputro, B. (2017). Development of Filtered Bispectrum for EEG Signal Feature Extraction in Automatic Emotion Recognition Using Artificial Neural Networks. *Algorithms*, *10*(2), 63. doi:10.3390/a10020063

Pushpalatha, S., & Pandya, J. (2014). Comparison of data models for hepatitis diagnosis - data mining technique. *International Journal of Advanced Research in Computer Science and Software Engineering*, *4*(1), 1092–1095.

Quero, Olmo, Aguilera, & Estévez. (2017). Real-Time Monitoring in Home-Based Cardiac Rehabilitation Using Wrist-Worn Heart Rate Devices. *Sensors, 17*(12).

Raamat, R., Talts, J., Jagomägi, K., & Länsimies, E. (1999). Mathematical modelling of non-invasive oscillometric finger mean blood pressure measurement by maximum oscillation criterion. *Medical & Biological Engineering & Computing*, *37*(6), 784–788.

Rafik, D., & Larbi, B. (2019). Autoregressive modeling based empirical mode decomposition (EMD) for epileptic seizures detection using EEG signals. *Traitement du Signal*, *36*(3), 273–279. doi:10.18280/ts.360311

Raghu, Sriraam, Gommer, Hilkman, Temel, Rao, Hegde, & Kubben. (2020). Cross-database evaluation of EEG based epileptic seizures detection driven by adaptive median feature baseline correction. *Clinical Neurophysiology, 131*(7), 1567-1578. doi:10.1016/j.clinph.2020.03.033

Rajaguru, H. (2019). Analysis of decision tree and k-nearest neighbor algorithm in the classification of breast cancer. Asian Pacific journal of cancer prevention. *APJCP, 20*(12), 3777. PMID:31870121

Rajkumar, E., & Romate, J. (2020). Behavioural Risk Factors, Hypertension Knowledge, and Hypertension in Rural India. *International Journal of Hypertension, 2020*, 1–7. doi:10.1155/2020/8108202 PMID:32231796

Rajput, Mohd, Shinde, Parathe, & Sahu. (2017). Design and implementaion of safety armband for women and children using ARM7. *International Journal of Engineering Technology Science and Research, 4*(4), 161-165.

Ramson, S. R. (2017). *Applications of wireless sensor networks—A survey. In 2017 international conference on innovations in electrical, electronics, instrumentation and media technology (ICEEIMT)*. IEEE.

Rangamani, A., Mukherjee, A., Basu, A., Arora, A., Ganapathi, T., Chin, S., & Tran, T. (2018). *Sparse Coding and Autoencoders*. Advance online publication. doi:10.1109/ISIT.2018.8437533

Rao, P. S., Kumar, A. S., Niyaz, Q., Sidike, P., & Devabhaktuni, V. K. (2021). Binary chemical reaction optimization based feature selection techniques for machine learning classification problems. *Expert Systems with Applications, 167*, 114169.

Rashid, B., & Rehmani, M. H. (2016). Applications of wireless sensor networks for urban areas: A survey. *Journal of Network and Computer Applications, 60*, 192–219. doi:10.1016/j.jnca.2015.09.008

Rattanyu, K., Ohkura, M., & Mizukawa, M. (2010). Emotion Monitoring from Physiological Signals for Service Robots in the Living Space. Institute of Control, Robotics and Systems, 580–583.

Rawat, K., Kumari, P., & Saha, L. (2021). COVID-19 vaccine: A recent update in pipeline vaccines, their design, and development strategies. *European Journal of Pharmacology, 892*, 173751. doi:10.1016/j.ejphar.2020.173751 PMID:33245898

Raza, M., Hussain, F. K., Hussain, O. K., Zhao, M., & Rehman, Z. (2019). A comparative analysis of machine learning models for quality pillar assessment of SaaS services by multi-class text classification of users' reviews. *Future Generation Computer Systems, 101*, 341–371. doi:10.1016/j.future.2019.06.022

Revanth, K. K., & Raja, N. S. M. (2019). Comprehensive SVM based Indian Sign Language Recognition. In *2019 IEEE International Conference on System, Computation, Automation and Networking (ICSCAN)*. IEEE. 10.1109/ICSCAN.2019.8878787

Rezaimehr, F., & Dadkhah, C. (2020). *A survey of attack detection approaches in collaborative filtering recommender systems. Artificial Intelligence Review*. Springer Netherlands. doi:10.100710462-020-09898-3

Ronneberger, O., Fischer, P., & Brox, T. (2015). U-Net: Convolutional Networks for Biomedical Image Segmentation. *LNCS, 9351*, 234–241. doi:10.1007/978-3-319-24574-4_28

Roshni, Sune, & Nerkar. (2018). Internet of Things Based Women Tracking And Security with Auto-defender System. *International Journal of Innovative Research in Computerand Communication Engineering, 6*(6), 63–68.

Rouse, I. L., Armstrong, B. K., & Beilin, L. J. (1983). The relationship of blood pressure to diet and lifestyle in two religious populations. *Journal of Hypertension, 1*(1), 65–72. doi:10.1097/00004872-198306000-00011 PMID:6681026

Royal, A., Mali, M. A., Kumar, V., Wagh, I. A., Bhushan, S., Mokal, A. N., Mehta, K., & Bhattacharya, S. (2021). Harnessing the potential of the primary healthcare facilities in India to respond COVID-19 pandemic: A scoping evidence-based research synthesis. *Journal of Family Medicine and Primary Care*, *10*(1), 116–121. doi:10.4103/jfmpc.jfmpc_1609_20 PMID:34017712

Rucco, Sorriso, Liparoti, Ferraioli, Sorrentino, Ambrosanio, & Baselice. (2018). Type and Location of Wearable Sensors for Monitoring Falls during Static and Dynamic Tasks in Healthy Elderly: A Review. *Sensors, 18*(5), 1-20.

Russell, J. A. (1980). A Circumplex Model of effect. *Journal of Personality and Social Psychology*, *39*(6), 1161–1178. doi:10.1037/h0077714

Rustam, F., Reshi, A. A., Aljedaani, W., Alhossan, A., Ishaq, A., Shafi, S., ... Rupapara, V. (2022). Vector mosquito image classification using novel RIFS feature selection and machine learning models for disease epidemiology. *Saudi Journal of Biological Sciences*, *29*(1), 583–594.

Sacks, F. M., Svetkey, L. P., Vollmer, W. M., Appel, L. J., Bray, G. A., Harsha, D., ... Karanja, N. (2001). Effects on blood pressure of reduced dietary sodium and the dietary approaches to stop hypertension (DASH) diet. *The New England Journal of Medicine*, *344*(1), 3–10. doi:10.1056/NEJM200101043440101 PMID:11136953

Saez, P., Peña, E., Martínez, M. A., & Kuhl, E. (2014). Computational modeling of hypertensive growth in the human carotid artery. *Computational Mechanics*, *53*(6), 1183–1196. doi:10.100700466-013-0959-z PMID:25342868

Said, Y., & Barr, M. (2021). Human emotion recognition based on facial expressions via deep learning on high-resolution images. *Multimedia Tools and Applications*, *80*(16), 25241–25253. doi:10.100711042-021-10918-9

Salakhutdinov, R., & Hinton, G. (2009). Deep Boltzmann Machines. *Proceedings of AISTATS 2009.*

Samala, R., Chan, H-P., Hadjiiski, L., Cha, K., & Helvie, M. (2016). *Deep-learning convolution neural network for computer-aided detection of microcalcifications in digital breast tomosynthesis*. doi:10.1117/12.2217092

Samala, R., Chan, H.-P., Hadjiiski, L., Helvie, M., Wei, J., & Cha, K. (2016). Mass detection in digital breast tomosynthesis: Deep convolutional neural network with transfer learning from mammography. *Medical Physics*, *43*, 6654. doi:10.1118/1.4967345]

Sarker, I. H. (2021). Machine learning: Algorithms, real-world applications and research directions. *SN Computer Science*, *2*(3), 1–21. doi:10.100742979-021-00592-x PMID:33778771

Sarker, I. H., Furhad, M. H., & Nowrozy, R. (2021). Ai-driven cybersecurity: An overview, security intelligence modeling and research directions. *SN Computer Science*, *2*(3), 1–18. doi:10.100742979-021-00557-0 PMID:33778771

Scherer, K. R. (2005). What are emotions? And how can they be measured? *Social Sciences Information. Information Sur les Sciences Sociales*, *44*(4), 695–729. doi:10.1177/0539018405058216

Schwartz, K., & Huff, B. (2010). *The story of Eli Lilly's open innovation journey—How one company developed a mature model*. PDMA Visions.

Sellwood, M. A., Ahmed, M., Segler, M. H. S., & Brown, N. (2018). Artificial intelligence in drug discovery. *Future Medicinal Chemistry*, *10*(17), 2025–2028. Advance online publication. doi:10.4155/fmc-2018-0212 PMID:30101607

Selvathi, D., & AarthyPoornila, A. (2017). *Performance analysis of various classifiers on deep learning network for breast cancer detection*. doi:10.1109/CSPC.2017.8305869

Shaffer, F., Shearman, F., Meehan, S., & Zachary. (2016). The Promise of Ultra-Short-Term (UST) Heart Rate Variability Measurements. *Psychology*. doi:10.5298/1081-5937-44.3.09

Sheffield. (2017). The Global Impact of Respiratory Disease. In *Forum of International Respiratory Societies* (2nd ed.). European Respiratory Society.

Shetty. (2010). https://www.narayanahealth.org/blog/respiratory-diseases-causes-symptoms-preventive-measures/

Shin, Y., Lee, S., Ahn, M., Cho, H., Jun, S. C., & Lee, H.-N. (2015, August). Noise robustness analysis of sparse representation based classification method for non-stationary EEG signal classification. *Biomedical Signal Processing and Control*, *21*, 818. doi:10.1016/j.bspc.2015.05.007

Shu, Li, Wang, Mi, Li, & Ren. (2015). A Pressure Sensing System for Monitoring with Polymer-Based Pressure Sensors and an Anti-Interference Post Processing Heart Rate Circuit. *Sensors, 15*(2), 3224-35.

Sidhu, R. K., Kumar, R., & Rana, P. S. (2020). Machine learning based crop water demand forecasting using minimum climatological data. *Multimedia Tools and Applications*, *79*(19–20), 13109–13124. doi:10.100711042-019-08533-w

Simonyan, K., & Zisserman, A. (2014). *Very Deep Convolutional Networks for Large-Scale Image Recognition.* arXiv 1409.1556.

Singh, D. (2012). Human Emotion Recognition System. *International journal of Image. Graphics, and Signal Processing*, *8*(8), 50–56. doi:10.5815/ijigsp.2012.08.07

Singh, K., & Malhotra, J. (2022). *Smart neurocare approach for detection of epileptic seizures using deep learning based temporal analysis of EEG patterns. Multimed Tools Appl.* doi:10.100711042-022-12512-z

Singh, Y., & Chugh, U. (2013). Mutual Exclusive Distributive Clustering (MEDC) Protocol for Wireless Sensor Networks. *International Journal of Sensors, Wireless Communications and Control*, *3*(2), 101–107. doi:10.2174/2210327 90302140505100253

Sivakami, K., & Saraswathi, N. (2015). Mining big data: Breast cancer prediction using DT-SVM hybrid model. *International Journal of Scientific Engineering and Applied Science*, *1*(5), 418–429.

Sivaranjani, S., Ananya, S., Aravinth, J., & Karthika, R. (2021, March). Diabetes prediction using machine learning algorithms with feature selection and dimensionality reduction. In *2021 7th International Conference on Advanced Computing and Communication Systems (ICACCS)* (Vol. 1, pp. 141-146). IEEE.

Soleymani, M., Lichtenauer, J., Pun, T., & Pantic, M. (2012). A Multimodal Database for Affect Recognition and Implicit Tagging. *IEEE Transactions on Affective Computing*, *3*(1), 42–55. doi:10.1109/T-AFFC.2011.25

Sonkusare, S., Ahmedt-Aristizabal, D., Aburn, M. J., Nguyen, V. T., Pang, T., Frydman, S., Denman, S., Fookes, C., Breakspear, M., & Guo, C. C. (2019). Detecting changes in facial temperature induced by a sudden auditory stimulus based on deep learning-assisted face tracking. *Scientific Reports*, *9*(1), 4729. doi:10.103841598-019-41172-7 PMID:30894584

Soundariya, R. S., & Renuga, R. (2017). Eye movement based emotion recognition using electrooculography. *Proceedings of the 2017 Innovations in Power and Advanced Computing Technologies (i-PACT).*

Srivastava, N., Hinton, G., Krizhevsky, A., Sutskever, I., & Salakhutdinov, R. (2014). Dropout: A Simple Way to Prevent Neural Networks from Overfitting. *Journal of Machine Learning Research, 15*, 1929–1958.

Stamler, J., Elliott, P., Kesteloot, H., Nichols, R., Claeys, G., Dyer, A. R., & Stamler, R. (1996). Inverse relation of dietary protein markers with blood pressure. *Circulation*, *94*(7), 1629–1634. doi:10.1161/01.CIR.94.7.1629 PMID:8840854

Steinhelper, M. E., Cochrane, K. L., & Field, L. J. (1990). Hypotension in transgenic mice expressing atrial natriuretic factor fusion genes. *Hypertension*, *16*(3), 301–307. doi:10.1161/01.HYP.16.3.301 PMID:2144261

Subramanian, B. (2017). ECG signal classification and parameter estimation using multiwavelet transform. *Biomedical Research, 28*(7), 3187–3193.

Sun, M., Wang, F., Min, T., Zang, T., & Wang, Y. (2018). Prediction for High Risk Clinical Symptoms of Epilepsy Based on Deep Learning Algorithm. *IEEE Access: Practical Innovations, Open Solutions, 6*, 77596–77605. doi:10.1109/ACCESS.2018.2883562

Sun, W., Tseng, B., Zhang, J., & Qian, W. (2016). Enhancing deep convolutional neural network scheme for breast cancer diagnosis with unlabeled data. *Computerized Medical Imaging and Graphics, 57*. Advance online publication. doi:10.1016/j.compmedimag.2016.07.004

Suryavanshi, T., Lambert, S., Lal, S., Chin, A., & Chan, T. M. (2020). Entrepreneurship and Innovation in Health Sciences Education: A Scoping Review. *Medical Science Educator, 30*(4), 1797–1809. doi:10.100740670-020-01050-8 PMID:34457846

Syed, L., Jabeen, S., Manimala, S., & Elsayed, H. A. (2019). Data science algorithms and techniques for smart healthcare using iot and big data analytics. In *Studies in Fuzziness and Soft Computing* (Vol. 374). doi:10.1007/978-3-030-03131-2_11

Szegedy, C., Liu, W., Jia, Y., Sermanet, P., Reed, S., Anguelov, D., Erhan, D., Vanhoucke, V., & Rabinovich, A. (2015). Going deeper with convolutions. *The IEEE Conference on Computer Vision and Pattern Recognition (CVPR)*, 1-9. 10.1109/CVPR.2015.7298594

Szegedy, C., Vanhoucke, V., Ioffe, S., Shlens, J., & Wojna, Z. (2016). Rethinking the Inception Architecture for Computer Vision. *2016 IEEE Conference on Computer Vision and Pattern Recognition (CVPR)*, 2818-2826. 10.1109/CVPR.2016.308

Tahmooresi, M., Afshar, A., Rad, B. B., Nowshath, K. B., & Bamiah, M. A. (2018). Early detection of breast cancer using machine learning techniques. *Journal of Telecommunication, Electronic and Computer Engineering (JTEC), 10*(3-2), 21-27.

Takam, C. A., Samba, O., Kouanou, A. T., & Tchiotsop, D. (2020). Spark Architecture for deep learning-based dose optimization in medical imaging. *Informatics in Medicine Unlocked, 19*. doi:10.1016/j.imu.2020.100335

Theerthagiri, Jacob, Ruby, & Yendapalli. (2021). Prediction of COVID-19 Possibilities using K-NN Classification Algorithm. *International Journal of Current Research and Review, 13*(6).

Tiffin, N., Meintjes, A., Ramesar, R., Bajic, V. B., & Rayner, B. (2010). Computational analysis of candidate disease genes and variants for salt-sensitive hypertension in indigenous Southern Africans. *PLoS One, 5*(9), e12989. doi:10.1371/journal.pone.0012989 PMID:20886000

Tjhjadi, H., & Ramli, K. (2020). Noninvasive Blood Pressure Classification Based on Photoplethysmography Using K-Nearest Neighbors Algorithm: A Feasibility Study. *Information (Basel), 11*(2), 93. doi:10.3390/info11020093

Trivedi, S. K., Dey, S., & Kumar, A. (2018). Capturing user sentiments for online Indian movie reviews: A comparative analysis of different machine-learning models. *The Electronic Library, 36*(4), 677–695. doi:10.1108/EL-04-2017-0075

Turner, J. T., Page, A., Mohsenin, T., & Oates, T. (2014). *Deep belief networks used on high resolution multichannel electroencephalography data for seizure detection.* Presented at the AAAI Spring Symp.

University of Stanford. (n.d.). *Convolutional Neural Networks for Visual Recognition.* https://cs231n.github.io/convolutional-networks/

Upadhyay, D., Manero, J., Zaman, M., & Sampalli, S. (2020). Gradient boosting feature selection with machine learning classifiers for intrusion detection on power grids. *IEEE eTransactions on Network and Service Management, 18*(1), 1104–1116.

Usman, S. M., Khalid, S., & Bashir, S. (2021). A deep learning based ensemble learning method for epileptic seizure prediction. *Computers in Biology and Medicine, 136*. doi:10.1016/j.compbiomed.2021.104710

Valls, M. G., & Val, P. B. (2013). Usage of DDS data-centric middleware for remote monitoring and control laboratories. *IEEE Transactions on Industrial Informatics*, *9*(1), 567–574. doi:10.1109/TII.2012.2211028

Van Der Walt, S., Colbert, S. C., & Varoquaux, G. (2011). The NumPy array: A structure for efficient numerical computation. *Computing in Science & Engineering*, *13*(2), 22–30. doi:10.1109/MCSE.2011.37

Van Dooren, M., de Vries, J.J. & Janssen, J.H. (2012). Emotional sweating across the body: Comparing 16 different skin conductance measurement locations. *Physiology & Behavior*, *106*(2), 298-304.

Vanmarkenlichtenbelt, W., Daanen, H., Wouters, L., Fronczek, R., Raymann, R., Severens, N., & Vansomeren, E. (2006). Evaluation of wireless determination of skin temperature using iButtons. *Physiology & Behavior*, *88*(4-5), 489–497. doi:10.1016/j.physbeh.2006.04.026 PMID:16797616

Vapnik, V. (1999). *The nature of statistical learning theory*. Springer Science & Business Media.

Vidyaratne, L., Glandon, A., Alam, M., & Iftekharuddin, K. M. (2016). Deep recurrent neural network for seizure detection. *Proc. Int. Joint Conf. Neural Netw. (IJCNN)*, 12021207. 10.1109/IJCNN.2016.7727334

Vieluf, S., Reinsberger, C., El Atrache, R., Jackson, M., Schubach, S., Ufongene, C., Loddenkemper, T., & Meisel, C. (2020). Autonomic nervous system changes detected with peripheral sensors in the setting of epileptic seizures. *Scientific Reports*, *10*(1), 11560. doi:10.103841598-020-68434-z PMID:32665704

Vijayan, A. E., Sen, D., & Sudheer, A. P. (2015). EEG-Based Emotion Recognition Using Statistical Measures and Autoregressive Modeling. *Proceedings of the 2015 IEEE International Conference on Computational Intelligence & Communication Technology*, 587–591. 10.1109/CICT.2015.24

Vijayarani & Dayananda. (2015). Liver disease prediction using SVM and Naïve Bayes algorithms. *International Journal of Science, Engineering and Technology Research, 4*(4), 816-820.

Vijayarani & Deepa. (2015). Naïve Bayes Classification for Predicting Diseases in Haemoglobin Protein Sequences. *International Journal of Computational Intelligence and Informatics, 3*(4).

Villon, O., & Lisetti, C. (2006). A User-Modeling Approach to Build User's Psycho-Physiological Maps of Emotions using Bio-Sensors. *Proceedings of the ROMAN 2006–The 15th IEEE International Symposium on Robot and Human Interactive Communication,* 269–276.

Villon, O., & Lisetti, C. (2007). Toward Recognizing Individual's Subjective Emotion from Physiological Signals in Practical Application. *Proceedings of the Twentieth IEEE International Symposium on Computer-Based Medical Systems (CBMS'07)*, 357–362. 10.1109/CBMS.2007.112

Voulodimos, A., Doulamis, N., Doulamis, A., & Protopapadakis, E. (2018). Deep Learning for Computer Vision: A Brief Review. Computational Intelligence and Neuroscience. doi:10.1155/2018/7068349

Vyas, M. (2018). Artificial intelligence: The beginning of a new era in pharmacy profession. *Asian Journal of Pharmaceutics*.

Wallin, B. G., & Charkoudian, N. (2007). Sympathetic neural control of integrated cardiovascular function: Insights from measurement of human sympathetic nerve activity. *Muscle & Nerve*, *36*(5), 595–614. doi:10.1002/mus.20831 PMID:17623856

Walter, B., Wang, S., Chun-An, C., & Jr-Shin, L. (2020). Scientific Reports. Nature, 10(1). doi:10.103841598-020-65401-6

Wan, L., Zeiler, M., Zhang, S., Lecun, Y., & Fergus, R. (2013). *Regularization of Neural Networks using DropConnect*. Academic Press.

Wang, J., Ding, H., Azamian, F., Zhou, B., Iribarren, C., Molloi, S., & Baldi, P. (2017). Detecting Cardiovascular Disease from Mammograms With Deep Learning. *IEEE Transactions on Medical Imaging*. doi:10.1109/TMI.2017.2655486

Wang, J., Wang, H., He, J., Li, L., Shen, M., Tan, X., Min, H., & Zheng, L. (2015). Wireless sensor network for real-time perishable food supply chain management. *Computers and Electronics in Agriculture*, *110*, 196–207. doi:10.1016/j.compag.2014.11.009

Wang, K., Bai, X., Li, J., & Ding, C. (2010). A service-based framework for pharmacogenomics data integration. *Enterprise Information Systems*, *4*(3), 225–245. doi:10.1080/17517575.2010.498525

Wang, L., Da Xu, L., Bi, Z., & Xu, Y. (2013). Data cleaning for RFID and WSN integration. *IEEE Transactions on Industrial Informatics*, *10*(1), 408–418. doi:10.1109/TII.2013.2250510

Wang, N., & Lyu, M. R. (2015). Extracting and selecting distinctive eeg features for efficient epileptic seizure prediction. *IEEE Journal of Biomedical and Health Informatics*, *19*(5), 1648–1659. doi:10.1109/JBHI.2014.2358640 PMID:25248205

Wang, Y., Lv, Z., & Zheng, Y. (2018). Automatic Emotion Perception Using Eye Movement Information for EHealthcare Systems. *Sensors (Basel)*, *18*(9), 2826. doi:10.339018092826

Wangyang, W., Honghai, W., & Huadong, M. (2019). An AutoEncoder and LSTM-Based Traffic Flow Prediction Method. *Sensors (Basel)*, *19*(2946), 1–16. PMID:31277390

Wang, Z., Nie, F., Zhang, C., Wang, R., & Li, X. (2021). Joint nonlinear feature selection and continuous values regression network. *Pattern Recognition Letters*, *150*, 197–206.

Waterhouse. (2003). New horizons in ambulatory electroencephalography. *IEEE Engineering in Medicine and Biology Magazine*, *22*(3), 7480.

Webb, G., Fürnkranz, J., Hinton, G., Sammut, C., Sander, J., Vlachos, M., Teh, Y., Yang, Y., Mladenić, D., Brank, J., Grobelnik, M., Zhao, Y., Karypis, G., Craw, S., Puterman, M., & Patrick, J. (2010). *Deep Belief Networks*. doi:10.1007/978-0-387-30164-8_209

Wiig, S., Aase, K., Billett, S., Canfield, C., Røise, O., Njå, O., Guise, V., Haraldseid-Driftland, C., Ree, E., Anderson, J. E., & Macrae, C. (2020). Defining the boundaries and operational concepts of resilience in the resilience in the healthcare research program. *BMC Health Services Research*, *20*(1), 330. doi:10.118612913-020-05224-3 PMID:32306981

Wijsman, J., Grundlehner, B., & Liu, H., H. H. and J. P. (2011). Towards mental stress detection using wearable physiological sensors. In *2011 Annual International Conference of the IEEE Engineering in Medicine and Biology Society* (pp. 1798–1801). 10.1109/IEMBS.2011.6090512

Wild, C. (2014). *World cancer report 2014*. World Health Organization.

Williams, G. (2011). Descriptive and predictive analytics. In *Data Mining with Rattle and R* (pp. 171–177). Springer. doi:10.1007/978-1-4419-9890-3_8

Witten, I. H., & Frank, E. (2002). Data mining: Practical machine learning tools and techniques with Java implementations. *SIGMOD Record*, *31*(1), 76–77. doi:10.1145/507338.507355

Workman, P., Antolin, A. A., & Al-Lazikani, B. (2019). Transforming cancer drug discovery with Big Data and AI. *Expert Opinion on Drug Discovery*, *14*(11), 1089–1095. Advance online publication. doi:10.1080/17460441.2019.1637414 PMID:31284790

Wu, J., Sun, L., & Jafari, R. (2016). A Wearable System for Recognizing American Sign Language in Real-Time Using IMU and Surface EMG Sensors. IEEE Journal of Biomedical and Health Informatics, 20(5), 1281–1290. doi:10.1109/JBHI.2016.2598302

Wu, X., & V. K. (2009). *The top ten algorithms in data mining.* CRC Press.

Wu, X., & Kumar, V. (Eds.). (2009). *The top ten algorithms in data mining*. CRC press. doi:10.1201/9781420089653

Yacchirema, D., Suarez de Puga, J., Palau, C., & Esteve, M. (2018). Fall detection system for elderly people using Iot and Big Data. *Procedia Computer Science*, *130*, 603–610. doi:10.1016/j.procs.2018.04.110

Yadav, S., Soni, J., Porwal, S., Chauhan, V., Rashid, S., & Jain, A. (2020). Tally Education in Covid-19 Era: Impact on Health, Cancer Care and Education Sectors. *Asian Pacific Journal of Cancer Care*, *5*(S1), 95–99. doi:10.31557/apjcc.2020.5.S1.95-99

Yang, M. H., Kang, S. Y., Lee, J. A., Kim, Y. S., Sung, E. J., Lee, K. Y., Kim, J.-S., Oh, H. J., Kang, H. C., & Lee, S. Y. (2017). The effect of lifestyle changes on blood pressure control among hypertensive patients. *Korean Journal of Family Medicine*, *38*(4), 173. doi:10.4082/kjfm.2017.38.4.173 PMID:28775806

Yang, Y., & Liu, X. (1999). A re-examination of text categorization methods. *Proceedings of the 22nd Annual International ACM SIGIR Conference on Research and Development in Information Retrieval, SIGIR 1999*, 42–49. 10.1145/312624.312647

Yasin, Jilani, & Danish. (2011). Hepatitis-C classification using data mining techniques. *International Journal of Computer Applications*, *24*(3), 1-6.

Yuan, Y., Xun, G., Jia, K., & Zhang, A. (2017). *A multi-view deep learning method for epileptic seizure detection using short-time Fourier transform.* Presented at the 8thACMInt. Conf. Bioinf., Comput. Biol., Health Inform., Boston, MA. 10.1145/3107411.3107419

Yuan, X., Yuan, J., Jiang, T., & Ain, Q. U. (2020). Integrated long-term stock selection models based on feature selection and machine learning algorithms for China stock market. *IEEE Access: Practical Innovations, Open Solutions*, *8*, 22672–22685.

Zazzaro, Cuomo, Martone, Montaquila, Toraldo, & Pavone. (2019). EEG signal analysis for epileptic seizures detection by applying Data Mining techniques. *Internet of Things*. doi:10.1016/j.iot.2019.03.002

Zhang, L., & Wang, Z. (2006). Integration of RFID into wireless sensor networks: architectures, opportunities and challenging problems. In *2006 Fifth international conference on grid and cooperative computing workshops* (pp. 463-469). IEEE. 10.1109/GCCW.2006.58

Zhang, J., Chen, M., Zhao, S., Hu, S., Shi, Z., & Cao, Y. (2016). Relief-Based EEG Sensor Selection Methods for Emotion Recognition. *Sensors (Basel)*, *16*(10), 1558. doi:10.339016101558

Zhang, N., Ding, S., Zhang, J., & Xue, Y. (2017). An overview on Restricted Boltzmann Machines. *Neurocomputing*, *275*. Advance online publication. doi:10.1016/j.neucom.2017.09.065

Zhang, N., Gupta, A., Chen, Z., & Ong, Y. S. (2021). Evolutionary machine learning with minions: A case study in feature selection. *IEEE Transactions on Evolutionary Computation*, *26*(1), 130–144. doi:10.1109/TEVC.2021.3099289

Zhang, Q., Chen, X., Zhan, Q., Yang, T., & Xia, S. (2017). Respiration-based emotion recognition with deep learning. *Computers in Industry*, *92-93*, 84–90. doi:10.1016/j.compind.2017.04.005

Zhang, Q., Xiao, Y., Dai, W., Suo, J., Wang, C., Shi, J., & Zheng, H. (2016). Deep learning based classification of breast tumors with shear-wave elastography. *Ultrasonics, 72*. Advance online publication. doi:10.1016/j.ultras.2016.08.004

Zhang, Z., & Parhi, K. K. (2016). Low-complexity seizure prediction from ieeg/seeg using spectral power and ratios of spectral power. *IEEE Transactions on Biomedical Circuits and Systems, 10*(3), 693–706. doi:10.1109/TBCAS.2015.2477264 PMID:26529783

Zhao, Z., Chen, W., Wu, X., Chen, P. C. Y., & Liu, J. (2017). LSTM network: A deep learning approach for short-term traffic forecast. *IET Intelligent Transport Systems, 11*(2), 68–75. doi:10.1049/iet-its.2016.0208

Zhou, Y., Jiang, J., Cui, Y., & Wu, Q. (2009). Corin, atrial natriuretic peptide and hypertension. *Nephrology, Dialysis, Transplantation, 24*(4), 1071–1073. doi:10.1093/ndt/gfn727 PMID:19131349

About the Contributors

Rosy Madaan is a PhD in Computer Engineering department from YMCA University of Science & Technology, Faridabad. She has total of more than 16 years of teaching experience. She has worked in various engineering colleges and currently she is working as an Associate Prof. in CSE department, FET of Manav Rachna International Institute of Research and Studies. Her areas of interest are information retrieval, search engines, crawlers and question answering systems. She has many research papers/chapters published in reputed journals/SCIE/conferences and patents granted/published. She has served as session chair in various conferences. She has worked as Guest Editor in "Advances and Innovation in Digital Technologies", Recent Patents of Engineering, Bentham science.

Komal Kumar Bhatia is working as Professor and Dean in the Department of Computer Engineering at J. C. Bose University of Science and Technology, YMCA. He has a work experience of 19 years. He has guided many Ph.D. scholars. He has also guided more than seventy M.Tech. Dissertations. He has published more than a hundred research papers in reputed journals and conferences. He has served as session chair in several conferences and delivered many expert talks. He has many patents published/granted to his credit. His areas of interest include Information Retrieval Systems, Hidden Web and Web Mining. He is also a member of several Professional bodies at the National/International level.

Supriya P. Panda (MS, Ph.D. [BGSU,Ohio, USA]) is working as a professor (CSE) and HOD (CSE) at Manav Rachna International Institute of Research &Studies at Faridabad(India) since 2016. She started her stint at BITS, Pilani, Rajasthan, where she served for ten years and has over three decades of the academic experience across various organizations in India and abroad. She has numerous research papers in reputed national and international journals, guided scholars, and chapter books to her credit.

Vishal Jain is presently working as an Associate Professor at Department of Computer Science and Engineering, School of Engineering and Technology, Sharda University, Greater Noida, U. P. India. Before that, he has worked for several years as an Associate Professor at Bharati Vidyapeeth's Institute of Computer Applications and Management (BVICAM), New Delhi. He has more than 14 years of experience in the academics. He obtained Ph.D (CSE), M.Tech (CSE), MBA (HR), MCA, MCP and CCNA. He has authored more than 90 research papers in reputed conferences and journals, including Web of Science and Scopus. He has authored and edited more than 30 books with various reputed publishers, including Elsevier, Springer, Apple Academic Press, CRC, Taylor and Francis Group, Scrivener, Wiley, Emerald, NOVA Science and IGI-Global. His research areas include information retrieval, semantic web, ontology engineering, data mining, ad hoc networks, and sensor networks. He received a Young Active Member Award for the year 2012–13 from the Computer Society of India, Best Faculty Award for the year 2017 and Best Researcher Award for the year 2019 from BVICAM, New Delhi.

Payal Gulati is an Assistant Professor at Department of Computer Engineering, J.C. Bose University of Science & Technology, YMCA, Faridabad, India. She received her Ph.D. in 2013 from Maharishi Dayanand University, Rohtak, India and has over 14 years of experience. She has contributed more than 30 papers in reputed journals and conferences. She is also a reviewer in Springer and Oxford journals. Her subject of interests includes Data Analytics, Machine Learning, Predictive Analysis, Energy Research and Advances in Development of Sustainable Smart Cities. She has 4 patents granted to her credit.

* * *

Komal Arora is a budding biotechnologist, B. tech Biotechnology graduate with an aggregate of 9.14 CGPA, having an idea of applying mathematical concepts to find the biology solutions.

Vijayakumari B. completed BE at Institute of Road and Transport Technologies during the year 1997 and received ME (Communication Systems) from Thiagarajar College of Engineering, Madurai, during the year 2006. She has completed PhD in Medical Image Processing at Thiagarajar College of Engineering, Madurai during the year 2014 and is currently working as an Assistant Professor (SG) in the Department of ECE at Mepco Schlenk Engineering College, Sivakasi. She had done her Ph.D work in the title "Identification of Victim in Forensic Dentistry from Dental Images" Her research area includes Medical image processing and image analysis. To her credit, she had published 16 papers in peer reviewed and Science Citation Indexed Journals both national and international and 35 papers in conferences. She is a Life Member of Indian Society for Technical Education (ISTE) and The Institution of Electronics and Telecommunication Engineers (IETE) chapters.

Sonali Gupta did her Ph.D. (Information Retrieval) from the Department of Computer Engineering, YMCA University of Science & Technology, M. Tech. from the University School of Information Technology, Guru Gobind Singh Indraprastha University (GGSIPU), Delhi in 2008 and B.Tech in Computer Engineering from Maharishi Dayanand University, India in 2003. She is Currently Working as Assistant Professor in the Department of Computer Engg. at J.C Bose University of Science and Technology, YMCA, Faridabad, Since 2009 to till date. She is having a total of 17 years of teaching experience. Her area of research includes Data Mining, Web Information retrieval, Web Mining, Artificial intelligence & Soft computing.

Tanvi Gupta is working as an Assistant Professor in Manav Rachna International Institute of Research and Studies. Also have around 15 papers in international conferences and journals.

Kulwinder Kaur is an independent researcher. Her research area is related to image processing and machine learning.

Pooja Khurana is a professional academician with strong analytical skills seeking the position of Associate professor and researcher focusing in Biomathematical modeling; skilled with applying the concepts of statistics, numerical analysis and probability in building and simulation of mathematical model for improving healthcare.

Deepak Kumar pursued Master of Sciences from Jamia Millia Islamia University, New Delhi and pursued Ph. D. from IBS Khandri, Agra in 2006. He is currently working as Professor in MRIIRS, Faridabad, India. He has Published more than 55 research papers in reputed national and international journals including Springer and IEEE and it's also available online. He has more than 22 years of teaching experience.

Nitendra Kumar received a Ph. D (Mathematics) from Sharda University, Greater Noida, India and a Master of Science (Mathematics and Statistics) from Dr Ram Manohar Lohia Avadh University, Faizabad, India. He worked with many leading organizations like Sharda University, RIET, Greater Noida. Presently, he is an Assistant Professor at the IIMT College of Engineering, Greater Noida with interests in the Wavelets and Variants, Data Mining, Inverse Problems, Epidemic Modelling, Fractional Derivatives and Statistical Methods. He has more than 10 years of experience in his research areas. He has published many research papers in reputed journals and also published 4 books on engineering mathematics. He contributes to the research community by undertaking various volunteer activities in the capacity of editor for two edited books and as a conference Speaker.

Sushil Kumar did his PhD in Computer Engineering from J.C Bose University of Science and Technology, YMCA, Faridabad in July 2021, M.E in Computer Science & Engineering from National Institute of Technical Teachers' Training & Research, Chandigarh affiliated to Punjab University, Chandigarh and B.Tech in Computer Engineering graduated from N.I.T Kurukshetra (Deemed University) formally known as Regional Engineering College Kurukshetra in 2002. He is Currently Working as Assistant Professor in the Department of Computer Engg. at J.C Bose University of Science and Technology, YMCA, Faridabad, Since 28th Feb 2011 to till date. He is having a total of 18 years of teaching experience. His area of research includes Internet technologies, Information Retrieval System and Computer organization & Architecture. He has authored papers in various national and international journals.

Ramya M. is an experienced faculty and ex-program analyst with demonstrated history of working in various industry projects. Strong operational professional with a Master's degree focused in Information Technology.

Swapnaneel Sharma Mazumder is a currently pursuing an integrated masters course for engineering in Biotechnology from Amity Institute of Biotechnology, Amity University, Noida, Uttar Pradesh, India.

R. Nagarajan received his B.E. in Electrical and Electronics Engineering from Madurai Kamarajar University, Madurai, India, in 1997. He received his M.E. in Power Electronics and Drives from Anna University, Chennai, India, in 2008. He received his Ph.D in Electrical Engineering from Anna University, Chennai, India, in 2014. He has worked in the industry as an Electrical Engineer. He is currently working as Professor of Electrical and Electronics Engineering at Gnanamani College of Technology, Namakkal, Tamilnadu, India. He has published more than 70 papers in International Journals and Conferences. His research interest includes Power Electronics, Power System, Communication Engineering, Network Security, Soft Computing Techniques, Cloud Computing, Big Data Analysis and Renewable Energy Sources

Pooja completed her Ph.D. in Computer Science and Engineering from National Institute of Technology, Jalandhar. She is experienced professional with hands-on skills on Deep Learning, Machine Learning, Image Processing, Pattern Recognition, Natural Language Processing, Genetic Algorithms and Data Mining. Imparting customized learning modules on ML, DL, AI, Data analysis Image Processing and NLP to industry professionals and students, experience with varied datasets including financial data, healthcare data, HR data, Smart grid data and weather data. She has experience of around 14 years in teaching UGPG students of computer science engineering, mentoring M.Tech thesis and projects in the area of image processing, data mining, IoT, E-commerce, Network security, biometrics, wireless networks, and routine organizational administration.

Shabna R. M. is a UG student studying B.E (Electronics and Communication Engineering) at Mepco Schlenk Engineering College, Sivakasi. Her research area is Embedded systems.

Mritunjay Rai is working as an Assistant Professor in Department of Electronics and Communication at SRM University, Lucknow-Deva Road, Barabanki, UP. He is pursuingPh.D. from IIT-ISM Dhanbad. He has completed his B.Tech in ECE from Sri Ramswaroop Memorial College of Engineering and Management, Lucknow (SRMCEM) in 2009 and Master of Engineering (distinction) in Instrumentation and Control from Birla Institute of Technology-Mesra, Ranchi in 2013. His areas of interest lie in image processing, speech processing, Artificial Intelligence, machine learning, deep learning, Internet of Things (IoT)and robotics & automation. He has more than 9 years of working experience in research as well as academic. In addition, he has guided several UG and PG projects. He has published many research articles in reputed Journals published by IEEE, Inderscience, etc. He has reviewed many research papers of Journals and international/national conferences.

Probeer Sahw is a PhD research scholar at IIT(ISM) Dhanbad. He completed his M. Tech from Netaji Subhas Institute of Technology, University of Delhi, Delhi, India in 2014 and B. Tech from Guru Gobind Singh Indraprastha University, Delhi, India in 2011. He has more than 8 years of experience in academia. Currently, he is serving as an Assistant Professor in the Department of Electrical Engineering, Galgotias College of Engineering and Technology, Greater Noida, India. His research interests incudes image processing, drives, dc-dc converters, renewable energy, electric and hybrid vehicles.

Rohan Saini is an M.Tech student at J.C. Bose University of Science and Technology, YMCA (Formerly YMCA UST).

Kannadhasan Suriyan is working as an Assistant Professor in the department of Electronics and Communication Engineering in Cheran College of Engineering, Karur, Tamilnadu, India. He is currently doing research in the field of Smart Antenna for Anna University. He is ten years of teaching and research experience. He obtained his B.E in ECE from Sethu Institute of Technology, Kariapatti in 2009 and M.E in Communication Systems from Velammal College of Engineering and Technology, Madurai in 2013. He obtained his M.B.A in Human Resources Management from Tamilnadu Open University, Chennai. He obtained his PGVLSI in Post Graduate diploma in VLSI design from Annamalai University, Chidambaram in 2011 and PGDCA in Post Graduate diploma in Computer Applications from Tamil University in 2014. He obtained his PGDRD in Post Graduate diploma in Rural Development from Indira Gandhi National Open University in 2016. He has published around 18 papers in the reputed indexed international journals and more than 125 papers presented/published in national, international journal and conferences. Besides he has contributed a book chapter also. He also serves as a board member, reviewer, speaker, session chair, advisory and technical committee of various colleges and conferences. He is also to attend the various workshop, seminar, conferences, faculty development programme, STTP and Online courses. His areas of interest are Smart Antennas, Digital Signal Processing, Wireless Communication, Wireless Networks, Embedded System, Network Security, Optical Communication, Microwave Antennas, Electromagnetic Compatibility and Interference, Wireless Sensor Networks, Digital Image Processing, Satellite Communication, Cognitive Radio Design and Soft Computing techniques. He is Member of IEEE, ISTE, IEI, IETE, CSI, IAENG, SEEE, IEAE, INSC, IARDO, ISRPM, IACSIT, ICSES, SPG, SDIWC, IJSPR and EAI Community.

Manonmani T. is a Senior Assistant Professor, Department of Computer Science and Engineering, Mepco Schlenk Engineering College, Sivakasi.

Siva Sundari T. is a UG student studying B.E (Electronics and Communication Engineering) at Mepco Schlenk Engineering College, Sivakasi . Her research area is Embedded systems.

Padmesh Tripathi is working as an Associate Professor of Mathematics at IIMT College of Engineering, Greater Noida, UP. He received his Ph.D. degree from Sharda University, Greater Noida (India). He completed his Master's and Bachelor's degrees from University of Allahabad, Prayagraj. He has been teaching since last 20 years at graduate and post-graduate levels. He has published many research papers in reputed journals and presented many papers in national/international conferences. He has been granted funds from prestigious organizations like: Cambridge University, UK (twice); University of California, Los Angeles, USA; University of Eastern Finland, Kuopio, Finland; INRIA, Sophia Antipolis, France, etc. and he visited these organizations. In addition, he has been granted funds from CIMPA (UNESCO) France to participate in a research school at Erbyl, Iraq.He has been member of Society of Industrial and Applied Mathematics (SIAM), Philadelphia, USA (2011-19). He is life member of Science and Engineering Institute (SCIEI), Los Angeles, USA; Indian Society of Industrial and Applied Mathematics (ISIAM), India; Ramanujan Mathematical Society, India; Purvanchal Academy of Sciences, India; International Association of Engineers, UK. He is member of EURO working group on continuous optimization (EUROPT), Italy; Society for Foundations of Computational Mathematics, USA. His area of research interests are inverse problems, signal processing, optimization, data science, etc.

Nalini Tyagi is a well-known author and researcher in the field of image processing. She obtained her bachelor's degree (B.Tech.) from UP Technical University in Electronics and Instrumentation Engineering. Then she completed her master's (M.Tech.) from M.D. University, Rohtak in the Electronics and Communication Engineering. She has published original articles in reputed journals in the area of her studies. Her research interests include image processing, Deep Learning, Machine Learning.

Index

I

K

L

M

N

P

R

S

T

U

W

www.ingramcontent.com/pod-product-compliance
Lightning Source LLC
LaVergne TN
LVHW060305011026
849161LV00011B/2779
* 9 7 8 1 6 6 8 4 2 5 0 8 4 *